# RYPINS' INTENSIVE REVIEWS

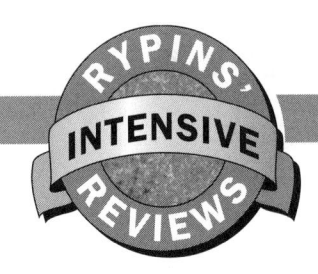

**Series Editor**

# Edward D. Frohlich, MD, MACP, FACC

Alton Ochsner Distinguished Scientist
Vice President for Academic Affairs
Alton Ochsner Medical Foundation
Staff Member, Ochsner Clinic
Professor of Medicine and of Physiology
Louisiana State University of Medicine
Adjunct Professor of Pharmacology and
Clinical Professor of Medicine
Tulane University School of Medicine
New Orleans, Louisiana

# RYPINS' INTENSIVE REVIEWS
## Pediatrics

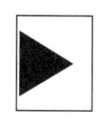

▶ **Margaret C. Heagarty, MD**
Professor of Pediatrics
Columbia University, College of Physicians and Surgeons
Director of Pediatrics
Harlem Hospital Center
New York, New York

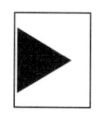

▶ **William J. Moss, MD, MPH**
Assistant Scientist
Division of Disease Control
Department of International Health
School of Hygiene and Public Health
Johns Hopkins University
Baltimore, Maryland

**Lippincott - Raven**
PUBLISHERS
Philadelphia • New York

Acquisitions Editor: Richard Winters
Developmental Editor: Mary Beth Murphy
Managing Editor: Susan E. Kelly
Manufacturing Manager: Dennis Teston
Associate Managing Editor: Kathleen Bubbeo
Production Services: P. M. Gordon Associates
Cover Designer: William T. Donnelly
Interior Designer: Susan Blaker
Design Coordinator: Melissa Olson
Indexer: M. L. Coughlin Editorial Services
Compositor: Lippincott–Raven Electronic Production
Printer: Courier/Kendallville

© 1997, by Lippincott–Raven Publishers. All rights reserved. This book is protected by copyright. No part of it may be reproduced, stored in a retrieval system, or transmitted, in any form or by any means—electronic, mechanical, photocopy, recording, or otherwise—without the prior written consent of the publisher, except for brief quotations embodied in critical articles and reviews. For information write **Lippincott–Raven Publishers, 227 East Washington Square, Philadelphia, PA 19106-3780.**

Materials appearing in this book prepared by individuals as part of their official duties as U.S. Government employees are not covered by the above-mentioned copyright.

Printed in the United States of America

**Library of Congress Cataloging-in-Publication Data**

Heagarty, Margaret C.
    Pediatrics / Margaret C. Heagarty, William J. Moss.
      p.  cm. — (Rypins' intensive reviews)
    Includes index.
    ISBN 0-397-51556-1
    1. Pediatrics–Outlines, syllabi, etc.  2. Pediatrics—
Examinations, questions, etc.  I. Moss, William J.  II. Title.
III. Series.
    [DNLM: 1. Pediatrics—examination questions.  WS 18.2 H433p 1997]
RJ48.3.H43 1997
618.92—dc21
DNLM/DLC                                                            97-3054
                                                                           CIP
for Library of Congress

Care has been taken to confirm the accuracy of the information presented and to describe generally accepted practices. However, the authors, editors, and publisher are not responsible for errors or omissions or for any consequences from application of the information in this book and make no warranty, express or implied, with respect to the contents of the publication.
    The authors, editors, and publisher have exerted every effort to ensure that drug selection and dosage set forth in this text are in accordance with current recommendations and practice at the time of publication. However, in view of ongoing research, changes in government regulations, and the constant flow of information relating to drug therapy and drug reactions, the reader is urged to check the package insert for each drug for any change in indications and dosage and for added warnings and precautions. This is particularly important when the recommended agent is a new or infrequently employed drug.
    Some drugs and medical devices presented in this publication have Food and Drug Administration (FDA) clearance for limited use in restricted research settings. It is the responsibility of the health care provider to ascertain the FDA status of each drug or device planned for use in their clinical practice.

9  8  7  6  5  4  3  2  1

# Preface

This volume represents the work of two pediatricians, one younger and one older. We have attempted to give the reader an overview of the important aspects of pediatrics that distinguishes it from other fields of medicine. Obviously, such a review text cannot cover the entire field of pediatric medicine in detail, but the authors hope that enough has been provided to whet the reader's appetite to seek further, more detailed information in the more encyclopedic texts readily available.

The authors share the common experience of working in an urban disadvantaged community in a public general hospital. This volume is dedicated to the children of this community, to whom the authors are devoted, as well as to all children who deserve and require informed and competent physicians to provide their medical care. We can only hope that this volume will make some small contribution to that effort.

Margaret C. Heagarty, MD
William J. Moss, MD, MPH

## Who Was "Rypins"?

Dr. Harold Rypins (1892–1939) was the founding editor of what is now known as the RYPINS' series of review books. Originally published under the title *Medical State Board Examinations,* the first edition was published by J. B. Lippincott Company in 1933. Dr. Rypins edited subsequent editions of the book in 1935, 1937, and 1939 before his death that year. The series that he began has since become the longest-running and most successful publication of its kind, having served as an invaluable tool in the training of generations of medical students. Dr. Rypins was a member of the faculty of Albany Medical College in Albany, New York, and also served as Secretary of the New York State Board of Medical Examiners. His legacy to medical education flourishes today in the highly successful *Rypins' Basic Sciences Review* and *Rypins' Clinical Sciences Review,* now in their 17th editions, and in the *Rypins' Intensive Reviews* series of subject review volumes. We at Lippincott–Raven Publishers take pride in this continuing success.

—*The Publisher*

# Series Preface

These are indeed very exciting times in medicine. Having made this statement, one's thoughts immediately reflect about the major changes that are occurring in our overall healthcare delivery system, utilization-review and shortened hospitalizations, issues concerning quality assurance, ambulatory surgical procedures and medical clearances, and the impact of managed care on the practice of internal medicine and primary care. Each of these issues has had a considerable impact on the approach to the patient and on the practice of medicine.

But even more mind-boggling than the foregoing changes are the dramatic changes imposed on the practice of medicine by fundamental conceptual scientific innovations engendered by advances in basic science that no doubt will affect medical practice of the immediate future. Indeed, much of what we thought of as having a potential impact on the practice of medicine of the future has already been perceived. One need only take a cursory look at our weekly medical journals to realize that we are practicing "tomorrow's medicine today." And consider that the goal a few years ago of actually describing the human genome is now near reality.

Reflect, then, for a moment on our current thinking about genetics, molecular biology, cellular immunology, and other areas that have impacted upon our current understanding of the underlying mechanisms of the pathophysiological concepts of disease. Moreover, paralleling these innovations have been remarkable advances in the so-called "high tech" and "gee-whiz" aspects of how we diagnose disease and treat patients. We can now think with much greater perspective about the dimensions of more specific biologic diagnoses concerned with molecular perturbations; gene therapy not only affecting genetic but oncological diseases; more specific pharmacotherapy involving highly specific receptor inhibition, alterations of intracellular signal transduction, manipulations of cellular protein synthesis; immunosuppresive therapy not only with respect to organ transplantations but also of autoimmune and other immune-related diseases; and therapeutic means for manipulating organ remodeling or the intravascular placement of stents. Each of these concepts has become inculcated into our everyday medical practice within the past decade. The reason why these changes have so rapidly promoted an upheaval in medical practice is continuing medical education, a constant awareness of the current medical literature, and a thirst for new knowledge.

To assist the student and practitioner in the review process, the publisher and I have initiated a new approach in the publication of *Rypins' Basic Sciences Review* and *Rypins' Clinical Sciences Review*. Thus, when I assumed responsibility to edit this long-standing board review series with the 13th edition of the textbook (first published in 1931), it was with a feeling of great excitement. I perceived that great changes would be coming to medicine, and I believed that this would be one ideal means of not only facing these changes head on but also for me personally to cope and keep up with these changes. Over the subsequent editions, this confidence was reassured and rewarded. The presentation for the updating of medical information was tremendously enhanced by the substitution of new authors, as the former authority "standbys" stepped down or retired from our faculty. Each of the authors who continue to be selected for maintaining the character of our textbook is an authority in his or her respective area and has had considerable pedagogic and formal examination experience. One dramatic recent example of the changes in author replacement just came about with the 17th edition. When I invited Dr. Peter Goldblatt to participate in the authorship of the pathology chapter of the textbook, his answer was "what goes around, comes around." You see, Dr. Goldblatt's father, Dr. Harry Goldblatt, a major contributor to the history of hypertensive disease, was the first author of the pathology chapter in 1931. What a satisfying experience for me personally. Other less human changes in our format came with the establishment of two soft cover volumes, the current basic and clinical sciences review volumes, replacing the single volume text of earlier years. Soon, a third supplementary volume concerned with questions and answers for the basic science volume appeared. Accompanying these more obvious changes was the constant updating of the knowledge base of each of the chapters, and this continues on into the present 17th edition.

And now we have introduced another major innovation in our presentation of the basic and clinical sciences reviews. This change is evidenced by the introduction of the *Rypins' Intensive Reviews* series, along with the 17th edition of *Rypins' Basic Sciences Review, Rypins' Clinical Sciences Review,* and the *Questions and Answers* third volume. These volumes are written to be used separately from the parent textbook. Each not only contains the material published in their respective chapters of the textbook, but is considerably "fleshed out" in the discussions, tables, figures, and questions and answers. Thus, the *Rypins' Intensive Reviews* series serves as an important supplement to the overall review process and also provides a study guide for those already in practice, preparing for specific specialty board certification and recertification examinations.

Therefore, with continued confidence and excitement, I am pleased to present these innovations in review experience for your consideration. As in the past, I look forward to learning of your comments and suggestions. In doing so, we continue to look forward to our continued growth and acceptance of the *Rypins'* review experience.

Edward D. Frohlich, MD, MACP, FACC

# Series Acknowledgments

In no other writing experience is one more dependent on others than in a textbook, especially a textbook that provides a broad review for the student and fellow practitioner. In this spirit, I am truly indebted to all who have contributed to our past and current understanding of the fundamental and clinical aspects related to the practice of medicine. No one individual ever provides the singular "breakthrough" so frequently attributed as such by the news media. Knowledge develops and grows as a result of continuing and exciting contributions of research from all disciplines, academic institutions, and nations. Clearly, outstanding investigators have been credited for major contributions, but those with true and understanding humility are quick to attribute the preceding input of knowledge by others to the growing body of knowledge. In this spirit, we acknowledge the long list of contributors to medicine over the generations. We also acknowledge that in no century has man so exceeded the sheer volume of these advances than in the twentieth century. Indeed, it has been said by many that the sum of new knowledge over the past 50 years has most likely exceeded all that had been contributed in the prior years.

With this spirit of more universal acknowledgment, I wish to recognize personally the interest, support, and suggestions made by my colleagues in my institution and elsewhere. I specifically refer to those people from my institution who were of particular help and are listed at the outset of the internal medicine volume. But, in addition to these colleagues, I want to express my deep appreciation to my institution and clinic for providing the opportunity and ambience to maintain and continue these academic pursuits. As I have often said, the primary mission of a school of medicine is that of education and research; the care of patients, a long secondary mission to ensure the conduct of the primary goal, has now also become a primary commitment in these more pragmatic times. In contrast, the primary mission of the major multidisciplinary clinics has been the care of patients, with education and research assuming secondary roles as these commitments become affordable. It is this distinction that sets the multispecialty clinic apart from other modes of medical practice.

Over and above a personal commitment and drive to assure publication of a textbook such as this is the tremendous support and loyalty of a hard-working and dedicated office staff. To this end, I am tremendously grateful and indebted to Mrs. Lillian Buffa and Mrs. Caramia Fairchild. Their long hours of unselfish work on my behalf and to satisfy their own interest in participating in this major educational effort is appreciated no end. I am personally deeply honored and thankful for their important roles in the publication of the Rypins' series.

Words of appreciation must be extended to the staff of the Lippincott–Raven Publishers. It is more than 25 years since I have become associated with this publishing house, one of the first to be established in our nation. Over these years, I have worked closely with Mr. Richard Winters, not only with the Rypins' editions but also with other textbooks. His has been a labor of commitment, interest, and full support—not only because of his responsibility to his institution, but also because of the excitement of publishing new knowledge. In recent years, we discussed at length the merits of adding the intensive review supplements to the parent textbook and together we worked out the details that have become the substance of our present "joint venture." Moreover, together we are willing to make the necessary changes to assure the intellectual success of this series. To this end, we are delighted to include a new member of our team effort, Ms. Susan Kelly. She joined our cause to ensure that the format of questions, the reference process of answers to those questions within the text itself, and the editorial process involved be natural and clear to our readers. I am grateful for each of these facets of the overall publication process.

Not the least is my everlasting love and appreciation to my family. I am particularly indebted to my parents who inculcated in me at a very early age the love of education, the respect for study and hard work, and the honor for those who share these values. In this regard, it would have been impossible for me to accomplish any of my academic pursuits without the love, inspiration, and continued support of my wife, Sherry. Not only has she maintained the personal encouragement to initiate and continue with these labors of love, but she has sustained and supported our family and home life so that these activities could be encouraged. Hopefully, these pursuits have not detracted from the development and love of our children, Margie, Bruce, and Lara. I assume that this has not occurred; we are so very proud that each is personally committed to education and research. How satisfying it is to realize that these ideals remain a familial characteristic.

Edward D. Frohlich, MD, MACP, FACC
New Orleans, Louisiana

# Introduction

## *Preparing for USMLE*

### UNITED STATES MEDICAL LICENSING EXAMINATION (USMLE)

In August 1991 the Federation of State Medical Boards (FSMB) and the National Board of Medical Examiners (NBME) agreed to replace their respective examinations, the FLEX and NBME, with a new examination, the United States Medical Licensing Examination (USMLE). This examination will provide a common means for evaluating all applicants for medical licensure. It appears that this development in medical licensure will at last satisfy the needs for state medical boards licensure, the national medical board licensure, and licensure examinations for foreign medical graduates. This is because the 1991 agreement provides for a composite committee that equally represents both organizations (the FSMB and NBME) as well as a jointly appointed public member and a representative of the Educational Council for Foreign Medical Graduates (ECFMG).

As indicated in the USMLE announcement, "It is expected that students who enrolled in U.S. medical schools in the fall of 1990 or later and foreign medical graduates applying for ECFMG examinations beginning in 1993 will have access only to USMLE for purposes of licensure." The phaseout of the last regular examinations for licensure was completed in December 1994.

The new USMLE is administered in three steps. Step 1 focuses on fundamental basic biomedical science concepts, with particular emphasis on "principles and mechanisms underlying disease and modes of therapy." Step 2 is related to the clinical sciences, with examination on material necessary to practice medicine in a supervised setting. Step 3 is designed to focus on "aspects of biomedical and clinical science essential for the unsupervised practice of medicine."

Today Step 1 and Step 2 examinations are set up and scored as total comprehensive objective tests in the basic sciences and clinical sciences, respectively. The format of each part is no longer subject-oriented, that is, separated into sections specifically labeled Anatomy, Pathology, Medicine, Surgery, and so forth. Subject labels are therefore missing, and in each part questions from the different fields are intermixed or integrated so that the subject origin of any individual question is not immediately apparent, although it is known by the National Board office. Therefore, if necessary, individual subject grades can be extracted.

Step 1 is a two-day written test including questions in anatomy, biochemistry, microbiology, pathology, pharmacology, physiology, and the behavioral sciences. Each subject contributes to the examination a large number of questions designed to test not only knowledge of the subject itself but also "the subtler qualities of discrimination, judgment, and reasoning." Questions in such fields as molecular biology, cell biology, and genetics are included, as are questions to test the "candidate's recognition of the similarity or dissimilarity of diseases, drugs, and physiologic, behavioral, or pathologic processes." Problems are presented in narrative, tabular, or graphic form, followed by questions designed to assess the candidate's knowledge and comprehension of the situation described.

Step 2 is also a two-day written test that includes questions in internal medicine, obstetrics and gynecology, pediatrics, preventive medicine and public health, psychiatry, and surgery. The questions, like those in Step 1, cover a broad spectrum of knowledge in each of the clinical fields. In addition to individual questions, clinical problems are presented in the form of case histories, charts, roentgenograms, photographs of gross and microscopic pathologic specimens, laboratory data, and the like, and the candidate must answer questions concerning the interpretation of the data presented and their relation to the clinical problems. The questions are "designed to explore the extent of the candidate's knowledge of clinical situation, and to test his [or her] ability to bring information from many different clinical and basic science areas to bear upon these situations."

The examinations of both Step 1 and Step 2 are scored as a whole, certification being given on the basis of performance on the entire part, without reference to disciplinary breakdown. The grade for the examination is derived from the total number of questions answered correctly, rather than from an average of the grades in the component basic science or clinical science subjects. A candidate who fails will be required to repeat the entire examination. Nevertheless, as noted above, in spite of the interdisciplinary character of the examinations, all of the traditional disciplines are represented in the test, and separate grades for each subject can be extracted and reported separately to students, to state examining boards, or to those medical schools that request them for their own educational and academic purposes.

This type of interdisciplinary examination and the method of scoring the entire test as a unit have definite advantages, especially in view of the changing curricula in medical schools. The former type of rigid, almost standardized, curriculum, with its emphasis on specific subjects and a specified number of hours in each, has been replaced by a more liberal, open-ended curriculum, permitting emphasis in one or more fields and corresponding deemphasis in others. The result has been rather wide variations in the totality of education in different medical schools. Thus, the scoring of these tests as a whole permits accommodation to this variability in the curricula of different schools. Within the total score, weakness in one subject that has received relatively little emphasis in a given school may be balanced by strength in other subjects.

The rationale for this type of comprehensive examination as replacement for the traditional department-oriented examination in the basic sciences and the clinical sciences is given in the National Board Examiner:

The student, as he [or she] confronts these examinations, must abandon the idea of "thinking like a physiologist" in answering a question labeled "physiology" or "thinking like a surgeon" in answering a question labeled "surgery." The one question may have been written by a biochemist or a pharmacologist; the other question may have been written by an internist or a pediatrician. The pattern of these examinations will direct the student to thinking more broadly of the basic sciences in Step 1 and to thinking of patients and their problems in Step 2.

Until a few years ago, the Part I examination could not be taken until the work of the second year in medical school had been completed, and the Part II test was given only to students who had completed the major part of the fourth year. Now students, if they feel they are ready, may be admitted to any regularly scheduled Step 1 or Step 2 examination during any year of their medical course without prerequisite completion of specified courses or chronologic periods of study. Thus, emphasis is placed on the acquisition of knowledge and competence rather than the completion of predetermined periods.

Candidates are eligible for Step 3 after they have passed Steps 1 and 2, have received the M.D. degree from an approved medical school in the United States or Canada, and subsequent to the receipt of the M.D. degree, have served at least six months in an approved hospital internship or residency. Under certain circumstances, consideration may be given to other types of graduate training provided they meet with the approval of the National Board. After passing the Step 3 examination, candidates will receive their Diplomas as of the date of the satisfactory completion of an internship or residency program. If candidates have completed the approved hospital training prior to completion of Step 3, they will receive certification as of the date of the successful completion of Step 3.

The Step 3 examination, as noted above, is an objective test of general clinical competence. It occupies one full day and is divided into two sections, the first of which is a multiple-choice examination that relates to the interpretation of clinical data presented primarily in pictorial form, such as pictures of patients, gross and microscopic lesions, electrocardiograms, charts, and graphs. The second section, entitled Patient Management Problems, utilizes a programmed-testing technique designed to measure the candidate's clinical judgment in the management of patients. This technique simulates clinical situations in which the physician is faced with the problems of patient management presented in a sequential programmed pattern. A set of some four to six problems is related to each of a series of patients. In the scoring of this section, candidates are given credit for correct choices; they are penalized for errors of commission (selection of procedures that are unnecessary or are contraindicated) and for errors of omission (failure to select indicated procedures).

All parts of the National Board examinations are given in many centers, usually in medical schools, in nearly every large city in the United States as well as in a few cities in Canada, Puerto Rico, and the Canal Zone. In some cities, such as New York, Chicago, and Baltimore, the examination may be given in more than one center.

The examinations of the National Board have become recognized as the most comprehensive test of knowledge of the medical sciences and their clinical application produced in this country.

# THE NATIONAL BOARD OF MEDICAL EXAMINERS

For years the National Board examinations have served as an index of the medical education of the period and have strongly influenced higher educational standards in each of the medical sciences. The Diploma of the National Board is accepted by 47 state licensing authorities, the District of Columbia, and the Commonwealth of Puerto Rico in lieu of the examination usually required for licensure and is recognized in the American Medical Directory by the letters DNB following the name of the physician holding National Board certification.

The National Board of Medical Examiners has been a leader in developing new and more reliable techniques of testing, not only for knowledge in all medical fields but also for clinical competence and fitness to practice. In recent years, too, a number of medical schools, several specialty certifying boards, professional medical societies organized to encourage their members to keep abreast of progress in medicine, and other professional qualifying agencies have called upon the National Board's professional staff for advice or for the actual preparation of tests to be employed in evaluating medical knowledge, effectiveness of teaching, and professional competence in certain medical fields. In all cases, advantage has been taken of the validity and effectiveness of the objective, multiple-choice type of examination, a technique the National Board has played an important role in bringing to its present state of perfection and discriminatory effectiveness.

Objective examinations permit a large number of questions to be asked, and approximately 150 to 180 questions can be answered in a $2\frac{1}{2}$-hour period. Because the answer sheets are scored by machine, the grading can be accomplished rapidly, accurately, and impartially. It is completely unbiased and based on percentile ranking. Of long-range significance is the facility with which the total test and individual questions can be subjected to thorough and rapid statistical analyses, thus providing a sound basis for comparative studies of medical school teaching and for continuing improvement in the quality of the test itself.

# QUESTIONS

Over the years, many different forms of objective questions have been devised to test not only medical knowledge but also those subtler qualities of discrimination, judgment, and reasoning. Certain types of questions may test an individual's recognition of the similarity or dissimilarity of diseases, drugs, and physiologic or pathologic processes. Other questions test judgment as to cause and effect or the lack of causal relationships. Case histories or patient problems are used to simulate the experience of a physician confronted with a diagnostic problem; a series of questions then tests the individual's understanding of related aspects of the case, such as signs and symptoms, associated laboratory findings, treatment, complications, and prognosis. Case-history questions are set up purposely to place emphasis on correct diagnosis within a context comparable with the experience of actual practice.

It is apparent from recent certification and board examinations that the examiners are devoting more attention in their construction of questions to more practical means of testing basic and clinical knowledge. This greater realism in testing relates to an increasingly interdisciplinary approach toward fundamental material and to the direct relevance accorded practical clinical problems. These more recent approaches to questions have been incorporated into this review series.

Of course, the new approaches to testing add to the difficulty experienced by the student or physician preparing for board or certification examinations. With this in mind, the author of this review is acutely aware not only of the interrelationships of fundamental information within the basic science disciplines and their clinical implications but also of the necessity to present this material clearly and concisely despite its complexity. For this reason, the questions are devised to test knowledge of specific material within the text and identify areas for more intensive study, if necessary. Also, those preparing for examinations must be aware of the interdisciplinary nature of fundamental clinical material, the common multifactorial characteristics of disease mechanisms, and the necessity to shift back and forth from one discipline to another in order to appreciate the less than clear-cut nature separating the pedagogic disciplines.

The different types of questions that may be used on examinations include the completion-type question, where the individual must select one best answer among a number of possible choices, most often five, although there may be three or four; the completion-type question in the negative form, where all but one of the choices is correct and words such as *except* or *least* appear in the question; the true-false type of question, which tests an understanding of cause and effect in relationship to medicine; the multiple true-false type, in which the question may have one, several, or all correct choices; one matching-type question, which tests association and relatedness and uses four choices, two of which use the word, *both* or *neither;* another matching-type question that uses anywhere from three to twenty-six choices and may have more than one correct answer; and, as noted above, the patient-oriented question, which is written around a case and may have several questions included as a group or set.

Many of these question types may be used in course or practice exams; however, at this time the most commonly used types of questions on the USMLE exams are the completion-type question (one best answer), the completion-type negative form, and the multiple matching-type question, designating specifically how many choices are correct. Often included within the questions are graphic elements such as diagrams, charts, graphs, electrocardiograms, roentgenograms, or photomicrographs to elicit knowledge of structure, function, the course of a clinical situation, or a statistical tabulation. Questions then may be asked in relation to designated elements of the same. As noted above, case histories or patient-oriented questions are more frequently used on these examinations, requiring the individual to use more analytic abilities and less memorization-type data.

For further detailed information concerning developments in the evolution of the examination process for medical licensure (for graduates of both U.S. and foreign medical schools), those interested should contact the National Board of Medical Examiners at 3750 Market Street, Philadelphia, PA 19104, USA; telephone number 215–590–9500.

## FIVE POINTS TO REMEMBER

To maximize chances for passing these examinations, the candidate should keep in mind a few commonsense strategies or guidelines.

First, it is imperative to prepare thoroughly for the examination. Know well the types of questions to be presented and the pedagogic areas of particular weakness, and devote more preparatory study time to these areas of weakness. Do not use too much time restudying areas in which there is a feeling of great confidence and do not leave unexplored those areas in which there is less confidence. Finally, be well rested before the test and, if possible, avoid traveling to the city of testing that morning or late the evening before.

Second, know well the format of the examination and the instructions before becoming immersed in the challenge at hand.

This information can be obtained from many published texts and brochures or directly from the testing service (National Board of Medical Examiners, 3750 Market Street, Philadelphia, PA 19104; telephone 215–590–9500). In addition, many available texts and self-assessment types of examination are valuable for practice.

Third, know well the overall time allotted for the examination and its components and the scope of the test to be faced. These may be learned by a rapid review of the examination itself. Then, proceed with the test at a careful, deliberate, and steady pace without spending an inordinate amount of time on any single question. For example, certain questions such as the "one best answer" probably should be allotted 1 to $1\frac{1}{2}$ minutes each. The "matching" type of question should be allotted a similar amount of time.

Fourth, if a question is particularly disturbing, note appropriately the question (put a mark on the question sheet) and return to this point later. Don't compromise yourself by so concentrating on a likely "loser" that several "winners" are eliminated because of inadequate time. One way to save this time on a particular "stickler" is to play your initial choice; your chances of a correct answer are always best with your first impression. If there is no initial choice, reread the question.

Fifth, allow adequate time to review answers, to return to the questions that were unanswered and "flagged" for later attention, and check every *n*th (e.g., 20th) question to make certain that the answers are appropriate and that you did not inadvertently skip a question in the booklet or answer on the sheet (this can happen easily under these stressful circumstances).

There is nothing magical about these five points. They are simple and just make common sense. If you have prepared well, have gotten a good night's sleep, have eaten a good breakfast, and follow the preceding five points, the chances are that you will not have to return for a second go-around.

Edward D. Frohlich, MD, MACP, FACC

# Contents

## Chapter 1
**History, Physical Examination, and Differential Diagnosis    1**

The Pediatric History    1
The Pediatric Physical Examination    2
Differential Diagnosis    3

## Chapter 2
**Growth and Development    5**

Normal Growth    5
Abnormal Patterns of Growth    9
Normal Development    10
Abnormal Development    14

## Chapter 3
**Nutrition and Metabolism    17**

Water Metabolism and Requirements    17
Electrolytes    18
Electrolyte Disorders    19
Acid-Base Disorders    20
Caloric Requirements    21
Vitamins    23

## Chapter 4
**Pregnancy, Labor, and Delivery of the Newborn    27**

Mortality Rate    27
Pregnancy and Its Effects on the Fetus    28
Labor and Delivery and the Effects on the Infant    32
Classification of the Newborn    34

## Chapter 5
**The Normal Newborn    39**

Neonatal Anatomy and Physiology    39

## Chapter 6
## Diseases of the Newborn    45

Cardiopulmonary Disorders    45
Hematologic/Hepatic Disorders    48
Gastrointestinal Disorders    52
Diseases of the Central Nervous System    54
Acquired Infections in the Newborn    55
Congenital Infections of the Newborn    56

## Chapter 7
## Infectious Diseases    61

General Principles of Pediatric Infectious Disease    61
Bacteremia and Sepsis    62
Scarlet Fever    63
Tuberculosis    64
Spirochetal Infection    65
Rickettsial Infection    66
Cat-Scratch Disease    66
Viral Infections    67
Parasitic Infections    70

## Chapter 8
## Disorders of the Respiratory System    73

Disorders of the Ears and Sinuses    73
Congenital Anomalies of the Respiratory Tract    74
Infections of the Respiratory Tract    75
Asthma    80
Cystic Fibrosis    81
Kartagener Syndrome    82
Alpha-1-Antitrypsin Deficiency    82
Sudden Infant Death Syndrome    83

## Chapter 9
## Genetic Disorders    85

Chromosomal Abnormalities    85

## Chapter 10
## Metabolic and Endocrine Disorders    89

Inborn Errors of Metabolism    89
Disorders of Amino Acid Metabolism    90
Peroxisomal Disorder    91
Sphingolipidoses    92
Disorders of Carbohydrate Metabolism    93
Glycogen Storage Diseases    94

Mucopolysaccharidoses    94
Thyroid Disorders    96
Adrenal Disorders    98
Disorders of the Pituitary Gland    99
Disorders of Puberty    100
Disorders of the Pancreas    102

## Chapter 11
# Hematologic and Malignant Disorders    105

Anemia    105
Iron Deficiency Anemia    105
Megaloblastic Anemias    107
Hemolytic Anemias    107
Pancytopenia    112
Thrombocytopenia    113
Hemophilias    113
Malignant Disorders    115
Leukemias    115
Lymphomas    117
Tumors of the Central Nervous System    118
Neuroblastoma    120
Wilms' Tumor    121
Rhabdomyosarcoma    121
Bone Tumors    122
Retinoblastoma    122
Histiocytoses    123

## Chapter 12
# Disorders of the Nervous System    125

Congenital Malformations of the Central Nervous System    125
Neurocutaneous Syndromes    126
Seizure Disorders    127
Movement Disorders    131
Infections of the Central Nervous System    131
Central Nervous System Trauma    134
Neuromuscular Disorders    134

## Chapter 13
# Cardiovascular Disorders    139

Congenital Heart Disease    139
Arrhythmias    145
Vasculitis    145

## Chapter 14
## Disorders of the Gastrointestinal System 149

Esophageal Foreign Bodies 149
Gastroesophageal Reflux 149
Pyloric Stenosis 150
Meckel's Diverticulum 150
Malrotation 151
Intussusception 151
Acute Appendicitis 152
Acute Gastroenteritis 152
Enzyme Deficiencies 153
Food Allergies 154
Crohn's Disease 154
Ulcerative Colitis 155
Indirect Inguinal Hernias 155

## Chapter 15
## Genitourinary and Renal Disorders 157

Genitourinary Disorders 157
Renal Disease 160

## Chapter 16
## Immunologic and Rheumatologic Disorders 167

Primary Immunodeficiencies 167
Acquired Immunodeficiencies 170
Rheumatologic Disorders 172

## Chapter 17
## Orthopedic Disorders 175

Congenital Anomalies 175
Infections of the Bones and Joints 178
Orthopedic Trauma 179
Skeletal Dysplasias 180

## Chapter 18
## Child Abuse and Neglect 181

## Chapter 19
## Ophthalmologic Disorders 183

Congenital Anomalies 183
Infections of the Eye 184

## Chapter 20
## Skin Disorders   187

Congenital Anomalies   187
Dermatitis   187
Vascular Lesions   189
Bacterial Skin Infections   190
Viral Skin Infections   191
Fungal Skin Infections   192
Parasitic Skin Infections   193

## Chapter 21
## Preventive Pediatrics   195

Dental Care   195
Poisoning   196
Automobile Accidents   197
Drowning   198
Burns   198
Childhood Immunizations   198

## Pediatrics Questions   203

## Pediatrics Answers and Discussion   267

## Pediatrics Must-Know Topics   297

## Index   309

# Chapter 1

# History, Physical Examination, and Differential Diagnosis

Children are growing, developing, and vulnerable organisms. This simple, if obvious, fact differentiates pediatrics from other areas of medicine. Although the field shares many concepts and approaches with all of medicine, it also requires special knowledge, skills, and attitudes.

## THE PEDIATRIC HISTORY

The structure of the pediatric history is similar to that of other branches of medicine; however, factors unique to children and their position within the family require special interviewing skills. With the exception of adolescents, the pediatric history is usually obtained from the parent or guardian rather than from the child. The parent may have concerns outside of the immediate medical problem which require the attention of the physician. The encounter with the parents also provides the physician with the opportunity to teach them about preventive pediatrics and the proper care of the child. Adolescents should be interviewed in the absence of the parent or guardian, even if a repeat history is necessary. History taking is an ongoing process, particularly for hospitalized children, with clarification and details continuously sought.

The **chief complaint** serves to focus the problem by clearly stating the child's age, sex, chronic medical conditions, and the most important signs and symptoms and their duration. This formulation serves to begin the process of generating a differential diagnosis, which is the primary goal of the pediatric history and physical examination. Secondary goals include the identification of other medical, familial, or social problems that require attention and intervention.

The **history of present illness** is a written narrative of the patient's illness and should have a coherent and logical flow, usually on a chronological basis. For infants, it is relevant to begin with the birth history. For children with chronic conditions, a brief history of this chronic condition should be recounted. The history of present illness should end with pertinent negative findings based on the differential diagnosis generated at this point.

The **past medical history** is a brief account of the child's medical history not described previously in the history of present illness. The past medical history should contain a description of the birth including the birth weight, chronic diseases or conditions, previous hospitalizations and surgery, fractures, and allergies to medications or foods.

A detailed **immunization history**, which should be part of every pediatric history, provides the basis for ensuring complete immunization at every medical encounter.

Details of the **dietary history** and **developmental history** are dependent on the age of the child and the medical problem. For infants, the dietary history should include the type of milk or formula and the amount and frequency of each feeding. Children with gastrointestinal or growth disturbances require more detailed dietary history. For preschool children, it is useful to divide the developmental history into gross motor, fine motor, language, and social development. School performance serves as a crude index of developmental achievement. Adolescents should be asked about school performance, drug use, and sexual activity.

The **family history** should provide a picture of the position of the child within the family and potential for inherited medical conditions. The **social history** provides a description of the family and its social and economic position within the community. Information about parental employment, housing conditions, and medical insurance provides important insights into the context of the child's health.

The **review of systems** is an attempt at the end of the pediatric history to uncover medical problems that have not been addressed previously. In contrast to adults, most children do not have multiple medical problems. However, the review of systems can be useful in detecting vision and hearing problems, dental problems, enuresis, and behavioral problems.

# THE PEDIATRIC PHYSICAL EXAMINATION

The skills required to examine a child are unique to pediatrics. First, the physician must enlist the cooperation and trust of the child. Useful techniques include speaking gently and approaching the child in a nonthreatening manner. The young child is often best examined on the parent's lap. To allow the child to feel comfortable with the examiner, it is best to begin by first touching the hands or feet. Once the child is calm and cooperative, auscultation of the **chest and heart** should be performed, followed by examination of the **abdomen**. The examination of the **head, neck, throat,** and **tympanic membranes** should be the final phase of the examination. Examination of the middle ear is not complete unless pneumatic otoscopy or insufflation is performed.

Some aspects of the pediatric physical examination require special attention. Measurement of **vital signs** should be part of every physical examination. With the exception of body temperature, the vital signs vary markedly with the age of the child (Table 1-1).

Proper measurement of **blood pressure** in children requires that the blood pressure cuff length be 80% to 100% of the circumference of the arm and that the arm be held at the level of the heart. The first Korotkoff sound marks the systolic blood pressure and the fourth Korotkoff sound (the change in tone) marks the diastolic pressure (in adults it is the loss of sound, the fifth Korotkoff sound, that marks the diastolic pressure). In children, the blood pressure in the legs is normally 10 mm Hg *higher* than in the arms.

**Anthropometric measurements** (**weight**, **height**, and **head circumference** in children less than age 3) are also a routine part of the pediatric physical examination. These measurements should be plotted on appropriate growth curves and compared with previous measurements. The head circumference is obtained by measuring the head in its widest diameter, including the most prominent part of the occiput through the area just above the supraorbital ridges of the forehead.

The **general appearance** of the ill child is of considerable importance in assessment. It is valuable to carefully observe the child while taking the history before the actual examination. The level of activity and interaction with the environment may provide important clues to the severity of illness, the neurodevelopmental status of the child, and the quality of the mother-child interaction.

**Signs of respiratory distress** include tachypnea, retractions, and nasal flaring, even in the absence of auscultatory findings. Many children will have cardiac murmurs that are caused by minor turbulence of blood flow rather than by structural cardiac defects. Because these murmurs, which are called **innocent** or **functional**, have no clinical significance, the parents and child should be reassured that these are benign findings. Characteristic innocent murmurs include Still's murmur, a musical murmur due to turbulence in the left ventricular outflow tract, best heard at the cardiac apex; peripheral pulmonic stenosis heard in the back of neonates; and venous hums, audible at the base of the heart, which disappear in the supine position.

## DIFFERENTIAL DIAGNOSIS

**Clinical reasoning** involves the generation of a list of hypotheses, the differential diagnosis, which then is altered and narrowed as information from the history, physical examination, and laboratory evaluation is obtained. The process of generating a differential diagnosis begins with the chief complaint. The list of hypotheses directs

# PEDIATRICS

**TABLE 1-1. Normal Vital Signs in Children**

### Age-Specific Heart Rates in Children (beats/minute)

| Age | 2% | Mean | 98% |
|---|---|---|---|
| <1 day | 93 | 123 | 154 |
| 1–2 days | 91 | 123 | 159 |
| 3–6 days | 91 | 129 | 166 |
| 1–3 weeks | 107 | 148 | 182 |
| 1–2 months | 121 | 149 | 179 |
| 3–5 months | 106 | 141 | 186 |
| 6–11 months | 109 | 134 | 169 |
| 1–2 years | 89 | 119 | 151 |
| 3–4 years | 73 | 108 | 137 |
| 5–7 years | 65 | 100 | 133 |
| 8–11 years | 62 | 91 | 130 |
| 12–15 years | 60 | 85 | 119 |

### Age-Specific Respiratory Rates in Children (breaths/minute)

| Age/Years | Boys | Girls |
|---|---|---|
| 0–1 | 31+–8 | 30+–6 |
| 1–2 | 26+–4 | 27+–4 |
| 2–3 | 25+–4 | 25+–3 |
| 3–4 | 23+–3 | 24+–3 |
| 4–5 | 22+–2 | 22+–2 |
| 5–6 | 21+–2 | 21+–2 |
| 6–7 | 20+–3 | 21+–3 |
| 7–8 | 20+–3 | 20+–2 |
| 8–9 | 19+–2 | 20+–2 |
| 9–10 | 19+–2 | 19+–2 |
| 10–11 | 19+–2 | 19+–2 |
| 11–12 | 19+–3 | 19+–3 |
| 12–13 | 19+–3 | 19+–2 |
| 13–14 | 19+–2 | 18+–2 |
| 14–15 | 18+–2 | 18+–3 |

*From* The Harriet Lane Handbook, *13th ed., pp. 101 and 335.*

further questioning. Modification of the differential diagnosis then directs the physical examination and the choice of laboratory studies. Physicians must keep an open mind to additional diagnostic possibilities, and not so readily adhere to a single diagnosis. Failure to do so may result in a critical oversight.

# Chapter 2

# Growth and Development

The hallmark of any professional concerned with the health and welfare of children is a profound understanding of and interest in children's growth and development.

## NORMAL GROWTH

Growth is defined as the process by which the human body increases in size as a result of an increase in the size and/or the number of the body's cells. Children do not grow at the same rate throughout childhood. The most rapid period of growth occurs during the embryonic and fetal period, during which the fetus grows from a single cell at conception to about 3300 grams (7½ pounds) at birth. Although infants obviously grow in size, the actual rate of growth decreases during the first 3 years of life. From the age of 3 years until the onset of puberty, children's rate of growth remains relatively steady. At puberty, the rate of growth again increases. Various organs show different patterns of growth throughout childhood. The central nervous system (CNS) grows rapidly in the first few years of life, whereas lymphoid tissue attains maximal growth during the early school years.

### Weight

The average newborn in the United States weighs about 3400 grams, with a normal range of 2500 to 4600 grams. Newborns may lose as much as 10% of their birth weight immediately following birth because of the loss of extracellular fluid, but they should regain their birth weight by 10 to 14 days of life. Normal full-term infants who gain an average of approximately 30 grams (1 ounce) a day during the first 5 to 6 months of life will double their birth weights by 5 to 6 months of age and triple their birth weights by 1 year of age. After the first year, weight gain averages about 2 to 3 kilograms (4 to 6 pounds) yearly. At 2.5 years, the birth weight is quadrupled. Subcutaneous tissue is maximum at 9 months of age. The following formulas provide a method of estimating average weight in children:

3 to 12 months of age: weight (in pounds) = age in months + 11
2 to 12 years: weight (in pounds) = (age in years × 5) + 18

## Height

Growth in stature progresses less rapidly than weight. The average newborn measures about 51 cm (20 inches) in length with a range of 46 to 56 cm. The length increases approximately 25 to 30 cm (10 to 12 inches) in the first year of life. After the first year, gain in height averages 6 to 8 cm (2.5 to 3.5 inches) yearly. The birth length usually doubles by 3 to 4 years of age, and it triples by 13 years of age. The eventual adult height can be approximated by doubling the value of the child's height at about 2 years of age. An estimate of the height of children between the ages of 2 to 12 years can be calculated using the following formula:

Height in inches = (age in years × 2) + 32

## Head Circumference

Increases in head circumference parallel the rapidly growing CNS. The newborn's head circumference averages approximately 35 cm, with a range of 32.6 to 37.2 cm. During the first year of life, the head circumference normally increases by about 10 to 12 cm (4 to 5 inches); during the second year of life, the head circumference increases only 2 cm (1 inch). The brain reaches adult size at about 12 years of age.

In general, a normal 7-month-old infant has a head circumference of 17 inches (43 cm); a 19-month-old child has a head circumference of 19 inches (48 cm); and a 5-year-old has a head circumference of about 20 inches (51 cm).

## Growth Charts

Serial measurements of these parameters of growth in populations of normal children provide the clinician with **standards** against which to measure the individual child. Several growth charts have been developed for this purpose. The most commonly used, prepared by the United States National Center for Health Care Statistics and derived from American children of different ethnic and socioeconomic backgrounds, presents height, weight, and head circumference growth curves for children of various ages and sex. Growth charts for weight-for-height and height velocity are also available and provide additional information in assessing the child with abnormal growth. Often the **pattern of growth** rather than a single measurement is more instructive. Over a period of time, a child should follow the same pattern on the growth curve; any significant deviation from this pattern suggests serious organic disease or a noxious environmental influence.

## Teeth

In most children, the first deciduous teeth erupt between 5 to 9 months of age in the following sequence: lower central incisors, upper central incisors, upper lateral incisors, and lower lateral incisors. Most children have six to eight teeth by 1 year of age. Eight more teeth erupt during the second year of life, including the first deciduous molars, canines, and second deciduous molars. The first permanent molars usually erupt during the seventh year of life as the deciduous teeth begin to shed, roughly following the order of their appearance, at a rate of four teeth each year. The second permanent molars erupt at about age 14 years.

## Sinuses

At birth, the maxillary and ethmoid sinuses are small and the frontal and sphenoidal sinuses undeveloped. The sphenoidal sinuses develop by 3 years of age and the frontal sinuses by 3 to 7 years of age.

## Bone Age

Since the ossification centers of the bones form at different and predictable ages, radiographic examination of the hands and feet provides an estimate of the child's bone age. Five ossification centers are usually present at birth: the calcaneus, cuboid, talus, the distal end of the femur, and the proximal end of the tibia. Until the age of 6 years, with the aid of the following formula, a radiograph of the wrist will assist in the determination of the child's bone age:

Age in years + 1 = number of ossification centers in the wrist

## Adolescence and Puberty

Adolescence is characterized by a consistent pattern of pubertal development. **Puberty**, the period between the first appearances of the adult genital configuration and the end of somatic growth, is characterized by **rapid growth** and by the development of **secondary sex characteristics**. The timing of puberty varies in females and males, but the development of secondary sexual characteristics follows a predictable pattern. This development is categorized by stages (sexual maturity ratings or Tanner stages) that mark the development of primary and secondary sexual characteristics: pubic hair and breast development in girls and pubic hair and genitalia enlargement in boys. In girls, the sexual maturity ratings of breast and pubic hair development occur in parallel. In boys, genital staging usually precedes staging of pubic hair, with testicular enlargement being the first sign of puberty. Peak height velocity is better correlated with sexual maturity rating than with chronological age. Table 2-1 provides the Tanner stages of secondary sexual characteristic for males and females.

The onset of puberty occurs earlier in girls than in boys. In the United States, in girls, the average age when puberty begins is 10.5 years, with a range between 8 to 13 years; in boys, the average onset of puberty is 12 years, with a range between 9 and 14 years. The age at menarche, the onset of menstruation, varies considerably, but in the United States it is usually about 12 to 13 years, with a range of 10 to 16.5 years. The majority of menstrual cycles in the first year or two after menarche are anovulatory.

Each stage of adolescence is associated with characteristic psychological, social, and cognitive development. The peer group forms an important set of relationships that powerfully influence the adoles-

### TABLE 2-1.
### Tanner Stages of Pubertal Development

**Females**

|  |  |
|---|---|
| Stage I | Preadolescent female |
| Stage II | Sparse, straight pubic hair along medial border of labia |
| | Breast and papilla slightly elevated with increased areolar diameter |
| Stage III | Increased amounts of darker pubic hair that begins to curl |
| | Breast and areola enlarged |
| Stage IV | Pubic hair is coarse and curly and abundant |
| | Breast areola and papilla form secondary mound |
| Stage V | Pubic hair in adult configuration forming feminine triangle and extending to medial surfaces of thighs |
| | Breasts have mature nipples and areola becomes part of the general contour of the breast |

**Males**

|  |  |
|---|---|
| Stage I | No pubic hair |
| | Preadolescent penis and testis |
| Stage II | Scant, long, light pubic hair |
| | Slight enlargement of penis with enlarged scrotum |
| Stage III | Small amount of dark curling pubic hair |
| | Longer penis and larger testis |
| Stage IV | Pubic hair resembles adult configuration but less in amount |
| | Larger penis with increase in breadth and size of glans penis and larger darkened scrotum |
| Stage V | Adult distribution of pubic hair that extends to medial surface of the thighs |
| | Adult size penis and testis |

cent's behavior. Cigarette smoking, drug and alcohol use, and sexual activity are all strongly influenced by the peer group as well as by the family. The need for achieving self-identity and independence often manifests itself in risky behavior and rebellion against authority. The concrete thinking of early adolescence is replaced by abstract reasoning by late adolescence.

# ABNORMAL PATTERNS OF GROWTH

## Malnutrition and Failure to Thrive

Kwashiorkor (protein deficiency), marasmus (energy deficiency), and marasmic kwashiorkor (combined deficiency) are the most extreme forms of **protein-energy malnutrition** (**PEM**). Children with severe PEM are prone to life-threatening infections, electrolyte disturbances, hypothermia and other nutritional deficiencies (vitamin A, iron).

Failure to thrive and growth retardation are among the most common presenting signs of serious disease in children. **Failure to thrive** is a term usually reserved for infants who show significantly diminished growth. The term **growth retardation** is usually reserved for older children. Children with chronic conditions such as sickle cell disease, cystic fibrosis, chronic infection (human immunodeficiency virus [HIV]), congenital heart disease, hypopituitarism, and chronic renal failure have diminished growth velocity and often fail to thrive.

## Nonorganic Failure to Thrive

Nonorganic failure to thrive, which is due to profound psychosocial disturbances, may be a manifestation of child abuse. The diagnosis is made by excluding obvious organic causes and a careful investigation of the child's environment, particularly the interaction between the child and the mother or primary caretaker. Removal of the child from the home environment and provision of adequate caloric intake are both diagnostic and therapeutic.

## Obesity

Childhood obesity may persist into adulthood, predisposing a person to hypertension, diabetes and hyperlipidemia. Obesity in childhood is associated with an increase in both adipocyte size and number. Rare causes of obesity in childhood include Prader-Willi syndrome and Laurence-Moon-Biedl syndrome. Such abnormalities, however, are usually associated with decreased height for age.

## Short Stature

The causes of short stature are many, but important diagnostic considerations include inflammatory bowel disease, chronic renal failure, Turner syndrome, and growth hormone deficiency. These organic causes of short stature must be distinguished from constitutional growth delay, a variant of normal growth with delayed puberty but eventual normal adult height, and from genetic or familial short stature. Comparison of skeletal maturation (bone age) with height age and chronologic age assists in distinguishing these patterns of growth.

## Microcephaly

Microcephaly may be either genetic or acquired. Genetic microcephaly may be associated with chromosomal abnormalities (trisomies 21 and 18 and cri du chat syndrome) and is usually present at birth. The causes of acquired microcephaly, which may be either intrauterine or postnatal, include congenital infections, maternal alcohol use, and hypoxic-ischemic encephalopathy.

## Hydrocephalus

Hydrocephalus, **excess accumulation of cerebrospinal fluid** (CSF), is a significant cause of an increased head circumference and is classified as either obstructive or nonobstructive (communicating). Obstructive hydrocephalus is due to obstruction of the flow of CSF in the CNS. Such structural abnormalities include stenosis of the aqueduct of Sylvius or compression of the fourth ventricle. Compression of the fourth ventricle occurs in the Chiari malformation and the Dandy-Walker cyst. Obstructive hydrocephalus can be treated by placement of a ventriculoperitoneal shunt.

Nonobstructive or communicating hydrocephalus results from the failure of absorption of CSF by the arachnoid villi and can be caused by subarachnoid hemorrhage and meningitis.

Macrocephaly in the absence of hydrocephalus can occur with Sotos' syndrome and certain inborn errors of metabolism.

# NORMAL DEVELOPMENT

Development may be defined as a continuous, progressive, and sequential process by which a child's level of function becomes more complex. This gradual progression of function, which reflects the gradual maturation of the CNS, proceeds in a cephalocaudad, proximodistal direction. Although the child's developmental process is assessed clinically at discrete points in time, in fact, the process continues throughout life in a general sequence and pattern that does not vary a great deal among normal children.

For the purposes of assessment, this developmental process can be classified into categories of gross motor, fine motor, language and social development. **Gross motor** developmental tasks include those that involve the large muscle groups of the trunk and extremities; **fine motor** tasks involve those of the small muscles of the body, specifically, the hands; **language** development refers to the growth of language and communicative skills; **social** development is defined as that involving interpersonal and social skills. Physicians caring for children should have a working knowledge of the common developmental milestones and the ages at which they are expected in normal children. Common developmental milestones from infancy to the preschool period are summarized in Tables 2-2 through 2-5.

## Psychosocial Development

Several theories are useful in understanding the stages of psychosocial development. Sigmund Freud first described stages of psychosocial development using his psychoanalytic theory. This theoretical analysis has been further elaborated by Erik Erikson, Anna Freud, and others.

### Freud

As applied to children, Freudian psychosocial development includes the following stages.

1. The **oral stage** is from birth to about 18 months and is characterized by the infant's great sensitivity to oral sensations and gratifications. At the outset, the infant cannot differentiate

**TABLE 2-2.**

**Developmental Milestones: Gross Motor Development**

| Activity | Age (months) |
| --- | --- |
| Sits with support | 3–4 |
| Sits alone | 7–8 |
| Stands alone for a few seconds | 12–13 |
| Walks unassisted | 12–15 |
| Climbs on furniture | 24 |
| Walks up stairs one step at a time | 24 |
| Rides tricycle | 36 |

**TABLE 2-3. Developmental Milestones: Fine Motor Development**

| Activity | Age (months) |
|---|---|
| Grasp reflex | At birth |
| Intentional reaching | 4–5 |
| Palmar grasp | 6–8 |
| Pincer grasp | 9–10 |
| Builds a six-block tower | 24 |
| Builds a three-block bridge | 36 |
| Reproduces a cross with a crayon | 36 |

between himself and the outer world, but over time develops the ability to distinguish between himself and those, usually the mother, who gratify his oral needs.

2. The **anal stage** is from 18 months to about 3 years when the child focuses on pleasures from the anal region principally during defecation. During this stage of development, the child gradually develops control over his impulses.
3. The **phallic stage**, from 3 to 5 years, is characterized by an interest in and focus upon the genital region. During this stage, the child begins to differentiate between the sexes.
4. The **latency stage** is between 5 years and adolescence and is characterized by Freud as a quiet period between the phallic stage and the next stage, the genital stage.
5. The **genital stage** occurs during adolescence and is characterized by the development of more mature relationships with those of the opposite sex.

**TABLE 2-4. Developmental Milestones: Language Development**

| Activity | Age |
|---|---|
| Indistinct throat noises | 3–5 weeks |
| Cooing | 10–12 weeks |
| Single and multiple syllables | 6–8 months |
| Two-word phrases | 36 months |
| Six- to seven-word phrases | 48 months |

### TABLE 2-5.
### Developmental Milestones: Social Development

| Activity | Age |
| --- | --- |
| Social smile | 4–6 weeks |
| Smiles at self in mirror | 6 months |
| Responds to word "no" | 8 months |
| Becomes frightened with strangers | 8–10 months |
| Knows own gender | 24–30 months |
| Plays in parallel | 24–36 months |

*Erikson*

Erik **Erikson**, who elaborated this basic Freudian theory, also described six stages of psychosocial development. These stages are described as positive and negative attributes, depending on whether the stage has been mastered.

1. **Basic trust versus mistrust**, the stage from birth to 18 months, is characterized by the development of trust that someone, usually the mother, will supply the infant's basic needs. Through the consistent gratifications of these needs the infant learns to trust others in the outside world.
2. **Autonomy versus shame and doubt**, the stage from 18 months to 3 years, involves the gradual development of self-control and independence. During this stage, the child begins to learn to delay gratification in the interest of more important goals.
3. **Initiative versus guilt**, between the ages of 36 months to 5 years, is characterized by the child's active planning and undertaking tasks. During this stage, the child also develops an active fantasy life with which he copes with fears and conflicts.
4. **Industry versus inferiority**, between the age of 5 to 12 years, is the stage during which the child begins preparation for adult work. During this stage, the child begins to enjoy work and develop a sense of accomplishment.
5. **Identity versus role confusion** begins during adolescence and is characterized by a consolidation of the adolescent's sense of his own unique personality and character.

*Piaget*

In addition to Freud and Erikson, Jean **Piaget** is an important theorist of child development, principally in the area of cognitive development. He also divides the developmental process into stages.

1. The **sensorimotor period** from birth to 2 years is characterized by the infant's interactions with the environment as governed

by his overt sensory and physical actions. Over a period of time, the infant gradually develops a sense of internal representation, which permits the development of the sense that objects outside himself have a separate and independent existence. Piaget calls this milestone object concept.
2. The **preoperational period** from 2 to 7 years of age is characterized by egocentrism, that is, the child's view is the only possible one. During this phase, thoughts and events are equally real to the child. The child's logic at this stage is correlational, that is, two events that happen at the same time are caused by each another.
3. The **concrete operational stage** from age 7 to 11 years is characterized by the gradual development of inductive logic, that is, the ability to generalize from specifics to general conclusions.
4. The **formal operational stage** after the age of 11 years is characterized by the final development to adult modes of thinking, which involves inductive logic, the application of a general principle to a specific instance.

Just as significant deviation in growth can signal either serious disease or environmental problems, so, too, does a significant deviation in a child's developmental progress.

# ABNORMAL DEVELOPMENT

The physician has available a variety of **developmental screening tests** that can be used to assess the developmental level of infants and children. The Denver Developmental Screening test, a simple and reliable test that can be used in children from birth to 6½ years, involves testing a series of milestones in the gross motor, fine motor, personal-social, and language domains.

The Goodenough draw-a-man test, which is especially useful for preschool children, involves giving the child a blank 8″ by 11″ sheet of paper and a pencil and asking the child to "draw a man, the best man you can." The draw-a-man test is scored by counting the number of body parts the child draws. These types of developmental tests are useful clinical screening instruments, but formal psychometric testing is required to confirm the diagnosis of developmental delay.

## Mental Retardation

**Developmental disability** results from a complex interaction of biological, environmental, familial and social factors. Mental retardation, a limitation in measured intelligence and adaptive behavior, ranges from borderline to profound and is characterized by delayed

### TABLE 2-6.
### Major Causes of Mental Retardation

**Chromosomal abnormalities**
    Fragile X syndrome
    Trisomies
    Cri du chat syndrome and other chromosomal deletions

**Congenital anomalies**
    Hydrocephalus
    Anencephaly
    Craniosynostosis

**Inborn errors of metabolism**
    Hypoglycemia
    Phenylketonuria and other disorders of amino acid metabolism
    Urea cycle defects
    Adrenoleukodystrophy
    Lipid storage diseases
    Galactosemia and other disorders of carbohydrate metabolism
    Mucopolysaccharidoses
    Disorders of purine and pyrimidine metabolism

**Diseases of the endocrine system**
    Congenital hypothyroidism

**Neurologic diseases**
    Cerebral palsy
    Neurocutaneous syndromes
    Infantile spasms and other epilepsy syndromes
    Duchenne muscular dystrophy and myotonic dystrophy
    Rett syndrome

**Infections of the CNS**
    Congenital cytomegalovirus infection
    Congenital rubella infection
    Congenital toxoplasmosis virus infection
    Meningitis and encephalitis
    Human immunodeficiency virus infection

**Hypoxia**
    Intrapartum asphyxia
    Periventricular leukomalacia
    Carbon monoxide poisoning

**Toxins**
    Fetal alcohol syndrome
    Hyperbilirubinemia and kernicterus
    Lead poisoning

**Head injuries**

**Child abuse and neglect**

achievement of developmental milestones. About 3% of the general population have an intelligence quotient (IQ) less than two standard deviations below the mean (less than 68) and are classified as mentally retarded.

Most children with mental retardation are mildly affected and are defined as **educable**. This group will function at about the fifth-grade level and as adults can manage unskilled or semiskilled occupations. Moderately retarded children (IQ between 51 and 36) who are defined as **trainable** will be able to dress themselves, feed themselves and be toilet trained. As adults, they require supervision but can function in a sheltered workshop setting. Only about 5% are so **severely retarded** (IQ below 35) that they are totally dependent and require custodial care.

Chromosomal abnormalities, recognizable syndromes, metabolic disorders, toxins (lead), and congenital infections are important causes of mental retardation. A classification of the major causes of mental retardation is found in Table 2-6.

## Cerebral Palsy

Cerebral palsy refers to a group of **nonprogressive disorders of motor function** due to abnormalities of the brain in its early development. Cerebral palsy is classified by the extremities involved (monoplegia, hemiplegia, diplegia, and quadriplegia) and the type of neurologic dysfunction (spastic, hypotonic, dystonic, and athetotic). Children with cerebral palsy frequently have epilepsy and cognitive impairment, although many children with cerebral palsy have normal intelligence. Infants born prematurely are at greater risk of cerebral palsy, as are full-term infants with congenital malformations and low-birth weight. Evidence is poor that cerebral palsy is related to problems during delivery or low Apgar scores.

# Chapter 3

# Nutrition and Metabolism

Because adequate nutrition is a prerequisite for normal growth and development in children, physicians must not only understand the physiologic requirements of the growing child but must also be able to translate these requirements into a diet consonant with the family's prevailing culture. The basic requirements of any diet include water, calories (in the form of carbohydrate, fat, and protein), vitamins, and minerals (Table 3-1).

## WATER METABOLISM AND REQUIREMENTS

The percentage of body water, specifically extracellular water, decreases with age. Equilibrium between extracellular fluid and intracellular fluid is maintained by the movement of water in response to osmotic gradients. Changes in osmolality, as occur with low intravascular protein concentration, result in an increase in interstitial fluid, edema, and ascites.

**TABLE 3-1.**

**Average Daily Nutritional Requirements for Infants and Children**

| Age | Calories | Protein (g) | A ($\mu$g) (RE) | D ($\mu$g) | C (mg) | Fe (mg) | Ca (mg) |
|---|---|---|---|---|---|---|---|
| 0–6 months | 115/kg | 13 | 375 | 7.5 | 30 | 6 | 400 |
| 6–12 months | 105/kg | 14 | 375 | 10 | 35 | 10 | 600 |
| 1–3 years | 1300 | 16 | 400 | 10 | 40 | 10 | 800 |
| 4–6 years | 1700 | 24 | 500 | 10 | 45 | 10 | 800 |
| 7–10 years | 2400 | 28 | 700 | 10 | 45 | 10 | 800 |

Columns A–C are Vitamins; Fe and Ca are Minerals.

Adapted from Recommendations of the Food and Nutrition Board, National Academy of Science National Research Council, revised, 1989.

Water requirements vary directly with the body's metabolic rate, and estimates of water requirements are based on this relationship. At basal conditions, obligatory **water requirements** are estimated to be **100 mL/100 calories metabolized**. A tripartite, linear relationship is then assumed between metabolic rate and body weight, resulting in the following estimation of water requirements:

100 mL/kg for the first 10 kg of body weight
50 mL/kg for the next 10 kg of body weight
20 mL/kg for additional kg of body weight

For example, an estimate of water requirements for a 9-kg child is 900 mL/day; for a 15-kg child, 1250 mL/day; and for a 22-kg child, 1540 mL/day.

The assumption that metabolic rate is proportional to body weight, however, is not always reasonable; for example, these estimates are not valid for neonates and premature infants whose metabolic rates and water requirements are significantly higher. Significant physical activity, increase in body temperature, sweating, tachypnea, and types of renal impairment (e.g., impaired concentrating ability) also increase water requirements.

**Body surface area** is better correlated with metabolic rate than body weight. For children who weigh more than 10 kg, water requirements may be estimated as 1500 mL/m$^2$/day.

# ELECTROLYTES

For the child with normal renal function and in the absence of abnormal electrolyte loss (as found in cystic fibrosis), a normal, varied diet provides sufficient sodium and potassium for growth. Daily requirements for **sodium and potassium** increase with age and body weight. Sodium requirements range from 120 to 500 mg/day, and potassium requirements range from 500 to 2000 mg/day. Serum concentrations do not reflect total body sodium or potassium, although total body sodium may be estimated using the body weight, volume of distribution (0.6 to 0.7), and serum sodium concentration.

Standard **parenteral solutions** for short-term hydration of hospitalized infants and children provide both sodium and dextrose. After determining that the child has normal renal function, potassium is usually added. The concentration of sodium in standard solutions ranges from 38 to 77 mEq/L. Normal saline, used for rapid volume replacement, has a sodium concentration of 154 mEq/L. Parenteral solutions containing 5% dextrose provide sufficient glucose to prevent significant protein catabolism over several days.

## Oral Fluid Therapy for Dehydration

Oral fluid therapy for the dehydration caused by acute gastroenteritis is divided into two phases: **rehydration** and **maintenance hydration**. Rehydration, which is used to replenish extracellular volume depletion, usually requires 4 to 6 hours and is best accomplished using a rehydration solution containing 75 to 90 mEq/L of sodium. Maintenance hydration and replacement of ongoing losses is accomplished using a solution containing 40 to 60 mEq/L of sodium. Because of a sodium cotransport system that facilitates the absorption of sodium and water and remains intact in gastroenteritis, both types of solution should contain glucose or a low molecular weight carbohydrate. Vomiting is not a contraindication to oral fluid therapy, and breast-feeding should not be discontinued. In the therapy of dehydration secondary to acute gastroenteritis, feeding should be reintroduced as early as the completion of the rehydration phase.

The degree of dehydration is classified as **mild, moderate, or severe**. These three degrees correspond approximately to 5%, 10%, and 15% loss of body weight. In older children and adults, these degrees correspond to 3%, 6%, and 9% loss of body weight. Assessment of the degree of dehydration is based on a number of clinical signs and symptoms including mucous membranes, tears, skin turgor, anterior fontanelle, and behavior. More refined assessment of the degree of dehydration requires comparison of predehydration and postdehydration weights and cannot be based on clinical assessment alone.

# ELECTROLYTE DISORDERS

## Sodium

**Hypernatremia** may result from salt poisoning, improper preparation of infant formulas, abnormal renal losses of water (diabetes insipidus), or as a consequence of gastroenteritis (hypernatremic dehydration). Too rapid correction of hypernatremia may cause cerebral edema and seizures. **Hyponatremia** results from either sodium depletion or water intoxication. Excessive sodium losses occur through the kidneys, skin (cystic fibrosis), or gastrointestinal tract (hyponatremia dehydration). Demyelination of the brain stem is a rare sequela of too rapid correction of hyponatremia.

## Potassium

**Hyperkalemia** results from excessive oral or parenteral intake or impaired renal excretion. Marked hyperkalemia can cause ventricular fibrillation and death. **Hypokalemia** usually results from urinary losses, as in diuretic use and Bartter syndrome, or gastrointestinal losses, as found in pyloric stenosis. Clinical manifestations include muscle weakness and cardiac arrhythmias.

### Glucose

**Hyperglycemia** is the cardinal manifestation of diabetes mellitus, but transient hyperglycemia may occur as a result of a significant sympathetic nervous system response. **Hypoglycemia** can have profound effects on the developing child because of the brain's critical requirement for glucose as its energy source. Sequelae of prolonged hypoglycemia include mental retardation and seizures. The causes of hypoglycemia in children include hyperinsulinism, hormone deficiencies, glycogen storage diseases, disorders of gluconeogenesis, toxins, and liver disease. Newborns small for gestational age and those born to diabetic mothers are especially vulnerable to hypoglycemia.

## ACID-BASE DISORDERS

The blood pH, the negative log of the hydrogen ion concentration, is normally maintained within a narrow range by the kidney and buffer systems. **Acidosis** and **alkalosis** refer to processes that affect the blood pH. **Acidemia** refers to an abnormally low blood pH (less than 7.36) and **alkalemia** to an abnormally high blood pH (greater than 7.46).

Acid-base disorders are classified as either **metabolic** or **respiratory** and as **simple** or **mixed**. Three measurements are necessary to interpret acid-base abnormalities: blood pH, $PCO_2$, and the bicarbonate level. Standard acid-base machines calculate the bicarbonate level using the Henderson-Hasselbalch equation based on measurement of the pH and $PCO_2$.

### Metabolic Acidosis

Simple metabolic acidosis is characterized by a **low bicarbonate level and blood pH**. The body attempts to compensate partially for metabolic acidosis by lowering the $PCO_2$ through hyperventilation. However, these compensatory mechanisms will not completely maintain a normal blood pH.

The causes of metabolic acidosis are usefully classified on the basis of changes in the **anion gap**. The anion gap indicates the amount of unmeasured anions in the blood and is calculated according to the formula:

$$\text{Anion gap} = [Na] - ([Cl] + [HCO_3])$$

in which [Na] represents the serum sodium concentration, [Cl] the serum chloride concentration, and [HCO$_3$] is the serum bicarbonate concentration. The normal anion gap is 8 to 12 mEq/L. The causes of metabolic acidosis with an increased anion gap include ketoacidosis, lactic acidosis, and toxins (methanol). The causes of metabolic acidosis with a normal anion gap include diarrhea and renal tubular acidosis.

## Metabolic Alkalosis

Simple metabolic alkalosis is characterized by an **elevation of the serum bicarbonate level and pH**. **Hypoventilation**, the compensatory mechanism, results in a **slight rise in PCO$_2$**. The causes of metabolic alkalosis include protracted vomiting (as in pyloric stenosis), adrenal disorders (hyperaldosteronism and Cushing syndrome), and Bartter syndrome.

## Respiratory Acidosis and Alkalosis

Simple respiratory acidosis and alkalosis reflect disturbances in pulmonary function. Respiratory acidosis occurs when there is diminished ventilation, as in central nervous system (CNS) depression, neuromuscular disorders, or obstructive diseases of the lung (asthma, bronchiolitis). Respiratory alkalosis occurs as a result of increased ventilation, as in anxiety, salicylate toxicity, hypoxemia, and fever. If prolonged, the kidney can partially compensate for the respiratory acidosis or alkalosis by modifying the bicarbonate concentration.

# CALORIC REQUIREMENTS

The daily caloric requirements for children vary with their age, stage of growth, activity level, fecal loss, and basal metabolic needs of the child. The **average daily caloric requirement** is about **100 to 120 kcal/kg**. During the growth spurt of adolescence, daily caloric requirements increase. Caloric requirements can be estimated using body weight or surface area.

Because deficits or excesses in caloric intake will be reflected in the child's pattern of growth, plotting the child's heights and weights on a standard growth chart is the best method of determining whether the child's caloric needs are being met.

# Infant Feeding

**Breast-feeding** is the preferred method for feeding most infants. Human milk has many advantages. It is available in an uncontaminated form so that the danger of gastrointestinal infection is reduced. Human colostrum and milk contain antibodies against bacterial and viral pathogens, most importantly secretory IgA. Secretory IgA in human milk is directed against the pathogens in the maternal-infant environment, does not harm normal gastrointestinal flora, and does not cause a harmful inflammatory reaction. Breast milk also contains phagocytic cells, iron binding lactoferrin, and a factor that promotes the growth of nonpathogenic flora, all of which protect the infant against infection. Human milk contains more carbohydrates and less than half the protein of cow's milk. Moreover, the protein in breast milk is more easily digested because it produces a smaller, softer curd. In short, human milk is the complete food that provides the infant with almost all of the nutrients required for the first 6 to 12 months of life.

The iron stores in full-term infants, as well as the absorption of iron from breast milk, are sufficient for the first 4 months of life. Beyond that age, **iron** should be added to the diet through iron supplements and the gradual introduction of iron-containing solid foods. Since breast milk does not contain sufficient vitamin D to prevent nutritional rickets, breast-fed infants should receive **400 IU of vitamin D daily**. The fluoride content of human milk is also low, and breast-fed infants should receive 0.25 mg of fluoride daily, although supplementation may be delayed until 6 months of age.

Some **drugs**, such as laxatives, anticoagulants, radioactive agents, atropine, quinine, nicotine, caffeine, and tetracycline, are **transferred** in varying amounts from the maternal circulation to **breast milk**. Oral contraceptives, steroids, diuretics, and most sedatives should also be prescribed cautiously because of the danger of maternal transfer to breast milk. Most antineoplastic agents, cyclosporin, ergotamines, and drugs of abuse (cocaine, heroin) are contraindicated during breast-feeding.

Because human immunodeficiency virus (HIV)-infected women may transmit HIV to their infants through breast milk, in developed countries where alternative milk-based formulas are readily available, infants of these women should not be breast-fed. However, because in underdeveloped countries the dangers of malnutrition and infection outweigh the danger of HIV transmission, the World Health Organization has recommended that HIV-infected women in these countries continue to breast-feed their infants.

Although the merits of breast-feeding seem obvious, most infants in the United States continue to be fed **commercially prepared infant formulas**. Most of these preparations are based on cow's milk that has been treated to make the protein more digestible. As in human milk, lactose is the major carbohydrate. Infant formulas contain either vegetable oils or a mixture of animal and vegetable fats and essential fatty acids. They are also fortified with vitamins and iron. The most commonly used commercial preparations are isocaloric (20 calories/ounce), but preparations of higher caloric content are available.

Previously, formulas based on evaporated milk, a concentrated form of cow's milk, were the most common form of cow's milk formula in the United States. With the advent of easy-to-use, commercially prepared infant formulas, the use of evaporated milk declined dramatically. Nevertheless, an evaporated milk formula remains an inexpensive and safe cow's milk formula for healthy infants. Because evaporated cow's milk contains a higher solute load than human milk, it should be diluted to decrease the effects of a high solute load on an immature kidney of the very young infant. Sugar is added to raise the formula's caloric content to the level of 20 calories per ounce. Unlike commercially prepared infant formulas, an evaporated milk formula does not contain supplemental iron. Therefore, infant's fed by this method should have supplemental iron by means of iron containing solid foods.

Most newborns must be fed, by breast or bottle, at 2 to 3 hour intervals. As infants become older, the intervals between feedings lengthen. By 6 to 8 weeks of age, most infants will have established a feeding schedule so that they can sleep as much as 6 hours per night.

The introduction of **solid food** should be delayed until the infant's developmental level is such that the infant can coordinate swallowing and has reasonable head control, usually at **4 to 6 months of age**. Single-ingredient solid foods should be introduced one at a time, at weekly intervals to allow for the identification of food intolerance. Iron-fortified cereals are often recommended as the introductory solid food.

A few infants do not tolerate milk-based infant formulas and require alternate preparations. The two most commonly used alternate formulas are **soy** formulas and **protein hydrolysate** formulas. Soy-based formulas are lactose free and may be used for infants with lactase deficiency, galactosemia and true IgE mediated milk intolerance. Soy-based formulas should not be used routinely following acute gastroenteritis.

The protein in protein hydrolysate formulas consists of amino acids and peptides. Most protein hydrolysate formulas do not contain lactose, and fat is in the form of easily absorbed medium-chain triglycerides. This type of formula is reserved for children with true milk protein intolerance and deficiencies of intestinal enzymes; however, cost and unsavory taste limit their use.

# VITAMINS

Vitamins are a group of organic substances not synthesized by the human body but essential as catalysts of cellular metabolism and thus for normal growth. Since the body does not manufacture vitamins, small amounts must be included in the diet. Some are soluble in fat and are ingested in dietary fat (vitamins A, D, E, and K), and some are water soluble (vitamin B complex and C).

## Vitamin Imbalances

### Vitamin A Deficiency

In the United States, vitamin A deficiency is rare in otherwise healthy children but may occur in children with malabsorption syndromes and with liver or pancreatic diseases. However, in developing countries vitamin A deficiency represents a major public health problem. In those countries, when administered to an entire community, vitamin A supplementation has been shown to reduce mortality from measles and to reduce childhood mortality rates.

Classically, vitamin A deficiency is characterized by loss of the eye's adaptation to darkness, resulting in night blindness. Drying of the conjunctiva and cornea eventually results in corneal clouding and blindness. Growth failure, mental retardation, and hyperkeratosis of the skin and mucous membranes may also occur.

### Hypervitaminosis A

Chronic hypervitaminosis A is characterized by growth failure, irritability, tender swelling of bones, hair loss, and seborrhea. Acute ingestion of toxic amounts of vitamin A may cause the syndrome of pseudotumor cerebri with signs and symptoms of increased intracranial pressure: irritability, drowsiness, vomiting, bulging fontanelles, and papilledema.

### Vitamin D Deficiency

Vitamin D deficiency, or **rickets**, is characterized by the failure in mineralization of osteoid tissue, typically at the end of long bones. The clinical manifestations of rickets include craniotabes, a thinning and softening of the skull; delayed closure of the fontanelles; widening of the distal ends of the long bones (particularly wrists) and ribs, caused by abnormal ossification of the epiphyseal plates; bowing and distortion of the lower extremities; and fractures.

Nutritional rickets is relatively rare in the United States because most milk and many foods are fortified with vitamin D. Infants who are exclusively breast-fed into the second year of life are at risk; thus, breast-fed infants should receive vitamin D supplementation. The treatment of nutritional rickets includes therapeutic doses of vitamin D as well as appropriate changes in the child's diet.

Rickets may also occur in children with impaired absorption of vitamin D or impaired metabolism of vitamin D, calcium, or phosphorous. The disease is also associated with severe chronic renal failure, chronic liver disease, and chronic anticonvulsant therapy (phenobarbital, phenytoin), which interferes with vitamin D metabolism.

*Hypervitaminosis D*

Infants given excessive amounts of vitamin D develop a **toxic syndrome** characterized by anorexia, growth failure, constipation, polyuria, polydipsia, soft tissue calcification, and elevated serum levels of calcium.

*Vitamin K Deficiency*

Typically, vitamin K deficiency occurs in the presence of disorders of gastrointestinal fat malabsorption, when the bacterial flora of the gastrointestinal tract has been disrupted transiently in the newborn period or by the prolonged administration of antibiotics. The condition is characterized by a **decrease in Factor II** (prothrombin) and **Factor VII** of the coagulation cascade, resulting in prolongation of the prothrombin time and hemorrhage. Factors IX and X are also vitamin K dependent.

Prophylactic intramuscular administration of 1.0 mg of oil-soluble vitamin K at the time of birth will prevent the transient vitamin K deficiency in the full-term newborn but is less effective in the premature infant.

*Vitamin E Deficiency*

Because vitamin E is available in vegetable oils and cereals, its deficiency is rare in normal children. But deficiency may occur in children with chronic malabsorption. Vitamin E supplementation prevents severe neuropathy in children with biliary atresia and muscle weakness in children with cystic fibrosis.

*Water-soluble Vitamin Deficiency*

Deficiencies of water-soluble vitamins are also rare in the United States in otherwise healthy children. Signs of **beriberi** (thiamine deficiency) include peripheral neuritis, myalgias, and congestive heart failure. Children with **pellagra** (niacin deficiency) classically manifest dermatitis, diarrhea, and dementia.

**Scurvy**, vitamin C deficiency, causes a defect in the formation of collagen, and in its classic form is characterized by swollen, painful joints; bleeding from the mucous membranes; spongy, friable gingiva with loosening of teeth; and impaired healing of wounds. The diagnosis of scurvy is usually confirmed by typical roentgenographic findings in the distal shaft of the long bones, particularly the knee. Children with scurvy improve rapidly with the addition of vitamin C preferably in the form of 100 to 200 mg of ascorbic acid given orally or parenterally.

**Pyridoxine** (vitamin B6) deficiency may result in myoclonic seizures in infants. Deficiencies of both **folic acid** and **vitamin B12** cause megaloblastic anemia. Folic acid deficiency can occur in children fed goat's milk. Vitamin B12 deficiency, which includes neurologic manifestations as well as anemia, can occur in children with pernicious anemia (absence of gastric intrinsic factor) and following surgical resection of the terminal ileum due to necrotizing enterocolitis.

## Mineral Imbalances

### Calcium

Calcium in serum is found either in the form of complexes with anions bound to protein (albumin) or free ionic calcium. Free ionic calcium is of particular physiologic importance. **Hypoalbuminemia** is associated with a low total serum calcium, but the ionized calcium may be normal. **Alkalemia** will decrease the amount of ionized calcium, and **acidemia** will increase ionized calcium levels.

**Hypocalcemia** occurs with vitamin D deficiency, hypoparathyroidism, and elevated serum phosphate levels. Tetany is the most prominent symptom of hypocalcemia. **Hypercalcemia** occurs with hyperparathyroidism, hyperthyroidism, hypervitaminosis D, and in children who are immobilized for prolonged periods for conditions such as fractures of the femur.

### Magnesium and Trace Elements

**Hypomagnesemia**, also a cause of tetany and seizures, occurs with gastrointestinal malabsorption or hypoparathyroidism. **Hypermagnesemia** is rare except in severe renal failure and infants born to mothers who received magnesium sulfate as treatment for preeclampsia. **Zinc** deficiency is characterized by growth retardation, hypogonadism, dermatitis, diarrhea, and impaired wound healing. Excess accumulation of **copper**, particularly in the liver, occurs in Wilson's disease (hepatolenticular degeneration). Deficiency of **selenium** is associated with cardiomyopathy.

# Chapter 4

# Pregnancy, Labor, and Delivery of the Newborn

## MORTALITY RATE

The **infant mortality rate**, defined as the number of deaths per 1000 live births of infants less than the age of 1 year, is often used as an index of the health status of children. The **neonatal mortality rate** is defined as the number of deaths per 1000 live births of newborns less than 28 days of life. In the United States in 1900, when the infant mortality rate was 162.9 per 1000 births, infectious causes accounted for most infant deaths. In the first 60 years of the twentieth century, scientific advances in control of infections, infant nutrition, improved sanitation, and better environmental conditions resulted in a steady decline in these rates in industrialized countries.

By the last decade of the twentieth century in the United States, most deaths during the first year of life are related to prematurity and low birth weight. Advances in the understanding of the physiology of sick and well newborns have transformed the clinical management of premature and low-birth-weight infants. Such techniques as electronic fetal monitoring, ultrasonography, methods for determination of acid base balance, phototherapy for hyperbilirubinemia, exchange transfusions, the use of newborn respirators and techniques of hyperalimentation have greatly improved the survival of low-birth-weight infants. The development of regional perinatal centers, where high-risk women and newborns have access to tertiary medical care, has also contributed to improved perinatal and infant mortality rates.

Despite these advances, in the United States considerable discrepancy remains in infant mortality rates among different social classes and ethnic groups. For example, the infant mortality rates of African Americans is substantially higher than that of white infants.

# PREGNANCY AND ITS EFFECTS ON THE FETUS

Because the mother and fetus represent a single physiologic unit, any serious maternal disease or condition can affect the developing fetus. **Adverse outcomes of pregnancy** are associated with low maternal socioeconomic and educational status; lack of prenatal care; poor maternal nutrition; drug, alcohol, or cigarette use; multiple pregnancies; and the presence of such maternal diseases as diabetes mellitus, hypertension, or sexually transmitted infections. In the presence of these maternal factors spontaneous abortion, congenital malformations, intrauterine growth retardation, mental retardation, or premature delivery may result.

**Extremes of maternal age** are also associated with increased neonatal mortality and abnormalities in the newborn. Early adolescence (females younger than 15 years of age) is associated with perinatal complications. Extremes of maternal age (older than 40 years of age) are also associated with an increased perinatal morbidity and mortality. Specifically, the incidence of chromosomal abnormalities, especially trisomies, is associated with advanced maternal age.

## Maternal Diabetes Mellitus

Maternal diabetes mellitus, especially if poorly controlled, is associated with the delivery of infants that are large for gestational age. However, women in whom the vascular complications of diabetes are well advanced tend to deliver small infants with intrauterine growth retardation.

Infants of diabetic mothers are at considerable risk for the development of **neonatal hypoglycemia**. Most newborns with hypoglycemia are asymptomatic, with the glucose level reaching the nadir at 1 to 3 hours after birth. Symptoms of hypoglycemia include irritability, lethargy, poor feeding, temperature instability, and seizures. If these symptoms appear later in an infant of a diabetic mother, they may be the consequence of **hypocalcemia** rather than hypoglycemia.

Because they tend to be larger at birth, infants of diabetic mothers have an **increased incidence of birth injuries**. Infants of diabetic mothers are several times more likely to develop respiratory distress syndrome, hyperbilirubinemia, and polycythemia. They also have an increased incidence of congenital birth anomalies, including cardiac malformations, lumbosacral agenesis, and small left colon syndrome.

## Maternal Systemic Lupus Erythematosus

Infants born to mothers with systemic lupus erythematosus (**SLE**) may develop the syndrome of neonatal lupus erythematosus. The majority (50% to 60%) of mothers are asymptomatic at the time of delivery but have anti-Ro and anti-La antibodies. The syndrome is characterized by a photosensitive skin rash and congenital heart block. The rash, which may begin hours to days after birth, resolves at about 6 months of age when the maternal IgG antibodies disappear from the infant's circulation. **Complete congenital heart block**, which occurs in about half of all cases of infants with neonatal lupus erythematosus, is permanent and may result in bradycardia, congestive heart failure, or hydrops fetalis.

## Toxemia of Pregnancy

**Preeclampsia**, a syndrome of maternal hypertension, edema, and proteinuria during pregnancy, causes vasculitis of the placenta and thus chronic intrauterine fetal hypoxia resulting in intrauterine growth retardation. Moreover, a chronically hypoxic fetus does not tolerate labor well and may develop intrapartum fetal distress, meconium aspiration and asphyxia.

**Eclampsia**, which is defined as a syndrome that includes the symptoms of preeclampsia with the addition of maternal seizures, places not only the mother but also her infant at very high risk. These newborns are very vulnerable to intrauterine asphyxia or fetal death.

## Twin and Multiple Pregnancies

Twin and multiple pregnancies result in a higher risk of complications for both the mother and infants. The perinatal mortality rate is higher for twins than singletons, in large part because twins are often delivered prematurely. **Fetal-fetal transfusion** causes one twin to become plethoric while the second twin will be small and anemic.

## Maternal Use of Medication

Both the type of medication and the timing of ingestion determine the effect on the pregnancy (Table 4-1). **Teratogenic drugs** taken during the period of **organogenesis** may result in abortion or congenital malformations. Medications taken late in pregnancy also may affect the newborn infant. For example, sulfonamides can cross the placenta, displace bilirubin from its binding site on albumin, and cause hyperbilirubinemia and kernicterus.

## Maternal Substance Abuse

Maternal substance abuse can have profound effects on the fetus and neonate. **Heroin** or **methadone** use results in symptoms of drug withdrawal: tremors, hyperirritability, high-pitched cry, poor feed-

### TABLE 4-1.
### Maternal Drug Use and Its Effect on the Fetus

| Drug | Effect |
| --- | --- |
| Angiotensin-converting enzyme (ACE) inhibitors | Skull abnormalities |
| Antineoplastic agents | Spontaneous abortion, multiple congenital anomalies, growth retardation |
| Carbamazepine | Growth retardation, craniofacial abnormalities |
| Cocaine | Spontaneous abortion, prematurity, abruptio placentae, growth retardation, hyperirritability, cerebral infarction |
| Coumadin | Midface hypoplasia, CNS malformation, mental retardation, shortened digits, bone abnormalities |
| Diethylstilbestrol | Adenocarcinoma of the vagina, genitourinary abnormalities in boys |
| Ethanol | Growth retardation, mental retardation, facial abnormalities, absent philtrum, congenital heart disease |
| Heroin | Growth retardation, narcotic withdrawal |
| Isotretinoin | Congenital anomalies involving the CNS, heart, and eyes |
| Magnesium sulfate | Neuromuscular depression |
| Phenytoin | Growth retardation, microcephaly, mental retardation, hypoplastic nails, congenital heart disease |
| Propylthiouracil | Goiter, hypothyroidism |
| Sulfonamides | Hyperbilirubinemia, kernicterus |
| Tetracycline | Enamel dysplasia, bone abnormalities |
| Thalidomide | Phocomelia |
| Valproic acid | Neural tube defects, mental retardation, congenital heart disease |

ing, and, occasionally, seizures. The symptoms of methadone withdrawal are similar to those of heroin but can be delayed in onset (at 2 to 6 weeks) and are often more severe and prolonged than in heroin withdrawal. Infants born to mothers who use heroin are frequently small for gestational age.

**Cocaine** use during pregnancy results in an increased frequency of spontaneous abortion, premature labor, and abruptio placentae. Infants exposed to cocaine in utero suffer from intrauterine growth retardation. Cerebral infarction and intracranial hemorrhage are rare but serious complications of intrauterine cocaine exposure. The long-term neurologic and cognitive outcomes of intrauterine cocaine exposure are unknown.

## Maternal Alcohol Use

The **fetal alcohol syndrome** is a pattern of **malformation** and **functional abnormalities** found in infants born to women who drink heavily throughout pregnancy. Features of the syndrome vary in severity with the amount of alcohol consumed. Characteristics of the fetal alcohol syndrome include growth retardation, facial abnormalities (short palpebral fissures, epicanthal folds, maxillary hypoplasia, and thin upper lip), cardiac abnormalities (septal defects), limb abnormalities, and delayed development and mental retardation. Extreme maternal alcohol use results in spontaneous abortion.

## Maternal Nutrition

The nutritional status of the mother is reflected in her prepregnancy weight, her weight gain during pregnancy, and in the birth weight of the newborn. The demands of pregnancy require an average of an additional 300 kcal per day. Iron supplementation is recommended for most pregnant women during the second and third trimester. **Folic acid supplementation reduces the risk of neural tube defects** in women who have had a previous child with a neural tube defect. Because other data suggest that folic acid supplementation reduces the risk of neural tube defects in the general population, the United States Public Health Service has recommended that women of reproductive age take 0.4 mg of folic acid daily to prevent neural tube defects in their infants.

Excessive vitamin and mineral intake, however, can be harmful during pregnancy. For example, excessive intake of vitamin A during pregnancy is associated with congenital birth defects.

## Maternal Colonization with Group B Streptococcus

Group B streptococcus is one of the most common bacterial causes of **neonatal sepsis**. Although different strategies have been recommended for the screening of pregnant women for group B streptococcal colonization, women in premature labor, with premature rupture of membranes and with fever during labor, are at particularly high risk of transmitting group B streptococcus to their infant. Chemoprophylaxis of mothers at high risk or known to be colonized with group B streptococcus is indicated.

## Fetal Assessment

Several techniques are available to assess the fetus, including ultrasonography (growth and anatomy), fetoscopy (facial and limb anomalies), amniocentesis (karyotype, genetic disorders, fetal maturity, alpha-fetoprotein determination, enzyme analyses), chorionic villus biopsy (karyotype, genetic disorders, enzyme analyses), and maternal serum alpha-fetoprotein (twins, neural tube defects, trisomies).

Examination of **amniotic fluid** can be used to assess **fetal lung maturity**. The concentration of lecithin, produced by type II fetal alveolar cells, equals that of sphingomyelin until the middle of the third trimester. Lung maturity is indicated by a lecithin to sphingomyelin ratio of 2:1 and correlates with a greatly diminished probability of respiratory distress syndrome.

### Polyhydramnios and Oligohydramnios

**Polyhydramnios**, which is defined as excessive amniotic fluid, is associated with a variety of neonatal complications including such congenital anomalies as anencephaly, duodenal atresia, tracheoesophageal atresia, and trisomy 21. **Oligohydramnios**, or an abnormally small amount of amniotic fluid, is also associated with a variety of congenital anomalies and increased perinatal risk. Such conditions as pulmonary hypoplasia and the development of such compression conditions as club feet are found with oligohydramnios. Ultrasonography is used to diagnose both of these conditions.

## LABOR AND DELIVERY AND THE EFFECTS ON THE INFANT

### Prolonged Rupture of the Membranes

Prolonged rupture of the membranes (**PROM**) prior to delivery (usually longer than 18 to 24 hours) is associated with an increased risk of maternal **chorioamnionitis** and may lead to **neonatal sepsis**. Although the risk is relatively low, the mortality associated with neonatal sepsis is high. For this reason, some obstetricians consider PROM an indication for immediate delivery by induction or cesarean section. However, if the membranes rupture early in the third trimester of pregnancy, the risks of prematurity and its complications must be weighed against the risk of intrapartum infection.

### Other Risk Factors during Labor

**Abruptio placentae**, the premature separation of the placenta during labor, and **placenta previa**, the abnormal placement of the placenta in the region of the cervical opening, are both causes of serious complications of labor that place both the infant and mother at high risk. Precipitous labor and delivery, of less than 3 hours duration, are also associated with increased perinatal risk.

### Premature Labor

**Prematurity** is the leading cause of perinatal mortality in the United States. The management of women in premature labor remains one of the most difficult tasks for the obstetrical and neonatology team. Risk factors for premature labor include prior history of a preterm delivery, incompetent cervix, multiple gestation, and premature rupture of the membranes.

Maternal hydration and tocolytic agents such as magnesium sulfate or sympathomimetic agents (ritodrine or terbutaline) have been used to suppress uterine contractions prior to 34 weeks gestation. Corticosteroids are commonly administered to women in premature labor to decrease the newborn's risk of respiratory distress syndrome.

## Intrapartum Asphyxia

Asphyxia, a general term describing the condition of fetal hypercarbia, hypoxemia, and acidemia, is commonly due to **uteroplacental insufficiency**. Sampling of capillary blood from the fetal scalp permits the determination of fetal pH; a pH of less than 7.25 demonstrates a significant degree of acidosis usually caused by fetal hypoxia, and a pH less than 7.20 is an indication for early delivery.

Electronic fetal monitoring during labor permits the demonstration of prolonged fetal bradycardia (less than 120 beats/min) and fetal tachycardia (greater than 160 beats/min), both of which suggest fetal hypoxia or other serious fetal conditions. **Fetal distress** is not always characterized by changes in fetal heart rate, but different patterns of fetal heart rate often provide a useful, noninvasive measure of hypoxemia. Periodic fetal cardiac decelerations or variability of the fetal cardiac rate may also signal fetal distress or intrapartum asphyxia. The presence of meconium in the amniotic fluid is an additional sign of fetal distress.

These signs of fetal distress — hypoxemia and acidemia — require prompt delivery of the fetus. However, only prolonged and severe fetal hypoxemia can produce brain damage, with resulting intellectual and motor abnormalities. In addition to damage to the central nervous system, intrapartum asphyxia can damage other organ systems including the kidneys, heart, intestines, and liver.

## Birth Injuries

Birth injuries from trauma during labor and delivery are more common in premature infants, large-for-gestational age infants, breech presentations, and in children of women with cephalopelvic disproportion.

**Caput succedaneum**, which is edema of the presenting newborn scalp, characteristically crosses suture lines. The edema resolves spontaneously in several days. **Cephalhematomas** are areas of subperiosteal hemorrhage; they do not cross suture lines because of the periosteal membrane. The breakdown of the pooled blood may result in hyperbilirubinemia. Cephalhematomas may take several weeks to months to resolve and can calcify.

Excessive traction on the head, neck, and shoulders causes **brachial plexus palsies**. In **Erb-Duchenne paralysis**, which results from injury to the fifth and sixth cervical nerves, the arm is held in adduction and internal rotation. The Moro reflex is absent on the side of the affected arm. **Klumpke paralysis**, which affects the hand, is due to injury to the seventh and eighth cervical nerves and the 1st thoracic nerve. **Clavicular fractures**, which are the most frequent fractures during delivery, may result in large callus formation during the healing process.

# CLASSIFICATION OF THE NEWBORN

## Apgar Score

The Apgar score, a technique for the immediate evaluation in the delivery room of a newborn's general condition, is based on assessment of the newborn's cardiac rate, respiratory effort, muscle tone, reflex irritability, and color (Table 4-2). The Apgar score is commonly determined at **1- and 5-minute intervals immediately after birth**. Most normal, full-term newborns have an Apgar score ranging from 8 to 10. This simple scoring system ranks each of the five criteria equally; however, heart rate and respiratory effort best represent the newborn's physiologic status. A low Apgar score at 1 minute of life indicates the need to resuscitate the infant; however, resuscitation should not be delayed or be dependent on the Apgar score. The Apgar score at 5 minutes, when compared with the score at 1 minute, indicates the effectiveness of the resuscitative effort and the need for further resuscitation. The Apgar score should not be used as evidence of asphyxia, nor should it be used to predict subsequent cerebral palsy or neurologic outcome. Factors that influence the Apgar score include maternal sedation or analgesia, the newborn's gestational age, and cardiac, pulmonary, or neurologic diseases in the infant.

## Gestational Age

Gestational age is defined as the number of weeks from the first day of the last normal menstrual period to the date of delivery. Although gestational age can be calculated from the mother's report of the date of her last menstrual period (LMP), these histories are frequently inaccurate. **Ultrasound** examination at less than 20 weeks gestation can be used to confirm the expected date of delivery.

Systems based on physical and neurologic signs found on examination of the newborn have been devised to estimate gestational

**TABLE 4-2. Apgar Score for Rapid Clinical Assessment of Newborns**

| Criteria | Score 0 | Score 1 | Score 2 |
|---|---|---|---|
| Heart rate | Absent | <100 | >100 |
| Respiratory rate | Irregular | Slow | Good |
| Muscle tone | Limp | Some flexion of extremities | Active motion |
| Reflex irritability (nose suctioning) | Response | Grimace | Cough or sneeze |
| Color | Blue, pale | Extremities blue | Pink |

*Adapted from* The Harriet Lane Handbook, *13th ed., p. 280.*

age. A commonly used version of these scoring systems is found in Figure 4-1.

By definition, **full-term** infants are those born between 38 to 42 weeks of gestation, **postterm** infants are those born after 42 weeks of gestation, and **preterm** infants are those of less than 38 weeks gestation.

A growth chart that displays the standards for weight, length and head circumference for infants of a variety of gestational ages is provided in Figure 4-2.

**Appropriate-for-gestational age (AGA) infants** fall within the 10th and 90th percentiles for weight for their gestational age. **Small-for-gestational age (SGA) infants** rank below the 10th percentile for their gestational age. **Large-for-gestational age (LGA) infants** rank above the 90th percentile for their gestational age. **LGA infants**, often born to mothers with diabetes mellitus or obesity, have a **higher incidence of birth injuries and congenital anomalies**, particularly congenital heart disease. Neonatal mortality rates decline steadily as the birth weight approaches 4000 grams, but increase again in LGA infants.

**Low-birth-weight infants** (less than 2500 grams) represent either preterm gestations or infants suffering from intrauterine growth retardation. **Intrauterine growth retardation** may be caused by abnormalities of the fetus itself (chromosomal disorders, chronic infections, congenital abnormalities), placental abnormalities (placentitis, placental separation), maternal malnutrition, chronic maternal disease (hypertension, renal disease, sickle cell anemia), and multiple or twin births.

**Very-low-birth-weight infants** (those weighing less than 1500 grams) are often premature births. Low-birth-weight, premature

## NEUROMUSCULAR MATURITY

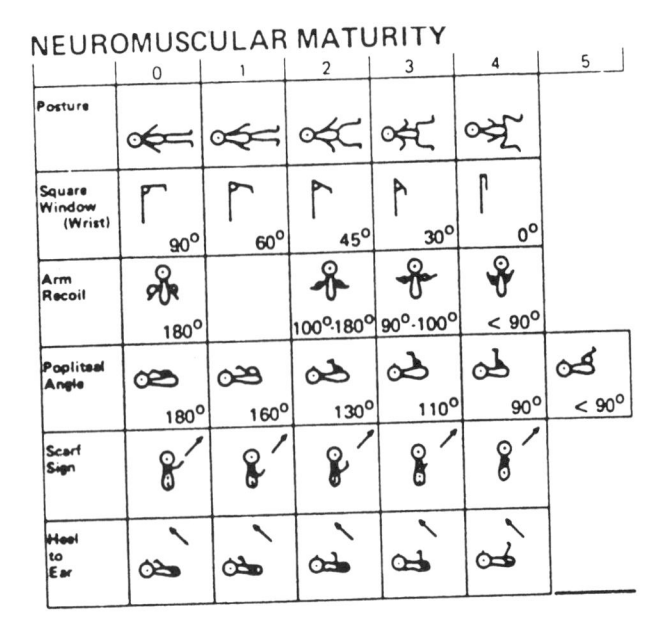

| | 0 | 1 | 2 | 3 | 4 | 5 |
|---|---|---|---|---|---|---|
| Posture | | | | | | |
| Square Window (Wrist) | 90° | 60° | 45° | 30° | 0° | |
| Arm Recoil | | 180° | | 100°-180° | 90°-100° | < 90° |
| Popliteal Angle | 180° | 160° | 130° | 110° | 90° | < 90° |
| Scarf Sign | | | | | | |
| Heel to Ear | | | | | | |

## MATURITY RATING

| Score | Wks |
|---|---|
| 5 | 26 |
| 10 | 28 |
| 15 | 30 |
| 20 | 32 |
| 25 | 34 |
| 30 | 36 |
| 35 | 38 |
| 40 | 40 |
| 45 | 42 |
| 50 | 44 |

## PHYSICAL MATURITY

| | 0 | 1 | 2 | 3 | 4 | 5 |
|---|---|---|---|---|---|---|
| SKIN | gelatinous red, transparent | smooth pink, visible veins | superficial peeling &/or rash, few veins | cracking pale area, rare veins | parchment, deep cracking, no vessels | leathery, cracked, wrinkled |
| LANUGO | none | abundant | thinning | bald areas | mostly bald | |
| PLANTAR CREASES | no crease | faint red marks | anterior transverse crease only | creases ant. 2/3 | creases cover entire sole | |
| BREAST | barely percept. | flat areola, no bud | stippled areola, 1–2 mm bud | raised areola, 3–4 mm bud | full areola, 5–10 mm bud | |
| EAR | pinna flat, stays folded | sl. curved pinna, soft with slow recoil | well-curv. pinna, soft but ready recoil | formed & firm with instant recoil | thick cartilage, ear stiff | |
| GENITALS Male | scrotum empty, no rugae | | testes descending, few rugae | testes down, good rugae | testes pendulous, deep rugae | |
| GENITALS Female | prominent clitoris & labia minora | | majora & minora equally prominent | majora large, minora small | clitoris & minora completely covered | |

Apgars _____ 1 min _____ 5 min
Age at Exam _____ hrs
Race _____ Sex _____
B.D. _____
LMP _____
EDC _____
Gest. age by Dates _____ wks
Gest. age by Exam _____ wks
B.W. _____ gm. _____ %ile
Length _____ cm. _____ %ile
Head Circum. _____ cm. _____ %ile
Clin. Dist. None _____ Mild _____
Mod. _____ Severe _____

**Figure 4-1.**
Assessment of gestational age, University of Cincinnati. (From Ballard J, Kazmaler K, Driver M. Simplified assessment of gestational age. *Pediatr. Res.* 1977;11:374.)

infants are at risk for respiratory distress syndrome, recurrent apnea, hypoglycemia, anemia, hyperbilirubinemia, intraventricular hemorrhage, necrotizing enterocolitis, and bacterial sepsis. Infants with intrauterine growth retardation have medical problems related to the underlying etiology of their growth retardation. They are also at increased risk of asphyxia, meconium aspiration, hypoglycemia, and polycythemia.

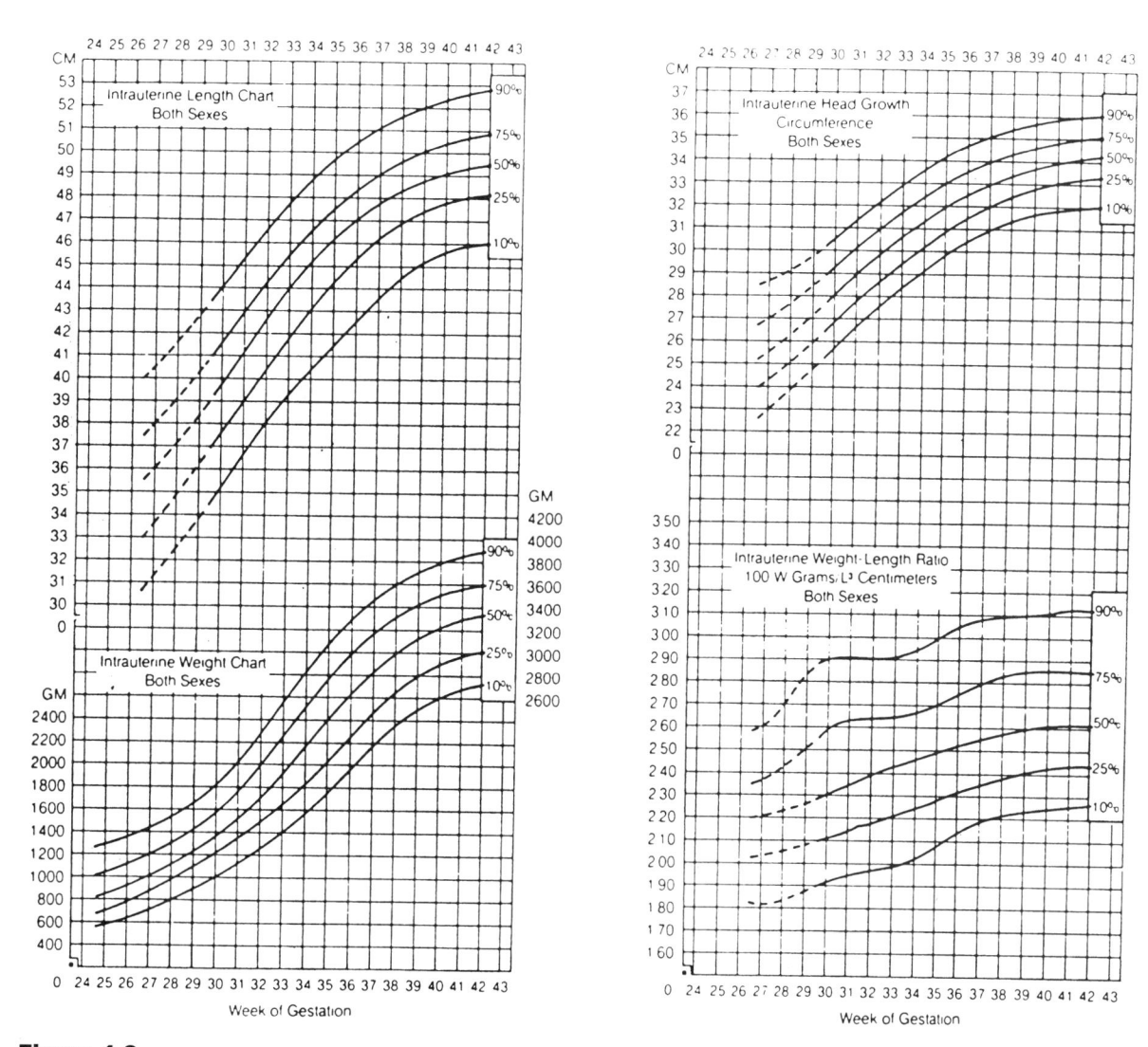

**Figure 4-2.**
Intrauterine growth curves for length, head circumference, and weight for singleton births in Colorado. (From Lubchenco L, Hansman C, Dressler M, et al. Intrauterine growth in length and head circumference as estimated from live births at gestational ages from 26 to 42 weeks. *Pediatrics* 1966;37:403. Copyright, American Academy of Pediatrics, 1966.)

# Chapter 5

# The Normal Newborn

The normal newborn has a large head, a round ruddy face, and a relatively small jaw. The chest is round and the abdomen prominent. The arms and legs are short in proportion to the length of the trunk. The normal **full-term infant** often maintains a **flexed posture** mirroring the position in utero; the extremities of premature and ill infants are frequently limp and held in extension. In the normal newborn, the liver and spleen are often palpable at or just below the costal margins, and the kidneys frequently can be felt by deep palpation of the abdomen.

## NEONATAL ANATOMY AND PHYSIOLOGY

The newborn's anatomy and physiology show certain developmental immaturities important in their care and management.

### Skin

The newborn's skin is anatomically immature; the epithelial layer is relatively thin, and the sweat and sebaceous glands are incompletely developed. Because of this thin epithelial layer, the newborn more readily loses heat and water. The loss of heat is exacerbated by the high surface area to body mass ratio.

Several different benign skin lesions are commonly found in the newborn infant. **Capillary hemangiomata**, "stork bites," are bluish-red areas in the skin commonly found at the nape of the neck, the bridge of the nose, and the eyelids. **Mongolian spots** are bluish-black discolorations found in the area of the sacrum and back. **Erythema toxicum** is a common vesiculopustular rash with a red base that occurs on the face, trunk, and limbs. The pustules contain eosinophils. **Miliaria** ("prickly heat") is a small vesicular eruption on the face, often with an erythematous reaction that results from plugging of eccrine ducts and sweat retention. **Milia** are small 1- to 2-mm white or yellow papules that occur on the nose, chin, and forehead.

**Acrocyanosis** is a transient, bluish discoloration of the hands and feet that does not signify systemic hypoxemia. These lesions, which fade and disappear with time, require no therapy.

## Umbilical Cord

The normal umbilical cord contains two umbilical arteries, one umbilical vein and remnants of the allantois, the omphalomesenteric duct, and Wharton jelly. A single umbilical artery should prompt the search for other congenital anomalies. The normal umbilical cord usually sloughs and heals in the first 2 weeks of life. The routine care of the neonatal umbilical cord includes application of an antimicrobial agent (triple dye, bacitracin) to prevent infection.

## Head

Because the bones of the newborn's skull are not fused, significant molding can occur as a result of engagement of the head within the birth canal. The skull of the normal newborn has two soft spots or fontanelles, which are points of juncture of several bones that are not yet ossified but are connected with fibrous tissue. The **posterior fontanelle**, located at the juncture of the occipital and parietal bones, usually closes by 6 to 8 weeks of life. The diamond-shaped **anterior fontanelle**, located in the midline and quite variable in size, usually closes anywhere from 9 to 18 months of age.

Children with congenital hypothyroidism may have a delay in the closure of the fontanelles. Any lesion causing increased intracranial pressure will cause bulging of the fontanelles.

The external auditory canal is short and straight, and the thick tympanic membrane is positioned at an oblique angle. **Epstein pearls** are benign small white papules found on the hard palate due to accumulations of epithelial cells. The **normal newborn can fixate and respond to changes in light**; the visual acuity of the newborn is estimated to be about 20/400.

## Respiratory System

At birth, the infant's cardiorespiratory system undergoes enormous changes that permit the newborn to take the first breath and to convert from the fetal to the adult cardiovascular system within minutes. Prior to birth, the airways are filled with fetal lung fluid, which contains surfactant, a phospholipid substance produced by type II alveolar cells beginning at 20 weeks gestation. At birth, fetal lung fluid is quickly removed and replaced by an equal volume of air. Surfactant remains to line the air-fluid interface of the alveoli and to reduce the surface tension that opposes lung expansion. Without pulmonary surfactant, a residual volume of air cannot be maintained and atelectasis develops. **Deficiency of surfactant results in the respiratory distress syndrome.**

Newborn infants breathe almost exclusively through diaphragmatic contraction. Consequently, the thorax recedes inward and the abdomen protrudes during inspiration. The newborn's respiratory rate is highly variable and may normally have a Cheyne-Stokes rhythm with short periods of apnea (5 to 10 seconds). Newborns breathe through their noses; nasal obstruction, as occurs with bilateral **choanal atresia**, can result in severe respiratory distress.

## Cardiovascular System

The **fetal circulation** is maintained by specific pressure relationships between the right and left sides of the heart. In the fetal circulation, the right-sided pressure (pulmonary) exceeds the left-sided pressure (systemic), allowing blood to flow from right to left through the foramen ovale and the ductus arteriosus. This **right-sided pressure elevation** depends on pulmonary vascular resistance caused by pulmonary arteriolar vasoconstriction. In contrast, left-sided pressure remains low in the fetal circulation because of the low resistance of the placental circulation.

At **birth**, these relationships reverse. With the clamping of the umbilical vessels, **left-sided** (systemic) **pressure rises** sharply, while the pulmonary artery pressure drops as the lungs expand with air. As the $PO_2$ rises, a prostaglandin-mediated pulmonary vasodilatation dramatically increases pulmonary blood flow. The elevated left arterial pressure closes the foramen ovale; the ductus arteriosus closes in response to a prostaglandin-mediated vasoconstriction.

Although these fetal vascular shunts (the foramen ovale and the ductus arteriosus) close functionally at birth, transient cardiac murmurs may be heard in the first few days of life because of delays in their structural closure. Most of these murmurs disappear within the first few weeks of life.

## Hematopoietic System

The newborn's red blood cells contain **hemoglobin F**, which during fetal life binds and transports oxygen at lower pressures than the hemoglobin found in adult red cells. The fetal total oxygen carrying capacity is also improved by an absolute increase in hemoglobin levels that range between 15 to 20 gm/dL. This high hemoglobin level falls rapidly, and by 2 to 3 months of age, the normal infant's hemoglobin is at a level of 9 to 13 gm/dL. This **physiologic anemia** represents a normal fall in hemoglobin, which is caused by decreased production of red blood cells by the bone marrow and requires no treatment. The hemoglobin level of the premature infant is lower than that of the full-term infant.

## Immunologic System

The neonatal immunologic system is immature; the cellular immune responses of chemotaxis, opsonization, phagocytosis, and killing are reduced. The newborn's humoral response is antigenically inexperienced and depends on maternal **IgG antibodies** that **cross the placenta** beginning at **20 weeks gestation**. An active transport system raises the infant's gamma globulin level above the mother's. IgM and IgA do not cross the placenta, but IgA is found in breast milk. Maternal IgG antibodies gradually disappear from the infant's circulation and are not detectable by 12 to 18 months of life. By 3 to 6 months of age, the infant's own humoral immune system begins to function.

Overwhelming infections in the neonate may be associated with a normal or low white blood cell count. The characteristic leukocytosis of the older child and adult may not be present.

## Renal System

Most normal newborns void within the first 12 hours of life, and many urinate shortly after birth. The newborn who fails to void after 24 hours should be evaluated. The neonatal renal system is also immature: The glomerular filtration rate is about one sixth that of adult values; the proximal tubules have a lower threshold for bicarbonate resorption; the kidney's concentrating capacity is about half that of an adult's function; and the excretion of inorganic phosphates and sulfates is limited.

A larger proportion of body weight exists as extracellular fluid in the newborn infant. In the first few days of life, this extracellular fluid is lost through diuresis, resulting in a decrease in body weight of 6% to 10%. Most infants will regain their birth weight by 2 weeks of age.

## Gastrointestinal System

The neonatal gastrointestinal system also exhibits several developmental immaturities. Because most gastrointestinal enzymes are present, the infant digests carbohydrates, fats, and proteins efficiently. However, pancreatic amylase is diminished; hence, starches are digested somewhat less well.

**Meconium**, a viscid greenish-black material found in the newborn's gastrointestinal tract, consists of a mixture of mucus, sloughed epithelial cells, bilirubin, and amniotic fluid. Infants usually pass meconium within the first 6 hours of life. Failure to pass meconium is found in infants with **imperforate anus**. Over a period of the first 4 to 5 days, meconium disappears from the bowel movements and is replaced by the yellowish stools of the milk-fed infant.

Because the liver is responsible for the conjugation and excretion of bilirubin and the newborn liver regularly shows immaturity of the enzymes of conjugation, particularly glucuronyl transferase, many infants are mildly jaundiced during the first few days of life. This "physiologic" **jaundice** approximates 5 to 6 mg/dL by the third day and falls to less than 2 mg/dL by the first week of life.

## Central Nervous System

The myelination of the central nervous system (CNS), incomplete at birth, continues throughout infancy and for the most part is complete within the first 2 years of life.

The normal newborn exhibits a variety of **primitive reflexes** that persist through the first few months of life. The **Moro** or startle reflex, in which the infant rapidly extends and then flexes the arms and legs in response to a sudden change in position or a loud noise, disappears by 3 to 6 months of life. The **rooting** reflex in which the infant turns toward the stimulation when touched on the cheek; the **grasp** reflex in which the infant will grasp a finger or object when placed in the palm; and the **tonic neck** reflex in which, when the infant's head is forcibly turned to one side, the arm on the side to which the face is turned extends and the opposite arm flexes, disappear within the first 6 to 12 months of life. Prolongation of these primitive reflexes beyond infancy suggests serious damage of the nervous system.

# Chapter 6

# Diseases of the Newborn

## CARDIOPULMONARY DISORDERS

### Respiratory Distress Syndrome

Respiratory distress syndrome (**RDS**), also called **hyaline membrane disease**, is a disease of preterm infants caused by a deficiency of surfactant in the distal airways, which results in severe atelectasis and reduced lung compliance. The incidence of the syndrome is inversely proportional to gestational age. This disease is a major cause of neonatal mortality, and, if untreated, can have a mortality rate as high as 75%.

RDS presents shortly after birth and tends to worsen in the first 12 to 24 hours with tachypnea, nasal flaring, grunting, intercostal, subcostal and supraclavicular retractions, and cyanosis. A typical diffuse ground-glass opacity with air bronchograms is found on chest radiograph. Infants with mild or moderate disease often show improvement within 3 to 4 days. Infants with severe disease may develop acidosis, apnea, pneumothorax, or interstitial emphysema. The early clinical picture can be confused with group B streptococcal sepsis.

The therapy for RDS, which is largely supportive, includes **assisted respiratory support**, particularly with **continuous positive airway pressure** (CPAP), meticulous control of blood pressure, correction of acid-base balance, careful monitoring, and nutritional support. CPAP, which prevents atelectasis by providing end expiratory pressure (5 to 10 cm of water pressure) to keep alveoli distended, does not necessarily require endotracheal intubation and may be delivered through nasal prongs. However, infants with severe disease require assisted **mechanical ventilation**. Nutritional support is provided through the intravenous administration of calories, electrolytes, and water (total parenteral nutrition or TPN).

The risk of severe RDS can be diminished by administering **corticosteroids** to pregnant women who are less than 32 to 33 weeks gestation and in whom delivery is imminent. **Surfactant administration**, either natural (human or animal) or synthetic, can be provided to high-risk infants to prevent the onset of RDS. Protocols usually call for multiple doses delivered through an **endotracheal tube** beginning immediately after birth. Surfactant has also been used to treat infants who develop respiratory distress syndrome. Clinical trials of surfactant therapy have shown a reduction in oxygen requirement, a reduction in the need for assisted ventilation, and the prevention of early barotrauma. However, the impact on long-term outcome, particularly on the incidence of bronchopulmonary dysplasia and on mortality rates, is less clear.

Complications of RDS may result either from the disease itself or from the therapy. Serious complications from endotracheal intubation, umbilical artery catheterization, and peripheral vein catheterization can arise. Anemia, pneumothorax, and persistent patent ductus arteriosus can result from the underlying pathogenesis of RDS in combination with aggressive therapy.

## Bronchopulmonary Dysplasia

Bronchopulmonary dysplasia (BOD) is a form of chronic lung disease that develops in infants treated for respiratory distress syndrome. However, newborns who for any reason require prolonged assisted ventilation with high concentrations of oxygen and high pressures are at risk for this complication.

Infants with BOD may develop cor pulmonale (right-sided heart failure) because of elevated pulmonary vascular resistance. The chest radiograph demonstrates a diffuse "bubbly" pattern of emphysema and fibrosis. The treatment of BOD includes respiratory support, oxygen, bronchodilators, steroids, diuretics, nutritional support, and meticulous management of respiratory infections.

## Transient Tachypnea of the Newborn

Transient tachypnea of the newborn is thought to be caused by a delayed resorption of fetal lung fluid and is characterized by the early onset of mild to moderate respiratory distress. The condition usually disappears within the first few days of life and is not nearly as severe as the respiratory distress syndrome with which it may be confused. Chest radiographs show prominent pulmonary vessels and fluid in the fissures of the lung.

## Meconium Aspiration Syndrome

**Meconium staining** of the amniotic fluid is usually triggered by fetal distress in term or postterm infants. Infants who aspirate meconium at delivery may develop respiratory distress and cyanosis so severe as to require **mechanical ventilation**. The condition may also be complicated by the development of a pneumothorax or pneumomediastinum. Suction of the airway at birth through an endotracheal tube may prevent the development of severe lung disease. Infants with severe meconium aspiration have a high mortality rate.

## Apnea

Apnea, a cessation of breathing for more than 10 to 15 seconds, may be **primary** (idiopathic) or **secondary** to a number of neonatal disorders. The secondary causes of apnea are listed in Table 6-1. Idiopathic apnea of prematurity is usually due to a combination of upper airway obstruction and immaturity of the respiratory center's response to hypercarbia and hypoxemia. Long periods of apnea (longer than 20 seconds) are often associated with bradycardia. Short periods of apnea respond to gentle stimulation of the infant. Longer periods of apnea, associated with significant bradycardia, require bag-mask ventilation with oxygen. Recurrent episodes can be prevented with CPAP

**TABLE 6-1.**
**Causes of Apnea in the Newborn**

**Infectious diseases**
  Sepsis
  Meningitis
**Diseases of the respiratory system**
  Hypoxemia
  Upper airway obstruction
  Respiratory distress syndrome
  Pneumothorax
  Pneumonia
  Atelectasis
**Diseases of the central nervous system**
  Intraventricular hemorrhage
  Hypoxic-ischemic encephalopathy
  Seizures
**Metabolic disorders**
  Hypoglycemia
  Hypocalcemia
**Hematologic disorders**
  Anemia
**Gastrointestinal disorders**
  Gastroesophageal reflux
  Bowel movement
**Extreme prematurity**

*Adapted from* Nelson Textbook of Pediatrics, *14th ed., Philadelphia: WB Saunders, p. 445.*

delivered by nasal prongs. Premature infants with idiopathic apnea may be treated with theophylline.

### Patent Ductus Arteriosus

**Failure of the closure** of the **ductus arteriosus** results in a reversal of blood flow through the patent ductus from the aorta to the low pressure pulmonary vascular system. This **shunting of blood** causes a widened pulse pressure and the classic "machinery" murmur. Large shunts can cause congestive heart failure and pulmonary hypertension.

A patent ductus arteriosus (**PDA**) in a premature infant is a result of gestational immaturity or hypoxia and is frequently associated with the respiratory distress syndrome. A PDA of this type often closes spontaneously. Because the local action of prostaglandins maintains an open ductus, indomethacin, a **prostaglandin inhibitor**, may be used to facilitate closure. A PDA in a term infant is the result of a defect of the ductus and requires surgical ligation and division.

### Persistent Fetal Circulation

Persistent fetal circulation (**PFC**), usually found in full-term or postmature infants, results from an **elevation of the pulmonary vascular resistance**, which causes a right-to-left shunt of blood through a patent ductus arteriosus and foramen ovale. PFC can be primary or secondary to various diseases of the newborn: asphyxia, meconium aspiration syndrome, pulmonary hypoplasia, group B streptococcal sepsis, polycythemia, or hypoglycemia. A preductal (right radial artery) and postductal (umbilical artery) oxygen gradient is consistent with right-to-left shunting through a patent ductus arteriosus.

The treatment of PFC includes mechanical ventilation, oxygen and vasodilators. Extracorporeal membrane oxygenation (ECMO), a form of cardiopulmonary bypass, has been used with some success to treat infants with severe PFC.

## HEMATOLOGIC/HEPATIC DISORDERS

### Neonatal Jaundice

Jaundice appears in newborns when the serum bilirubin exceeds 5 mg/dL. **Elevated levels of bilirubin** can be the result of increased hemolysis of red blood cells, of immature liver function, or of congenital obstructions of the biliary system. Hepatobiliary disease is suggested by an elevation of conjugated (direct-reacting) bilirubin in excess of 10% of the total serum bilirubin or 2 mg/dL. A classification of the common causes of jaundice in newborns is provided in Table 6-2.

## Physiologic Jaundice

Physiologic **hyperbilirubinemia** is an elevated level of unconjugated bilirubin that exceeds normal adult levels and is due to the normal

**TABLE 6-2. Causes of Neonatal Jaundice**

**Unconjugated hyperbilirubinemia**
- Isoimmune hemolysis
  - ABO incompatibility
  - Rh incompatibility
- Red cell membrane defects
  - Hereditary spherocytosis
- Erythrocyte enzyme defects
  - G6PD deficiency
  - Pyruvate kinase deficiency
- Polycythemia
  - Infant of a diabetic mother
  - Fetal transfusion
- Hepatic enzyme defects
  - Crigler-Najjar syndrome
  - Glucuronyl transferase deficiency type II

**Conjugated hyperbilirubinemia (cholestasis)**
- Infection
  - Sepsis
  - Viral hepatitis
- Metabolic disease
  - Disorders of carbohydrate metabolism (galactosemia)
  - Disorders of amino acid metabolism (tyrosinemia)
  - Disorders of lipid metabolism
- Endocrine diseases
  - Hypothyroidism
- Intrahepatic bile duct paucity
  - Alagille syndrome (arteriohepatic dysplasia)
  - Zellweger syndrome
- Extrahepatic
  - Biliary atresia
  - Choledochal cyst

hepatic immaturity in the conjugation of bilirubin. Physiologic jaundice usually peaks on the third day of life with bilirubin levels of 5 to 6 mg/dL. Physiologic hyperbilirubinemia must be distinguished from pathologic causes of jaundice.

## Breast-Milk Jaundice

Some breast-fed infants may also develop significant jaundice in the first few days of life. The breast milk of some mothers contains 5-beta pregnane-3 alpha, 20 beta idol, or nonesterified long chain fatty acids that inhibit the action of glucuronyl transferase hepatic conjugation. These infants are otherwise healthy.

In this situation, if breast-feeding is continued, the hyperbilirubinemia gradually decreases in many infants. If breast-feeding is discontinued for a day or so, the jaundice disappears and breast-feeding can be restarted without the reappearance of jaundice. In a few infants, the level of the hyperbilirubinemia may require phototherapy treatment.

## Hemolytic Disease of the Newborn

**Hemolytic disease** of the newborn is a common cause of jaundice and a rapidly rising unconjugated bilirubin level. The most common form, isoimmune hemolysis, is caused by incompatibilities between the mother's red blood cell antigens and the infant's red blood cell antigens. Hemolysis results from the destruction of fetal and neonatal red blood cells by maternal IgG antibodies that cross the placenta during pregnancy. These maternal antibodies develop as a result of maternal exposure to red cell antigens of a foreign blood group or Rh type. **Maternal sensitization** occurs during a fetal-maternal transfusion, during current or prior pregnancies, or from mismatched blood transfusions.

*Erythroblastosis fetalis* or Rh incompatibility occurs when an Rh-negative mother has an Rh-positive infant. In 90% of these infants, the offending **Rh factor** is the D blood group antigen. Erythroblastosis fetalis is less common in the African-American population than in the white population. The level of **hemolytic anemia** found in these infants varies, but severely affected infants are born with profound anemia, jaundice, and even signs of congestive heart failure. **Hydrops fetalis** is a term used to describe the most severe form of this condition in which the newborn presents with severe anemia, cardiovascular decompensation, and anasarca.

Laboratory evaluation of the infant will reveal anemia, reticulocytosis, unconjugated hyperbilirubinemia, and a positive direct Coombs' test.

The incidence of Rh hemolytic disease of the newborn has been reduced dramatically with the use of a potent **anti-Rh immune globulin** (RhoGAM) given to the Rh-negative mother immediately after birth of an Rh-positive infant.

## ABO Incompatibility

ABO incompatibility occurs when the mother and infant have an incompatibility of the **major blood groups**. In the most common situation, the mother has type O blood group, whereas the infant has either A or B blood group. In this, as in all isoimmune hemolytic anemias, the direct Coombs' test is weakly or moderately positive. This form of isoimmune hemolysis is usually less severe and less likely to require clinical intervention. In newborns, high levels of unconjugated bilirubin from any cause can result in the development of **kernicterus**, with resultant permanent neurologic damage or death. Kernicterus occurs when **unconjugated bilirubin is deposited in the brain**, particularly the basal ganglia and cerebellum. Clinical manifestations include opisthotonos, seizures, hearing loss, and choreoathetoid cerebral palsy.

The guidelines for the treatment of neonatal hyperbilirubinemia involve consideration of the indirect bilirubin level, the infant's gestational age, the cause of the hyperbilirubinemia, and the infant's age.

**Phototherapy**, the use of ultraviolet lights, depends on the absorption of radiant energy by the unconjugated bilirubin molecule, which makes it water soluble and allows its further metabolism and excretion by the kidney. If the level of unconjugated hyperbilirubinemia cannot be controlled by phototherapy, exchange transfusion of the infant is required.

## Hemorrhagic Disease of the Newborn

The most common hemorrhagic disease of the newborn is a transient **decrease in the vitamin K-dependent factors** II, VII, IX, and X, which occurs 48 to 72 hours after birth. This decrease in coagulation factors, especially in premature infants, may be so severe that spontaneous hemorrhage from the nose, gastrointestinal tract, or from the site of needle sticks or minor surgery (circumcision), may occur. Intracranial hemorrhage is a rare but serious complication.

**Vitamin K deficiency** is more severe in breast-fed infants and in those born to mothers receiving phenobarbital or phenytoin. Hemorrhagic disease of the newborn can be prevented by parenteral administration of 1 mg of vitamin K at birth.

# GASTROINTESTINAL DISORDERS

## Necrotizing Enterocolitis

Necrotizing enterocolitis (**NEC**) is a mucosal or transmucosal **intestinal necrosis** commonly of the distal ileum or proximal colon. Although the **etiology** of this condition is **unknown**, premature infants are at high risk. Polycythemia, early oral feeding, and gastrointestinal infection have also been implicated as contributing factors.

The infant with NEC develops abdominal distension, vomiting, and bloody stools. Abdominal radiographs may demonstrate **pneumatosis intestinalis**, a pathognomonic finding of intramural gas within the intestinal wall. The necrosis may result in bowel perforation, bacterial sepsis, and death.

Therapy for NEC involves careful acid-base and nutritional management coupled with broad antibiotic coverage. Many of these infants require surgical resection of the involved segment of intestine. Some infants who require surgery develop strictures at the site of the intestinal anastomosis. Infants with severe disease may require extensive bowel resection and develop short bowel syndrome, which is characterized by malabsorption and failure to thrive.

## Meconium Ileus

**Intestinal obstruction** due to a **meconium plug** may occur in several diseases: cystic fibrosis, congenital aganglionic megacolon (Hirschsprung's disease), small left colon syndrome in infants of diabetic mothers and infants whose mothers were treated with magnesium sulfate therapy for preeclampsia.

Many infants with these conditions will have an associated intestinal atresia, volvulus or stenosis. If the obstruction is severe, meconium peritonitis can result from a perforation of the intestine.

## Hirschsprung's Disease

**Congenital aganglionic megacolon**, or Hirschsprung's disease, is the most common cause of intestinal obstruction in neonates. Hirschsprung's disease is more common in males than females and is occasionally familial. Pathologically, there is absence of ganglion cells within the intestinal wall extending from the anus to the colon. The rectum and sigmoid colon are usually involved, although the abnormality can extend throughout the entire colon or be limited to the region of the anal sphincter.

Infants with the disease present with difficulty or delay in passing meconium, failure to thrive, and intestinal obstruction. Diarrhea may occur and can alternate with periods of constipation. **Entero-

**colitis** is a serious complication that can lead to severe dehydration and bowel perforation. Older children present with constipation present since birth, marked abdominal distention, fecal abdominal masses, and the absence of feces in the rectum.

The diagnosis is made by biopsy of the involved segment of colon. Barium enema shows a narrow, involved segment with an abrupt dilatation where normal colon begins.

**Surgical resection** of the involved colon is required. A preliminary colostomy is usually performed in the neonatal period, followed by a definitive surgical pull-through procedure later in infancy.

## Tracheoesophageal Atresia

Most infants with esophageal atresia also have a fistula connecting the trachea with the distal esophageal pouch. Other variations of this **congenital anomaly** include the "H" type, in which there is no esophageal atresia but a fistulous connection between the esophagus and the trachea.

Manifestations of esophageal atresia include excessive oral secretions, polyhydramnios, and the inability to pass a feeding tube into the stomach. Infants with a fistulous connection of the proximal esophageal pouch to the trachea choke on feedings. A fistulous connection of the distal esophageal pouch to the trachea results in abdominal distention.

Various other congenital anomalies are associated with tracheoesophageal atresias, including skeletal abnormalities of the spine and radius as well as urogenital anomalies.

A **tracheoesophageal fistula** represents a surgical emergency. Many of these children will develop postoperatively either strictures or stenosis at the site of the esophageal anastomosis or gastroesophageal reflux.

## Cleft Lip and Palate

**Cleft lip and palate**, due to a combination of genetic and nongenetic factors (multifactorial inheritance), may be associated with other congenital anomalies. Cleft lip and palate may exist separately or in combination and may vary in severity from small notches to extensive bony clefts. Affected children have difficulty feeding and are prone to recurrent otitis media, hearing loss, and speech defects. Therapy includes fitting of a prosthesis to aid feeding, corrective surgery, speech therapy, and proper dental care.

## The Umbilicus

Superficial infection of the umbilicus causes a moist area at the base, often with a mucoid discharge. The infection clears with alcohol cleansing. Deeper infection of the umbilicus, heralded by periumbilical erythema, is a serious infection of the newborn because of the potential for spread to the bloodstream or liver.

Persistent granulation tissues, a **granuloma**, resolves with cauterization with silver nitrate.

**Umbilical hernias**, due to incomplete closure of the umbilical ring, are common, especially in African-American children. Most umbilical hernias resolve within the first few years of life and do not require surgical intervention. Incarceration of intestine is rare. However, hernias that do not close by early school age should be repaired surgically.

An **omphalocele** is a protrusion of abdominal organs through the umbilicus without a covering of skin. Omphaloceles are associated with the Beckwith syndrome, which is characterized by intractable hypoglycemia, macrosomia, and an increased risk of malignant tumors.

# DISEASES OF THE CENTRAL NERVOUS SYSTEM

## Intraventricular Hemorrhage

Premature infants are at risk of intraventricular hemorrhage in the subependymal germinal matrix within the first 3 days of life. The **germinal matrix** is a highly vascular area of immature neurons and glial cells and is not present in the full-term infant. Bleeding may extend into the ventricles and result in ventricular dilatation.

Risk factors for intraventricular hemorrhage in the preterm infant include asphyxia, hypovolemia, hypertension, and respiratory distress syndrome. Severe hypoxic-ischemic injury results in **periventricular leukomalacia**, a necrosis of the periventricular white matter. Damage to the corticospinal tracts gives rise to a spastic diplegia.

The diagnosis of intraventricular hemorrhage and periventricular leukomalacia can be confirmed by ultrasonography through the open anterior fontanelle of the newborn.

## Retinopathy of Prematurity

Retinopathy of prematurity (**ROP**) is a spectrum of vascular **abnormalities of the retina**, including abnormal vascular proliferation, scarring, and retinal detachment. ROP occurs in premature infants in response to several injurious conditions, including hyperoxia, and occurs most frequently in very **sick premature infants**.

All infants weighing less than 1500 grams, and at especially high risk, should be screened at 6 to 9 weeks after birth. In most infants, the condition resolves spontaneously; however, cryotherapy is effective in preventing retinal detachment in infants with severe disease.

# ACQUIRED INFECTIONS IN THE NEWBORN

## Sepsis

Virtually any bacteria can cause sepsis in the neonate; however, the usual causative agents are those found in the maternal vaginal or gastrointestinal tract. The pattern of bacterial causes of neonatal sepsis has varied over the years. Previously, group A beta-hemolytic streptococcus and *Staphylococcus aureus* were major causes of infection in the newborn, but since the 1970s, **group B beta-hemolytic streptococci** have become a major problem. In addition, neonates are especially vulnerable to infections with such gram-negative organisms as *Escherichia coli* and such usually commensal organisms as *S. epidermidis*. The risk of neonatal sepsis is increased in premature infants, those who deliver after prolonged rupture of membranes, and those whose mothers have chorioamnionitis.

Neonatal sepsis may present with a fulminant course, resulting in death within hours, or it may present with vague, nonspecific symptoms. A variety of signs and symptoms may signal the presence of sepsis, including lethargy, poor feeding, jaundice, temperature instability, respiratory distress, or periods of apnea, abdominal distention, hypotonia, and altered cry. In the later stages of disease, infants will present with shock, coma, sclerema, purpura, severe respiratory distress, and renal failure.

Early onset group B streptococcal sepsis presents with respiratory distress, pneumonia, persistent fetal circulation, and septic shock; it may be indistinguishable from respiratory distress syndrome. Late onset group B streptococcal infection typically manifests as meningitis. However, group B streptococcal infection of the neonate can involve almost any organ. Infection with *Listeria monocytogenes* may resemble the clinical picture of group B streptococcal sepsis.

Because neonatal sepsis is commonly associated with more localized forms of infection, the presence of sepsis should alert the clinician to the possibility of meningitis, pneumonia, osteomyelitis, urinary tract infection, and necrotizing enterocolitis. Thus, in the face of symptoms and signs of possible sepsis, a complete evaluation including examination of the spinal fluid is required.

However, because no laboratory or radiographic finding is rapid or reliable enough to substitute for clinical judgment and because of the urgency of the situation, the treatment of neonatal sepsis is regularly begun before a causative organism is identified. **Broad**

**antibiotic coverage** to deal with both gram-negative (*E. coli*) and gram-positive (group B streptococcus) organisms is commonly employed until a definitive bacteriologic diagnosis can be made.

## Conjunctivitis

Conjunctivitis in the newborn is commonly due to inflammation from prophylactically administered silver nitrate drops or to infection with *Neisseria gonorrhoeae* or *Chlamydia trachomatis*. The etiologic agent can sometimes be distinguished by the timing of infection: Inflammation from silver nitrate occurs within the first day of life; infection with gonococcus typically occurs on days 2 to 5; and infection with chlamydia on between 5 to 14 days of life. However, Gram stain and culture of the exudate and antigen detection for chlamydia should be performed. Gonococcal conjunctivitis is a serious infection, and, if untreated, can progress to corneal ulceration and deeper infection of the globe.

The use of **neonatal ocular prophylaxis** has significantly reduced the incidence of gonococcal conjunctivitis. Topical 1% silver nitrate, 0.5% erythromycin, or 1% tetracycline are considered equally effective. However, neither silver nitrate nor topical antibiotics have been demonstrated consistently to prevent ocular infection with chlamydia. Since some infants exposed to chlamydia will later develop an afebrile pneumonitis, newborns with chlamydia conjunctivitis may be given prophylactic oral erythromycin to prevent this complication.

## Neonatal Tetanus

Neonatal tetanus is caused by the neurotoxin tetanospasmin produced by *Clostridium tetani*, which infects the umbilical stump. The incubation period is 5 to 14 days. Affected infants develop difficulty in sucking and swallowing. Generalized hypertonicity, spasms, and opisthotonos follow. Treatment is with tetanus immune globulin (TIG), penicillin G, and muscle relaxants. In developing countries where neonatal tetanus is common, the fatality rate is very high. Because of the maternal transfer of antibodies to the infant during pregnancy, neonatal tetanus can be prevented by the administration of the tetanus toxoid vaccine to all girls or women prior to pregnancy. Proper newborn umbilical hygiene can also prevent this disease.

## CONGENITAL INFECTIONS OF THE NEWBORN

Screening for congenital infections should be based on specific exposures and clinical syndromes. Routine serologic screening for

TORCH infections (**t**oxoplasmosis, **o**ther viruses, **r**ubella, **C**MV, **h**erpes) is of no value and should not be performed. Maternal screening during pregnancy for syphilis, hepatitis B, human immunodeficiency virus (HIV), and rubella antibodies are part of proper antenatal care.

## Syphilis

Because women with syphilis can infect their fetus at any point during their pregnancy, all women should be tested for syphilis at least once during pregnancy and at the time of delivery. Every infant should also be tested for syphilis at birth.

**Congenital infection** with syphilis causes fetal death in 40% of infected infants. Symptoms of early congenital syphilis begin within the first 2 years of life. The infant with early congenital syphilis will present with failure to thrive, hepatosplenomegaly, generalized lymphadenopathy, jaundice, a variety of rashes including a characteristic maculopapular rash of the palms and soles, moist lesions of the mucous membranes, profuse nasal discharge ("snuffles"), bone lesions, anemia, and thrombocytopenia.

Manifestations of **late congenital syphilis**, which develop over the first two decades of life, include frontal bossing, anterior bowing of the tibia (saber shins), peg-shaped central incisors (Hutchinson teeth), saddle nose deformity, linear scars around the mouth and anus (rhagades), corneal scarring, and deafness.

The diagnosis of congenital syphilis is made by physical examination, radiographic examination of the long bones, quantitative nontreponemal serologic test for syphilis such as Venereal Disease Research Laboratory (VDRL) and rapid plasma reagin (RPR), and analysis of the cerebrospinal fluid (CSF) for VDRL, cells, and protein. Measurement of specific antitreponemal antibodies, particularly IgM, may also be useful. Infants with proven or highly probable congenital syphilis should be treated with penicillin G.

## Herpes Simplex

**Perinatal infection** of the newborn with herpes simplex virus, usually type 2, can result in systemic infection, including the liver and central nervous system (CNS); localized encephalitis; or skin and mucous membrane involvement, including keratitis and chorioretinitis. The risk of perinatal herpes simplex infection is much higher in women with primary infection than in those with recurrent infection.

The diagnosis is confirmed by culture of the virus from vesicles, nasopharynx, eyes, or body fluids. However, culture of the virus is difficult in infants with localized encephalitis. Neonates suspected of having herpes simplex infection should be treated promptly with acyclovir.

## Human Immunodeficiency Virus

Adverse outcomes of pregnancy are common in women infected with **HIV**. However, many confounding maternal variables make it difficult to establish a causal relationship. No pattern of embryopathy resulting from maternal HIV infection has been established, nor is there conclusive evidence that maternal HIV infection directly causes adverse perinatal outcome. Such complications of advanced maternal HIV infection as maternal infection (tuberculosis, toxoplasmosis) and malnutrition, as well as the presence of other sexually transmitted infections, can adversely affect the infant.

The rate of perinatal transmission of the virus from an infected woman to her fetus or infant varies with geographic areas but is in the range of 20% to 40%. The risk of perinatal transmission can be reduced significantly if the mother receives zidovudine during the third trimester and the infant is treated during the perinatal period.

## Cytomegalovirus

Most infants with congenital cytomegalovirus (CMV) infection are asymptomatic. Long-term sequelae, which may not be apparent at birth, include sensorineural hearing loss and learning disabilities. Severe **congenital infection** causes intrauterine growth retardation, microcephaly, periventricular calcifications, chorioretinitis, jaundice, hepatosplenomegaly, and purpura. The diagnosis of congenital infection is made by viral isolation, particularly from the urine or by a strongly positive test for serum IgM anti-CMV antibody. The isolation of the virus beyond 3 weeks of life does not distinguish intrauterine from postnatal infection. Perinatal infection can occur during delivery, from breast milk, or through blood transfusion.

## Varicella Zoster

**Maternal varicella-zoster infection** in the first or early second trimester may cause a congenital varicella syndrome, characterized by atrophy and scarring of the extremities. When the mother develops varicella within 5 days before delivery to 2 days after delivery, she has not yet developed protective antibodies to pass to the infant. For this reason, the newborn is at high risk for the development of severe varicella infection and death. These infants should receive **varicella-zoster immunoglobulin** (VZIG) immediately after birth to protect them from infection.

## Hepatitis B

Perinatal transmission of hepatitis B occurs in infants born to mothers who are positive for **hepatitis B e antigen**. Ninety percent of infants infected perinatally will develop chronic hepatitis B and are at increased risk for subsequent chronic active hepatitis, cirrhosis, and hepatocellular carcinoma.

All women should be screened for hepatitis B surface antigen during early and late pregnancy. Those infants whose mothers are positive should receive hepatitis B immune globulin within 12 hours of birth as well as the initial dose of the hepatitis B vaccine. The vaccination schedule for hepatitis B should be completed within the first 6 months of life.

## Rubella

Primary maternal rubella infection during pregnancy, which may be asymptomatic in as many as 50% of women, causes congenital rubella syndrome in their newborns. The effect on the fetus depends on the gestational age at time of infection. Congenital heart disease occurs when the gestational age is 9 to 12 weeks, congenital deafness occurs with infection before 16 weeks gestation.

The signs and symptoms of **congenital rubella syndrome** are protean and include hepatosplenomegaly, lymphadenopathy, radiographic changes of the femur and humerus (celery stalk lesions), sensorineural hearing loss, congenital heart disease (PDA, pulmonary artery stenosis, septal defects), cataracts, retinopathy, microcephaly, and mental retardation.

## Human Papillomavirus

Human papillomavirus is a **sexually transmitted** virus that causes genital **warts and neoplasms**. Human papillomavirus (types 6 and 11) can be transmitted to newborns, placing them at risk for the development of respiratory papillomatosis and resultant upper airway obstruction.

## Parvovirus B19

Maternal infection with human parvovirus B19, which infects the precursors of the erythroid cell line, may result in severe fetal anemia or death.

## Bacterial Vaginosis

Bacterial vaginosis is a condition in which the normal vaginal flora is replaced with anaerobic bacteria, *Gardnerella vaginalis* and *Mycoplasma hominis*. Infants born to women with bacterial vaginosis are at risk of preterm delivery.

## Toxoplasmosis

As with congenital CMV infection, most infants with congenital toxoplasmosis are asymptomatic. Long-term sequelae, which may not be apparent at birth, include mental retardation, learning disabilities, and visual impairment. Severe congenital toxoplasmosis causes hydrocephalus, microcephaly, cerebral calcifications, chorioretinitis, lymphadenopathy, hepatosplenomegaly, and thrombocytopenia.

The diagnosis is made by ophthalmologic examination for chorioretinitis and computerized tomography of the brain to identify intracranial calcifications. **Serologic diagnosis**, using Toxoplasma-specific IgM or IgA, should be performed by a reference laboratory. Because infants born to mothers with primary infection during pregnancy or with concurrent HIV infection are at high risk for congenital toxoplasmosis, empirical treatment should be considered.

# Chapter 7

# Infectious Diseases

## GENERAL PRINCIPLES OF PEDIATRIC INFECTIOUS DISEASE

### Fever

Fever seems to be an adaptive host response that augments the body's immunologic defense against infecting pathogens. In general, the *height of fever does not distinguish bacterial from viral infection*, although some studies suggest that bacterial infection is more likely with extremes of hyperpyrexia (greater than 41°C). Young children appear to tolerate fever better than adults, but some develop benign febrile seizures. The pattern of fever can be useful in establishing certain diagnoses and in monitoring response to therapy.

Fever should always prompt a careful search for serious bacterial infection in infants less than 2 to 3 months of age and in children immunocompromised for any reason: sickle cell anemia, nephrosis, primary immune dysfunction, or human immunodeficiency virus (HIV) infection. Children who present with **petechiae** and those with **indwelling catheters** (central venous or urinary catheters or cerebrospinal fluid [CSF] shunts) should also be examined carefully for the presence of bacterial infection. In these circumstances, if no source of infection is found, hospitalization, appropriate cultures, and empiric antibiotic therapy should be considered (Table 7-1).

Fever in an infant less than 2 to 3 months of age without an obvious cause of the fever beyond mild upper respiratory tract symptoms is a common problem. Because the early signs of **sepsis** in infants of this age may be subtle, even experienced pediatricians may not be able to distinguish febrile young infants with benign viral infections from those with serious bacterial infection. Because a *delay in the diagnosis of sepsis in young infants can be fatal*, many authorities recommend that febrile infants less than 2 to 3 months of age be treated for sepsis until proven otherwise. A complete blood count and cultures of the blood, urine, and CSF are obtained before the infant is treated with broad spectrum parenteral antibiotics for several days until the results of the bacterial cultures are available.

**TABLE 7-1.**

**Fever Syndromes in Children**

| Fever Syndromes | Age Group | Diagnostic Concerns | Laboratory Tests | Hospital Admission | Treatment |
|---|---|---|---|---|---|
| Rule out serious bacterial infection | 0–3 months | Sepsis, meningitis, UTI, pneumonia, benign viral illness | CBC, blood culture, CSF analysis, urine culture (CXR) | Yes | Empiric, parenteral antibiotics |
| Occult bacteremia | 3 months–2 years | Bacteremia, benign viral illness | CBC, blood culture, CSF analysis | In some cases (see text) | In some cases (see text) |
| Fever and petechiae | Any age | Meningococcemia, sepsis | CBC, blood culture, CSF analysis | Yes, if bacteremia suspected | Parenteral antibiotics for bacteremia |
| Seizure with fever | 9 months–5 years | Meningitis, febrile seizure | CSF analysis | Yes, if meningitis suspected | Parenteral antibiotics for meningitis |

*This table is meant to show different diagnostic possibilities in children with fever. It does not provide a comprehensive diagnostic or treatment plan for each of these fever syndromes. Febrile children who appear ill require hospitalization and empiric treatment with antibiotics. Children with a focal bacterial infection require treatment with antibiotics.*

*CBC = complete blood count; CSF = cerebrospinal fluid; CXR = chest radiograph; UTI = urinary tract infection*

## BACTEREMIA AND SEPSIS

**Bacteremia** refers to a situation in which bacteria enter the blood stream through local infections or through the gastrointestinal, genitourinary, or respiratory tracts. Common bacterial pathogens in children (pneumococci, *Haemophilus influenzae* type b, meningococcus) often first colonize in the nasopharynx and subsequently invade the blood stream. A viral upper respiratory tract infection may facilitate bacterial invasion of the blood stream. Bacteremia may present with catastrophic and fatal septic shock, or it may go undetected until such local infections as meningitis, osteomyelitis, or cellulitis present.

**Occult bacteremia,** a bacteremia without an obvious focus of infection, occurs most commonly in children between the ages of 3 to 24 months. However, most children in this age group who present with high fever probably have a viral infection (human herpesvirus 6 or an enterovirus) rather than a bacterial infection. The bacterial etiologic agent is usually *Streptococcus pneumoniae*, but *H. influenzae* type b, *Neisseria meningitidis*, and *Salmonella* species have also been isolated from children with occult bacteremia. Occult bacteremia may resolve without treatment, or it may progress to the development of such localized infections as meningitis, arthritis, or pneumonia.

The diagnosis of **occult bacteremia** is difficult because of the **absence of specific signs and symptoms**. Although most authorities use clinical assessment, height of fever, and total white cell count as clues to the probability of bacteremia, no combination of variables completely predicts the presence of bacterial infection.

The management of children with suspected occult bacteremia is controversial. A blood culture should be obtained in all suspected cases. If adequate home monitoring is assured, the child may be returned home without therapy but with clear instructions to the parents to return if the child's condition worsens. Some authorities recommend antibiotic prophylaxis with ceftriaxone, particularly if adequate home monitoring follow-up cannot be assured and if hospitalization is impossible or undesirable. Ill-appearing infants should always be hospitalized and treated with antibiotics.

If the blood culture shows the presence of **pneumococci**, the child should be evaluated immediately. Because pneumococcal occult bacteremia has a high rate of spontaneous resolution, if, on reevaluation, the child is afebrile, the child may be sent home again after a second blood culture is obtained.

Children who appear ill, continue to have fever, or have a bacterial blood culture containing a pathogen other than pneumococcus should be hospitalized for treatment with parenteral antibiotics.

Bacteremia frequently follows instrumentation of the respiratory, gastrointestinal, or genitourinary tracts. The possibility of such a transient bacteremia is the justification for antibiotic prophylaxis against bacterial endocarditis in children with heart disease.

## Meningococcemia

Acute **meningococcemia** is a fulminant bacteremia, due to *N. meningitidis*, that rapidly progresses to septic shock. The coexistence of **fever and petechiae** should always raise concern of serious bacterial infection, particularly meningococcemia. Children with meningococcemia develop petechiae, purpura, disseminated intravascular coagulation (DIC), hypotension, and renal failure. Antibiotic therapy should not be delayed in children suspected of having meningococcemia or septic shock.

## SCARLET FEVER

**Scarlet fever** is caused by infection with group A streptococci, which produce erythrogenic toxins. In addition to the signs and symptoms of streptococcal pharyngitis, children with scarlet fever have an erythematous, fine papular rash that has a sandpaper texture. The rash begins in the neck, axillae, and groin and progresses to involve the entire body. Desquamation occurs toward the end of the first week of illness. **Pastia lines** are areas in the antecubital fossa that do not blanch with pressure. The **white strawberry tongue** of scarlet fever is a white coating, seen in the first few days of illness, which later desquamates, creating the **red strawberry tongue**. The treatment for scarlet fever is penicillin.

# TUBERCULOSIS

**Tuberculosis** in children almost always results from primary infection with *Mycobacterium tuberculosis* rather than reactivation of latent disease as found in adults. Tuberculosis in a child indicates exposure to an adult with contagious disease and should prompt **identification and treatment of the source case**.

Most children infected with *M. tuberculosis* are asymptomatic and are only identified by a **positive tuberculin skin reaction**. Tuberculin skin testing consists of the *intradermal* injection of 5 tuberculin units of purified protein derivative. Children at high risk should be tested annually.

Definitions of a positive Mantoux skin test are given in Table 7-2. Previous immunization with bacillus Calmette-Guerin (BCG) vaccine does *not* alter these definitions. Approximately 10% of immunocompetent children with tuberculous infection do not have positive tuberculin skin tests; this figure is higher for immunocompromised children who are anergic.

The presence of clinical manifestations distinguishes tuberculous disease from tuberculous infection. Most children with disease present with hilar adenopathy with or without pulmonary parenchymal disease. In the absence of other signs or symptoms, a chest radiograph usually serves to distinguish children with the disease from those with infection. Because the sputum of children with pulmonary tuberculosis is usually negative for mycobacteria, either by acid-fast stain or culture, these children are noninfectious.

**Extrapulmonary tuberculosis**, including cervical adenitis, tuberculous meningitis, and miliary tuberculosis, occurs in approximately one quarter of cases of children with tuberculous disease. Infants and young children, particularly those who are immunocompromised or malnourished, are at risk of the serious and often fatal forms of miliary or tuberculous meningitis. Congenital tuberculosis is extremely rare.

Children with **tuberculous infection** (without evidence of disease) should receive **isoniazid prophylaxis** for 9 months. Prophylaxis greatly reduces the risk of reactivated tuberculous disease later in life.

### TABLE 7-2. Definition of a Positive Mantoux Skin Test in Children

**A reaction greater than or equal to 5 mm is POSITIVE in:**
- Children in close contact with persons who have known or suspected infectious tuberculosis
- Children suspected to have tuberculous disease, including those with clinical evidence or a consistent chest radiograph
- Children who are immunosuppressed or who have HIV infection

**A reaction greater than or equal to 10 mm is POSITIVE in:**
- Children younger than 4 years of age
- Children at risk of disseminated tuberculosis, including those with chronic diseases such as malnutrition, diabetes mellitus, chronic renal failure, and lymphoma
- Children born, or whose parents were born, in areas where tuberculosis is highly prevalent
- Children exposed to adults at risk of tuberculosis, including adults who are homeless, HIV-infected, intravenous drug users, including those who have been incarcerated or institutionalized or who live in poor, inner-city neighborhoods

**A reaction greater than or equal to 15 mm is POSITIVE in:**
- Children over 4 years of age with no risk factors

*Adapted from the AAP 1994 Red Book, p. 485.*

Children with **pulmonary tuberculosis** are usually treated with a 6-month regimen consisting of isoniazid, rifampin, and pyrazinamide for the first 2 months and isoniazid and rifampin for the remaining 4 months. In areas where isoniazid and rifampin resistance is prevalent, a fourth drug should be added to the regimen (usually ethambutol or streptomycin). Because hepatitis due to isoniazid is extremely rare in children, routine testing of liver function is not recommended.

## SPIROCHETAL INFECTION

### Lyme Disease

**Lyme disease**, caused by the spirochete *Borrelia burgdorferi*, is transmitted by the bite of ticks of the genus *Ixodes*. Lyme disease is the most common vector-borne disease in the United States. The incubation period, although variable, is usually 1 week.

Infected children may develop a characteristic annular rash at the site of the tick bite (**erythema chronicum migrans**), which is associated with fever, malaise, headache, and arthralgias. Disseminated infection occurs weeks to months later, and includes arthritis (usually large joints), neurologic disease (facial palsy, peripheral neuropathy), and heart disease (heart block, myocarditis).

The diagnosis should be based on clinical findings. Because serologic diagnosis is often problematic, serologic tests should be used only to support the clinical diagnosis. Amoxicillin or tetraycline is used to treat early Lyme disease. Patients with severe neurologic involvement, carditis, or persistent arthritis should be treated with ceftriaxone or parenteral penicillin.

Lyme disease is prevented by avoiding tick bites through the use of protective clothing and tick repellents. Although controversial, in specific circumstances some authorities recommend prophylactic antibiotics following tick bites.

## RICKETTSIAL INFECTION

**Rocky Mountain spotted fever** (RMSF), caused by *Rickettsia rickettsii* and transmitted by the bite of ticks, is *not limited* to the Rocky Mountain area but is found throughout the United States. Transmission is most common in the spring and winter, with an incubation period of approximately 1 week.

Infected children develop fever, headache, myalgia, vomiting, and a petechial rash, which usually begins on the wrists and ankles as erythematous macules and papules and evolves into a petechial eruption, which rapidly spreads to the trunk. The palms and soles are usually involved. Disseminated intravascular coagulation, shock, and multisystem involvement can ensue.

The diagnosis is established serologically by demonstrating a fourfold rise in antibody titer between acute and convalescent sera. Treatment is with tetracycline or chloramphenicol. As with Lyme disease, parents can help prevent RMSF in their children by dressing them appropriately, applying tick repellents, and inspecting them for the presence of ticks.

## CAT-SCRATCH DISEASE

**Cat-scratch disease**, which is caused by *Bartonella henselae*, follows the scratch of a healthy cat, usually a kitten. Lymphadenopathy develops approximately 2 weeks after the scratch but the incubation period is variable. Infected children develop regional lymphadenopathy, commonly axillary and epitrochlear lymphadenopathy. The diagnosis can be confirmed by Warthin-Starry silver impregnation stain of lymph node tissue, but biopsy is not necessary in all cases. A serologic test is available. Most cases resolve spontaneously within several months; antibiotics are reserved for children with severe disease and are of probable but unproven benefit.

# VIRAL INFECTIONS

## Measles

Measles, which is caused by an RNA virus of the paramyxovirus family, is **highly infectious** by person-to-person spread. In the United States, measles is more common in the winter and spring. The incubation period (to onset of rash) is approximately 2 weeks; infected children are contagious 4 days before the rash until 4 days after the appearance of the rash.

Children with measles have fever, conjunctivitis, coryza, cough, Koplik spots (small white spots on the buccal mucosa), and a generalized erythematous maculopapular rash. The complications of measles include otitis media, croup, pneumonia, diarrhea, and encephalitis and are more common in infants less than 1 year of age.

Although measles can be prevented with the live-attenuated **measles virus vaccine**, vaccine failure occurs in approximately 5% of children. Recent outbreaks of measles in the United States have prompted changes in the recommended immunization schedule to include the addition of a second dose of the vaccine.

**Immunocompromised children** who are exposed to measles should receive **immunoglobulin**, regardless of their immunization status, either to prevent or to lessen the severity of the disease. In developing countries, children with measles should be treated with vitamin A to reduce its morbidity and mortality. In the United States, immunocompromised or malnourished children or those with severe measles may also benefit from vitamin A treatment.

## Mumps

Mumps, caused by a paramyxovirus, is transmitted by the respiratory route. In the United States, mumps is more common in the winter and spring. The incubation period is 2 to 3 weeks; infected children are contagious several days before the onset of parotitis until 5 days after the appearance of the parotid swelling.

Children with mumps present with fever, malaise, anorexia, and swelling of the salivary glands, especially the parotids. On examination, diffuse **swelling of the parotid** gland, which obliterates the angle of the jaw, is found along with swelling and erythema of the opening of Stensen's duct in the buccal mucosa. However, mumps can be asymptomatic. Children with mumps often develop a mild meningoencephalitis with headache, vomiting, and a stiff neck. This complication rarely causes permanent sequelae. In postpubertal adolescent boys, mumps can cause orchitis. Mumps is usually diagnosed clinically, but serologic tests and tissue culture can be useful in problematic cases.

The disease can be prevented through the administration of the **live mumps vaccine** usually given in combination with measles and rubella vaccines (MMR).

## Rubella

Rubella, caused by an RNA virus of the *Togaviridae* family, is transmitted through nasopharyngeal secretions. The peak incidence of infection is late winter and early spring. The incubation period is 2 to 3 weeks; children are infectious several days before the appearance of rash to 1 week after the rash.

Children with rubella present with fever, suboccipital, posterior, auricular, and cervical lymphadenopathy, and a generalized erythematous maculopapular rash. Arthralgias and arthritis can occur, especially in girls. Rubella infection is often asymptomatic.

**Congenital rubella** following infection in pregnant women is the most serious complication of rubella infection. Tissue culture and serologic testing of acute and convalescent sera can be used to confirm the diagnosis in pregnant women and newborns. Rubella and congenital rubella can be prevented through immunization with the live rubella vaccine. Adolescent girls should not become pregnant within 3 months after receiving the vaccine.

## Roseola

Roseola, caused by infection with human herpesvirus 6 and a frequent cause of high fever in children between the ages of 6 months and 2 years, is transmitted though the respiratory route. Children with roseola typically present with high fever of several days duration, which is followed by a generalized erythematous macular rash that coincides with the cessation of fever.

### *Erythema Infectiosum*

*Erythema infectiosum*, or Fifth disease, is caused by parvovirus B19 and is contagious only before the onset of the typical rash. Children with this disease present with fever and a distinctive facial erythematous rash with a "slapped cheek" appearance. A lace-like, symmetric rash on the arms, trunk, and thighs may also be present.

Infection with parvovirus B19 in children with hemolytic anemias can also cause aplastic crises due to infection of erythrocyte precursors by the virus. Children with aplastic crises due to parvovirus B19 infection are contagious for several weeks. The diagnosis is confirmed by measurement of IgM antibodies to parvovirus B19. Adults with this infection may develop a transitory arthritis.

## Infectious Mononucleosis

Infectious mononucleosis is caused by a herpesvirus, **Epstein-Barr virus** (EBV), and is transmitted by close personal contact. The disease, which has no seasonal pattern, has an incubation period of between 30 to 50 days and may be contagious for many months. Young children frequently have asymptomatic infection or a nonspecific febrile illness.

Older children and adolescents classically present with fever, exudative pharyngitis, generalized lymphadenopathy, splenomegaly, and atypical lymphocytes on blood smear. Children with infectious mononucleosis who have been treated with ampicillin frequently develop a generalized erythematous rash.

The diagnosis is confirmed by serologic tests. Because nonspecific heterophile antibody tests are usually negative in children less than 4 years of age, specific EBV serologic tests, which commonly measure IgG and IgA antibodies against viral capsid antigen (VCA), must be used for diagnosis. Other EBV antigens useful for serologic diagnosis are early antigen (EA) and EBV nuclear antigens (EBNA). Corticosteroids have been used to treat children with severe infectious mononucleosis.

## Enteroviruses

Nonpolio enteroviruses frequently cause nonspecific febrile illnesses, upper respiratory tract infections, and viral exanthems in infants and children. Enteroviral infections have a seasonal pattern of summer and fall, with an incubation period of 3 to 6 days. Children may be infectious for several weeks.

Several distinct clinical syndromes are caused by enteroviruses. **Herpangina** is characterized by high fever and small erythematous vesicles and ulcers on the anterior tonsillar pillars. Children with **pleurodynia** present with fever and spasmodic pain of the chest or upper abdomen. Coxsackievirus A16 causes **hand-foot-mouth syndrome**, and is characterized by small ulcers on the tongue and buccal mucosa and vesicles on the hands and feet. The buttocks may also be involved. Coxsackieviruses B1-B5 cause **myocarditis** in infants and children. Enterovirus 70 causes **acute hemorrhagic conjunctivitis**. The diagnosis of enterovirus infection is confirmed by culture.

## Viral Hepatitis

Viral hepatitis follows infection with several distinct viruses.

### Hepatitis A Virus

Hepatitis A virus, an RNA picornaviral infection transmitted by the **fecal-oral route**, has an incubation period of 25 to 30 days. Most infants and young children infected with hepatitis A virus are either asymptomatic or have a nonspecific febrile illness. Older children characteristically present with fever, malaise, anorexia, nausea, and jaundice. The diagnosis is confirmed by serologic tests for anti-hepatitis A IgM and IgG antibodies. A vaccine for hepatitis A is available.

### Hepatitis B Virus

Hepatitis B is a DNA virus transmitted through **blood** or **body fluids**. Hepatitis B virus can be transmitted **perinatally**. Although most young children with hepatitis B infection are asymptomatic, infants or young children with hepatitis B infection are at high risk of developing chronic hepatitis B infection and subsequent **cirrhosis or hepatocellular carcinoma**. The diagnosis is confirmed serologically. The American Academy of Pediatrics recommends that all infants be immunized against hepatitis B. Other viral causes of hepatitis are hepatitis C and hepatitis E.

# PARASITIC INFECTIONS

## Pinworm

Pinworm, caused by infection with the nematode *Enterobius vermicularis*, is the **most prevalent nematode infection** in the United States. Children with pinworms can present with perianal pruritus, irritability, or loss of appetite. The diagnosis is made by applying transparent tape to the perianal region in the morning and examining the tape microscopically for the presence of eggs. Treatment is with pyrantel pamoate or mebendazole. Reinfection is common.

## Roundworm

Roundworm infection with the nematode *Ascaris lumbricoides* is acquired by ingestion of eggs from contaminated soil. Adult worms live in the small intestine. Most infected children are asymptomatic. Adult worms may occasionally be passed in the stool or vomitus. Intestinal obstruction is rare but can occur with heavy infection. The diagnosis is confirmed by examination of the stool for *Ascaris* eggs. Treatment is with pyrantel pamoate or mebendazole.

## Hookworm

Hookworm infection, caused by the nematodes *Ancylostoma duodenale* and *Necator americanus*, is a common cause of iron deficiency anemia in children from tropical, developing countries. Infection is acquired when filariform larvae in the soil penetrate the skin of bare foot children. The adult worms live in the small intestine and feed on intestinal mucosa and blood. Children with hookworm infection present with iron deficiency anemia, but severe infection can produce protein malnutrition. The diagnosis is confirmed by identification of the characteristic eggs in the stool. Treatment is with mebendazole or pyrantel pamoate and iron supplementation.

## Malaria

Malaria is a major cause of childhood morbidity and mortality in many parts of the world. Infection by one of the four important *Plasmodium* species is acquired from the bite of the female *Anopheles* mosquito. *Plasmodium falciparum*, which causes the most severe form of infection in children, can be fatal.

Symptomatic infected children have periodic fever, malaise, headache, myalgias, pallor, jaundice, and hepatosplenomegaly. Early in the course of disease, the characteristic cyclical fever pattern may not be present. Hemolysis can be so severe as to cause profound anemia. **Cerebral malaria**, caused by vascular obstruction of cerebral capillaries by infected erythrocytes, can result in the development of seizures, coma, and death. Other manifestations of malaria in children include pulmonary edema, renal failure, and the nephrotic syndrome. **Congenital malaria** resembles neonatal sepsis.

The diagnosis is confirmed by examination of thick and thin blood smears for malaria parasites. Treatment with antimalarials depends upon the *Plasmodium* species and the severity of illness. Unfortunately, chloroquine resistance is common in many parts of the world. Chemoprophylaxis can prevent malaria in travelers to endemic areas.

Children with sickle cell trait are protected against severe malaria. The presence of glucose-6-phosphate dehydrogenase deficiency (G6PD) and beta-thalassemia are also thought to be protective.

# Chapter 8

# Disorders of the Respiratory System

## DISORDERS OF THE EARS AND SINUSES

### Acute Otitis Media

Acute otitis media is characterized by inflammation and the accumulation of fluid in the middle ear. The most common **bacterial** causes are *Streptococcus pneumoniae*, nontypable *Haemophilus influenzae*, and *Moraxella catarrhalis*. The child with acute otitis media usually presents with a history of a viral upper respiratory infection, fever, otalgia, and irritability. On examination a **red, bulging tympanic membrane**, which does not move with pneumatic otoscopy, is observed. The bony landmarks behind the tympanic membrane are obscured. Children frequently have mild conductive hearing loss. An erythematous tympanic membrane is not sufficient to establish the diagnosis because crying and viral upper respiratory tract infections can cause erythema of the membrane.

Because the causative agent is rarely known, once the diagnosis is established such **broad spectrum antibiotics** as amoxicillin (with or without clavulanate), trimethoprim-sulfamethoxazole, or erythromycin-sulfisoxazole are usually prescribed empirically. Recurrent acute otitis media, three new episodes within 6 months, can be managed with prophylactic antibiotics. Tympanostomy tubes should be reserved for children who fail to respond to antibiotic prophylaxis or those who have persistent effusion with documented hearing loss. Adenoidectomy and particularly tonsillectomy should be avoided if possible, especially in young children.

Complications of acute otitis media include otitis media with residual or persistent effusion, mastoiditis, and cholesteatoma. Residual or persistent effusions can cause conductive hearing loss. There is some concern that language delay may result, although the evidence is not strong. Treatment options include observation, antibiotics, or antibiotics plus corticosteroids.

Children with **mastoiditis** that may involve the periosteum and bone present with fever, tenderness, and swelling of the mastoid prominence, and with the pinna of the ear pushed outward. The diagnosis is confirmed by computerized tomography of the mastoid. Therapy includes parenteral antibiotics, tympanocentesis, and mastoidectomy.

A **cholesteatoma** is a white, greasy collection of desquamated epithelium and keratin within the middle ear and can invade the surrounding tissue. On otoscopic examination a cholesteatoma appears as a white mass. Surgical removal is required.

## External Otitis Media

External otitis media is due to infection of the **auditory canal**, usually following some predisposing factor such as excessive moisture ("swimmer's ear") or trauma. *Pseudomonas aeruginosa* is the most common bacterial etiology, although a variety of gram-negative or gram-positive bacteria, viruses, and fungi can cause external otitis. Children present with **ear pain exacerbated by pressure on the tragus**. On otoscopic examination, a green, purulent discharge may be seen in the external canal; visualization of the tympanic membrane may be difficult because of the extreme tenderness of the canal. Treatment is topical antibiotics and corticosteroids.

## Sinusitis

Sinusitis, inflammation of the sinuses, probably occurs with most cases of viral nasopharyngitis. Acute purulent sinusitis should be suspected in children with severe or prolonged viral upper respiratory tract infection. *S. pneumoniae*, nontypable *H. influenzae*, and *M. catarrhalis* are the common bacterial pathogens. In addition to fever and purulent nasal discharge, children with acute sinusitis may have headache, localized facial tenderness, and periorbital edema. The complications of acute sinusitis include orbital cellulitis and cavernous sinus thrombosis. On radiographic examination, opacification of the sinuses with air fluid levels is found. Computerized tomography may be useful in difficult cases. Treatment is with **antibiotics**, usually trimethoprim-sulfamethoxazole or amoxicillin plus clavulanate. Complicated sinusitis requires drainage.

# CONGENITAL ANOMALIES OF THE RESPIRATORY TRACT

**Laryngomalacia** and **tracheomalacia** are congenital defects of the airway walls that cause collapse of the upper airway on inspiration and stridor in neonates. In severe instances, feeding may be compromised. The conditions resolve as the child grows.

Congenital abnormalities of the lung are rare but include **congenital lobar emphysema**, in which an emphysematous and distended lobe obstructs normal lung; **cystic adenomatoid malformation**, in which a cystic lobe obstructs normal lung; and **pulmonary sequestration**, nonfunctioning cystic lung tissue that receives a systemic, rather than pulmonary, blood supply.

# INFECTIONS OF THE RESPIRATORY TRACT

Respiratory tract infections are among the most common causes of illness in children. Because **airway resistance** is inversely proportional to the fourth power of the radius of the airway, infections causing narrowing of the airways, due to edema and inflammation, commonly provoke more severe disease in young infants.

## Acute Nasopharyngitis

Acute nasopharyngitis, or the **common cold**, is due to viral infection of the nose and pharynx. Rhinoviruses and coronavirus are common etiologic agents. Much less commonly, group A streptococcus can cause acute nasopharyngitis. Most frequent in the first 2 years of life, children have an average of five to eight episodes yearly. Children in day care and nurseries are at increased risk. Otitis media, sinusitis, and cervical adenitis are frequent complications. Although over-the-counter cold remedies are widely available and frequently used, most children with acute nasopharyngitis do not require pharmacologic therapy. *Aspirin should not be used* because of its association with Reye's syndrome in children with influenza virus or varicella infection.

## Pharyngitis and Tonsillitis

Pharyngitis and tonsillitis are commonly due to viral infection of the pharynx and tonsils. Adenoviruses, coxsackieviruses, and Epstein-Barr virus (infectious mononucleosis) are among the viruses that can cause pharyngitis.

## Group A Beta-Hemolytic Streptococcus

**Group A beta-hemolytic streptococcus** causes a small but significant proportion of cases of **pharyngitis** in children older than the age of 2 years. Children with streptococcal pharyngitis frequently have headache, cervical adenopathy, abdominal pain, vomiting and high fever. However, clinical findings cannot be used to distinguish streptococcal pharyngitis from viral pharyngitis; the diagnosis must be based on culture or rapid antigen detection methods for streptococcus. Because the antigen detection test has a low sensitivity, those with a negative test should also have a throat culture to confirm the diagnosis.

Children with documented streptococcal pharyngitis should be treated with **penicillin**. Complications of streptococcal pharyngitis include peritonsillar abscess, retropharyngeal abscess, poststreptococcal glomerulonephritis, and rheumatic fever. Early treatment prevents rheumatic fever but does not prevent **poststreptococcal glomerulonephritis**.

## Retropharyngeal Abscess

Retropharyngeal abscess is a disease found only in young children because of the **presence of a lymph node chain** between the posterior pharyngeal wall and the prevertebral space, which regresses by the age of 4 years. The infection frequently follows pharyngitis and is caused by group A beta-hemolytic streptococci, oral anaerobes, and *Staphylococcus aureus*.

A child with a retropharyngeal abscess presents with high fever, refusal to swallow, drooling, and respiratory distress. The diagnosis may be made by inspection, palpation, and lateral radiograph of the neck. Complications include rupture, aspiration, and local extension.

## Infectious Croup

Infectious croup is a syndrome caused by upper airway obstruction due to infection of the larynx and trachea. The spectrum of the syndrome ranges from laryngotracheobronchitis, epiglottitis, diphtheria, and bacterial tracheitis. The clinical picture is characterized by dyspnea, hoarseness, a brassy cough, and stridor. Infants and young children develop more severe disease because of their narrow upper airway. Many of these infectious processes also involve the lower airways.

## Spasmodic Croup

Spasmodic croup occurs in young children between the ages of 1 and 3, usually at night, and resolves within several hours. Children with spasmodic croup will often develop these symptoms recurrently with mild viral upper respiratory illnesses.

## Laryngotracheobronchitis

Laryngotracheobronchitis, the most common cause of croup, is a viral infection of both upper and lower airways. The signs and symptoms of croup may coexist with signs of lower respiratory tract disease such as wheezing and rales. Rhinitis and conjunctivitis are often present as well. Parainfluenza virus is the most common etiologic agent. Anterior-posterior radiographs of the upper airway show the classic "steeple" sign, due to narrowing of the airway at the level of the vocal cords from edema and inflammation.

## Epiglottitis

Epiglottitis, an infection of the larynx and epiglottis due to *H. influenzae* type b, is a severe and life-threatening pediatric disease. Usually found in children between the ages of 2 and 7 years, epiglottitis presents with fever, general signs of toxicity, the acute onset of inspiratory stridor, hoarseness, drooling and respiratory distress. Older children may sit leaning forward drooling with their mouths open. Respiratory failure due to airway obstruction can develop rapidly.

The **pharynx** of a child with these symptoms *should not be examined* unless the examiner is prepared to intubate or perform a tracheostomy immediately; stimulation of the posterior pharynx may cause immediate laryngeal obstruction and respiratory arrest. The diagnosis can be made by lateral radiograph of the neck in which the swollen, enlarged epiglottis, resembling a thumb, can be visualized. Children suspected of having epiglottitis should be accompanied by a physician capable of intubating the child at all times.

The treatment of children with epiglottitis is **parenteral antibiotic therapy**. These children may require several days of nasotracheal intubation. The incidence of epiglottitis has decreased following widespread immunization against *H. influenzae* type b.

## Diphtheria

Diphtheria, which is caused by a toxin produced by *Corynebacterium diphtheriae*, is characterized by the formation of a grey-white membrane in the nasopharynx and palate, the result of tissue necrosis and an inflammatory reaction. Removal of the membrane causes bleeding and serosanguinous or purulent nasal discharge and cervical adenopathy may be present. Downward extension of the diphtheritic membrane to the larynx will cause the signs and symptoms of croup. Respiratory tract obstruction can be fatal. Myocarditis and heart block are serious common complications that occur in the second week of illness. Transient cranial nerve palsies can occur several weeks after the onset of infection. The diagnosis is based on the clinical picture and confirmed by culture on special media.

Treatment is with equine antitoxin and antibiotics, penicillin or erythromycin. *Diphtheria can be prevented by administration of diphtheria toxoid vaccine.*

## Pertussis

Pertussis, or whooping cough, is a highly contagious clinical syndrome caused by a variety of agents including *Bordetella pertussis*, other *Bordetella* species and adenovirus. Pertussis can be divided into catarrhal, paroxysmal, and convalescent stages. The catarrhal stage is marked by nonspecific upper respiratory tract symptoms, including nasal discharge and low grade fever. The characteristic paroxysmal stage follows, during which **repetitive coughs** are **followed by an inspiratory whoop**. These episodes may be associated with cyanosis and vomiting. Marked lymphocytosis is common. Secondary bacterial pneumonia and seizures may complicate this stage. The convalescent stage begins after 4 to 6 weeks, although a cough may persist for months.

A special Bordet-Gengou media is required to culture *Bordetella*. Rapid diagnostic tests are also available. Early treatment (within 2 weeks of onset) with erythromycin is useful, however, the disease is not often recognized during this time. Later treatment with erythromycin may reduce infectivity but does not change the course of the disease. Immunization is protective.

## Bronchiolitis

Bronchiolitis is a winter or early spring viral infection of infants and small children. It usually is caused by respiratory syncytial virus (RSV), but other viral etiologic agents such as parainfluenza virus and adenovirus can also cause the disease.

A child with this condition presents with a history of a viral upper respiratory infection followed by the onset of respiratory distress and wheezing. On examination tachypnea, tachycardia, nasal flaring, intercostal retractions, prolonged expirations, and wheezing are found. In severe cases, cyanosis and prostration may be present. RSV may cause **apnea** in young infants. Arterial blood gas analysis demonstrates both hypoxemia and relative hypercarbia in relation to the degree of tachypnea. Chest radiograph shows hyperinflation.

The **treatment** of bronchiolitis is largely **supportive**. In young infants, the disease may be so severe as to require mechanical ventilation for respiratory failure. Bronchodilators are frequently used, but their efficacy has not been conclusively demonstrated. Treatment with the antiviral agent ribavirin remains controversial; it may be indicated in some infants with underlying pulmonary, cardiac, and immunodeficiency diseases, or in infants with severe disease.

# Pneumonia

Pneumonia in infants and young children is commonly due to viral agents such as **respiratory syncytial virus (RSV)**, parainfluenza viruses, and adenovirus. Rhinorrhea, wheezing, radiographic evidence of hyperinflation, and a family member with a respiratory tract infection are often found in a child with viral pneumonia. However, viral pneumonia may be difficult to distinguish from bacterial pneumonia.

## Bacterial Pneumonia

Bacterial pneumonia, in children, often follows a viral respiratory tract infection, and is due to *S. pneumoniae* in over 90% of cases. Characteristic features of pneumococcal pneumonia include high fever, leukocytosis, and lobar consolidation; however, the classic features may not be present in infants and young children. Lower lobe pneumonia can mimic an acute abdomen. One third of cases of children with pneumococcal pneumonia have bacteremia.

### *Haemophilus Influenzae*

*H. influenzae* type b pneumonia has a clinical picture resembling that of pneumococcal pneumonia, although the onset is frequently less abrupt. Other sites of invasive disease can occur simultaneously, and children with *H. influenzae* type b pneumonia not infrequently have concurrent meningitis.

## Staphylococcal Pneumonia

Staphylococcal pneumonia is unusual, but is more common in infants than older children. Empyema and pneumatoceles are features typically associated with staphylococcal pneumonia.

### *Mycoplasma Pneumoniae*

*Mycoplasma pneumoniae*, a common cause of pneumonia in older children and adolescents, presents with cough, fever, malaise, sore throat, and headache. The symptoms may persist for several weeks. The presence of cold hemagglutinins supports the diagnosis. Treatment is with erythromycin in young children; tetracycline may be used in adolescents.

### *Chlamydia Trachomatis*

*Chlamydia trachomatis* can cause an afebrile pneumonitis in very young infants. Cough and eosinophilia are prominent features. Infants with a history of chlamydial conjunctivitis in the newborn period, not treated with systemic erythromycin, are at high risk. Erythromycin is the treatment of choice.

### Hydrocarbon Pneumonia

Hydrocarbon pneumonia results from ingestion and aspiration of volatile hydrocarbon liquids, such as kerosene, gasoline, and furniture polish. Induction of vomiting and gastric lavage after ingestion of hydrocarbons is usually contraindicated because of the risk of further aspiration. The onset of the symptoms of cough, vomiting, and fever may be delayed as long as 6 hours after exposure.

## ASTHMA

Asthma remains the most frequent cause of hospitalization for children. One third of patients with asthma develop symptoms in the first year of life; most have developed symptoms by school age. Despite advances in the understanding of its pathogenesis and treatment, the morbidity and mortality of asthma in children has increased over the past two decades.

Asthma results from **increased airway responsiveness and inflammation**. Both **genetic and environmental factors** predispose to asthma. Airway responsiveness in children is increased by allergens, respiratory tract infections, and air pollutants, including cigarette smoke. Infants with bronchiolitis are at increased risk of developing asthma. Attacks of asthma in children may also be precipitated by sinusitis, gastroesophageal reflux, and exercise. The important role of inflammation in the pathogenesis of asthma, including the evidence that inflammation increases airway responsiveness, has led to the early use of corticosteroids. By inducing receptor production, **corticosteroids** may also increase the effectiveness of beta-adrenergic agents used to promote bronchodilatation.

Children with asthma present with tachypnea, tachycardia, cough, wheezing, retractions, and respiratory distress. The condition is often worse at night. With a severe asthma attack, that is, **status asthmaticus**, air movement may be so reduced that wheezing is not audible; the wheezing becomes apparent only as the child improves.

The **diagnosis** of asthma is usually made by the clinical presentation, family history, and response to therapy. Rarely, pulmonary function testing with methacholine challenge, exercise testing, or bronchodilator therapy is warranted. Children with asthma frequently have eosinophilia in both the blood and sputum; IgE levels are often elevated. Chest radiographs of children with asthma typically show hyperinflation and patchy areas of atelectasis.

The **treatment** of asthma varies with the severity of disease, but the elimination or reduction of exposure to known allergens is important for all children. Mild chronic asthma is treated with intermittent **inhaled $\beta_2$-agonists**; oral β-agonists may be used in infants unable to tolerate inhalation therapy.

Children with moderate asthma are treated with **cromolyn sodium**, β-agonists, and inhaled corticosteroids. Children with severe asthma may require oral corticosteroids.

Theophylline, once widely used for the treatment of asthma in children, may be added to the regimen of beta-agonists and corticosteroids in children with moderate and severe asthma, but it is no longer recommended as first-line therapy. Seizures and arrhythmias can occur with theophylline toxicity.

*Children with status asthmaticus require hospitalization and aggressive therapy* with bronchodilators, corticosteroids, oxygen, and pulmonary toilet.

Some evidence suggests that the overuse of β-agonists may be partly responsible for the increase in asthma mortality; persistent use should be monitored carefully. Long-term use of corticosteroids can cause growth retardation, weight gain, adrenal suppression, cataracts, hypertension, and osteoporosis. **Inhaled steroids** and **alternate-day oral therapy** reduce the likelihood of these complications.

## CYSTIC FIBROSIS

Cystic fibrosis is an **inherited multisystem disease** characterized by chronic lung disease, exocrine gland dysfunction, and malabsorption due to an apical membrane ion transport defect. The gene for cystic fibrosis is located on the long arm of chromosome 7 and is transmitted as an autosomal recessive trait. The cystic fibrosis gene codes for a cell membrane protein called cystic fibrosis transmembrane regulator (CFTR). Many genetic defects involving this locus have been described.

Uncommon in black children, cystic fibrosis has a general prevalence of about 1/2500 children of European ancestry. The disease varies in its severity; about half of the children with the condition present during infancy.

The child with cystic fibrosis commonly has symptoms of failure to thrive; recurrent pulmonary infections with chronic cough; chronic sinusitis; bulky, greasy stools; clubbing of the digits; and occasionally rectal prolapse or nasal polyps. Infants may present with meconium ileus.

Pulmonary colonization with *S. aureus* and *P. aeruginosa* are common. Colonization with *Burkholderia cepacia* is associated with more rapid pulmonary deterioration. Malabsorption can lead to vitamin deficiencies, particularly of vitamins E, A, and K. Cirrhosis of the liver, diabetes mellitus, male infertility, and cor pulmonale develop in children with cystic fibrosis who survive to adolescence and adulthood.

The diagnosis of cystic fibrosis is frequently based on the presence of **elevated sweat chloride levels** (greater than 60 mEq/L) with evidence of chronic pulmonary disease, documented pancreatic insufficiency, or a family history of the disease. Several other conditions are associated with elevated sweat chloride levels, including adrenal insufficiency and hypothyroidism.

The management of cystic fibrosis involves the use of **oral pancreatic enzymes** to enhance gastrointestinal absorption, supplemental water soluble vitamins, antibiotic therapy for pulmonary infections, chest physical therapy to promote postural drainage of respiratory secretions, genetic counseling, and support of the child and family in coping with this chronic disease. Many children with cystic fibrosis die during adolescence or early adulthood; the median duration of survival is increasing and now is approximately 30 years of age.

## KARTAGENER SYNDROME

**Kartagener syndrome**, also called primary ciliary dyskinesis, refers to a group of genetically heterogenous disorders of ciliary motility. Clinical manifestations, which reflect the ciliary dyskinesis, include chronic otitis media, sinusitis, bronchitis, and male infertility. Because of the role cilia play in embryogenesis, situs inversus is commonly present. Diagnosis is made by electron microscopy of affected cilia. Viral respiratory tract infections can also induce ciliary dyskinesis.

## ALPHA-1-ANTITRYPSIN DEFICIENCY

Alpha-1-antitrypsin deficiency is an antiprotease deficiency that results in the **early onset of emphysema**. Proteolytic enzymes, which are released by bacteria and leukocytes, cannot be degraded and destroy normal lung tissue. Some children develop neonatal cholestasis and childhood cirrhosis. Enzyme replacement therapy is available.

# SUDDEN INFANT DEATH SYNDROME

Sudden infant death syndrome (SIDS) refers to the sudden and unexpected death of an apparently healthy infant, usually at 2 to 3 months of age. Even autopsy fails to discover a cause of death. In the United States, the incidence of SIDS is approximately 1 to 2 per 1000 live births. Increased rates occur in boys, families living in poverty, families with a previous child who died of SIDS, and during the winter season. The association of SIDS with the prone sleeping position has led to recommendations that all infants be placed in the supine position.

SIDS probably represents a spectrum of disorders, and the diagnosis must be made by exclusion. No single pathologic or etiologic agent has been consistently associated, but considerable research on SIDS has focused on abnormal cardiorespiratory function, perhaps secondary to altered central nervous system control. Some children diagnosed as having SIDS probably have undetected inborn errors of metabolism, congenital arrhythmias (prolonged Q-T interval), other congenital anomalies, or are victims of child abuse.

Infants who appear to have suffered apnea or a cardiorespiratory arrest, and who recover or are resuscitated, are said to have an "apparent life-threatening event" (ALTE). Although of great concern to parents and physicians, it is unclear whether these infants are at high risk of SIDS. Because of the paucity of data demonstrating a relationship between ALTE and SIDS, home apnea monitoring is highly problematic.

# Chapter 9

# Genetic Disorders

## CHROMOSOMAL ABNORMALITIES

### Trisomy 21

Trisomy 21 (Down syndrome) occurs in approximately 1 in 800 live births. Most likely, half of all fetuses with trisomy 21 are spontaneously aborted early in pregnancy. As with other trisomies, **maternal nondisjunction during meiosis** with the resulting trisomy 21 in the fetus is associated with advanced maternal age. However, trisomy 21 can occur in younger women because of translocation or paternal nondisjunction. For the small percentage of women (less than 5%) whose children have translocation trisomy 21, the risk of recurrence in succeeding pregnancies is high.

Children with trisomy 21 have typical facies with prominent epicanthal folds, speckled irides (Brushfield spots), prominent tongue, and a small head with flattened occiput. Their extremities are characterized by poor muscle tone, short stubby feet with a widened space between the first and second toes, and short stubby hands with an incurred fifth finger and a palmar crease (a single line that extends across the breadth of the palm). Most exhibit growth and developmental retardation.

#### Congenital Heart Disease

Congenital heart disease occurs in approximately half of all cases of children with trisomy 21. The most common cardiac abnormalities are **endocardial cushion defects** and **ventricular septal defects**. Defects range from mild to severe, with the most severe being complete atrioventricular canal with a large defect of the atrioventricular septum and a single atrioventricular valve. Endocardial cushion defects are characterized by a superior axis on electrocardiogram. Children with trisomy 21 develop pulmonary vascular obstructive disease more rapidly than other children with septal defects, sometimes as early as 6 months of age. Duodenal atresia and imperforate anus are also associated with trisomy 21, and acute lymphocytic leukemia is more prevalent.

### Trisomy 18

Trisomy 18 occurs in approximately 1 in 8000 live births. Most infants with trisomy 18 are born small for gestational age, with the characteristic findings of fine facial features, low set ears, prominent occiput, unusual flexion deformity of the fingers, and rockerbottom feet. Other abnormalities include congenital heart disease (ventricular septal defects and patent ductus arteriosus), hernias, and mental retardation. Most children with trisomy 18 die in early infancy.

### Trisomy 13

Trisomy 13, which occurs in approximately 1 in 20,000 births, is characterized by microcephaly, mental retardation, failure to thrive, cleft lip, ocular defects, congenital heart disease, and polydactyly. As with trisomy 18, most children with trisomy 13 die in early infancy.

### Turner Syndrome

Turner syndrome occurs in approximately 1 in 3000 live births, but the vast majority end in spontaneous abortion. Turner syndrome can result from a number of different chromosomal abnormalities. Simple deletion of the short arm of the X chromosome results in the Turner syndrome phenotype. However, the most common chromosomal abnormality is a **single X chromosome** (45,X karyotype).

Girls with Turner syndrome present with short stature, webbed neck, low posterior hairline, broad chest, gonadal dysgenesis ("streak" gonads consisting of connective tissue), absent pubertal development, and primary amenorrhea. Newborns with Turner syndrome have edema of the dorsa of the hands and feet and excess skin on the neck. Congenital heart disease is common, including bicuspid aortic valve, aortic stenosis, and coarctation. Renal and urinary tract anomalies are also common, as is recurrent otitis media and hearing loss. Less severe phenotypic changes are found in girls with mosaicism, particularly 45,X/46,XX karyotype, which comprises approximately one quarter of cases of all girls with Turner syndrome.

The diagnosis of Turner syndrome and Turner mosaicism should be considered in **girls** with **short stature and primary amenorrhea**. The diagnosis is made by chromosomal analysis. Buccal smear determination of sex chromatin (Barr body) should *not* be used to establish the diagnosis of Turner syndrome. Therapy with growth hormone can improve final adult height, and estrogen replacement therapy can induce puberty.

### Noonan Syndrome

Noonan syndrome describes boys and girls with the clinical features of Turner syndrome but with a normal karyotype. In contrast to

Turner syndrome, mental retardation is common; pulmonary valve stenosis is the typical cardiac lesion.

## Mixed Gonadal Dysgenesis

Children with mixed gonadal dysgenesis, associated with 45,X/46,XY karyotype, may resemble girls with Turner syndrome. However, affected infants more commonly have ambiguous genitalia, and may even have phenotypic male genitalia. Affected children have short stature and are at risk of gonadal tumors (gonadoblastomas).

## Klinefelter Syndrome

Klinefelter syndrome, 47,XXY karyotype, occurs in approximately 1 in 1000 live male births. As with autosomal trisomies, Klinefelter syndrome results from **nondisjunction during meiosis** (two-thirds maternal); an increased risk occurs with advanced maternal age. Although behavioral, cognitive (mental retardation), and psychiatric symptoms may occur in early childhood, the diagnosis usually is not made until delayed puberty is recognized. Gynecomastia, small penis and testicular size, and infertility are common. More severe Klinefelter phenotypes occur with more than two X chromosomes (for example 48,XXXY karyotype). Testosterone replacement therapy can induce virilization.

## Other Sex Chromosome Abnormalities

Numerous other disorders of sex chromosomes have been identified. Boys with the **47,XYY karyotype,** occurring in 1 in 1000 newborn males, tend to be tall but have few other characteristic physical findings. Some may have attention deficit disorder and antisocial behavior. The **47,XXX karyotype**, occurring in 1 in 1000 newborn females, may also be associated with tall stature and behavioral and learning problems.

**Fragile X syndrome**, due to an expansion of nucleotide triplet repeats, refers to a propensity for chromosomal breaks on the long arm of the X chromosome and is a common cause of **mental retardation in boys**. Males with this syndrome also have large testicles. Heterozygotic females may also be mentally retarded.

## Chromosomal Deletions

**Cri du chat syndrome**, caused by a deletion of the short arm of **chromosome 5 (5p-),** is so named because affected young infants have cries that resemble that of a kitten. Mental retardation, microcephaly, hypertelorism, and low-set ears are common findings.

Deletion of the short arm of **chromosome 11 (11p-)** is associated with aniridia and Wilms' tumor. Deletion of the long arm of **chromosome 13 (13q-)** is associated with retinoblastoma.

## Single and Multifactorial Genetic Defects

**Single gene defects** are inherited as autosomal dominant, autosomal recessive, X-linked recessive, or X-linked dominant disorders. Many such defects, particularly autosomal dominant disorders, arise by spontaneous mutation; thus, the typical Mendelian family history may not be obtained.

**Multifactorial genetic defects** involve multiple genes in the context of environmental stimuli. They are responsible for many diseases of children, including cleft lip and asthma. The mode of inheritance for multifactorial genetic disorders is complex and variable.

An unusual type of single gene defect is found in several hereditary neurodegenerative diseases including Huntington's disease, myotonic dystrophy, spinal muscular atrophy, and Friedreich's ataxia, as well as fragile X syndrome, and involves trinucleotide repeats. In each case, the susceptibility gene contains repeated sequences of trinucleotides (CAG, coding for the amino acid glutamine, in Huntington's disease and spinal muscular atrophy). An increasing number of repeats in subsequent generations results in earlier age of onset and more severe symptoms (genetic anticipation).

## Mitochondrial Encephalomyelopathies

Mitochondrial encephalomyelopathies are due to genetic defects in mitochondrial DNA. The mode of inheritance of mitochondrial genetic disorders differs from Mendelian inheritance. Because mitochondrial DNA is passed from the mother to infant through the oocyte, affected fathers cannot transmit the trait but affected mothers can transmit to all children.

# Chapter 10

# Metabolic and Endocrine Disorders

## INBORN ERRORS OF METABOLISM

Inborn errors of metabolism describe a group of single gene defects that result in an alteration or interference with normal biochemical pathways. Hundreds of these relatively rare conditions have been described. Most of these disorders present during the neonatal period or early childhood; however, many affected infants appear normal at birth. These diseases, if not detected and treated promptly, can result in serious permanent damage, especially to the central nervous system (CNS). Suspicion should be raised by parental consanguinity and a family history of infant deaths.

Common signs and symptoms of inborn errors of metabolism include failure to thrive, developmental delay, lethargy, poor feeding, persistent vomiting, hepatomegaly, and seizures. Common laboratory findings include hypoglycemia, metabolic acidosis, hyperammonemia, and ketonuria.

Microtechniques using capillary blood have been devised that permit screening of newborns for the presence of many of these metabolic disorders. Most states in America require routine metabolic screening of newborns. All states require routine neonatal screening for phenylketonuria (PKU) and hypothyroidism. In addition, screening for other metabolic disorders such as galactosemia, maple syrup urine disease, and homocystinuria are required in many states.

The clinician faced with a child suspected of an inborn error of metabolism should begin with measurements of serum electrolytes, glucose, acid-base status, ammonia, and urinary ketones. Measurement of blood and urine amino acids and urine organic acids should also be considered. Measurement of specific metabolites is required to confirm the diagnosis.

# DISORDERS OF AMINO ACID METABOLISM

### Phenylketonuria

Phenylketonuria (**PKU**) is an inborn error of metabolism in which the enzyme phenylalanine hydroxylase, required to metabolize the essential amino acid phenylalanine, is absent. The disease is inherited as an autosomal recessive trait with an incidence of about 1 in 10,000. Somewhat less common in African Americans and more common in Ashkenazi Jews, PKU is a condition that can be detected by newborn screening, but the screening test should not performed until the infant has been fed several milk feedings containing phenylalanine.

Children with PKU **appear normal at birth**, but gradually develop fair skin, light hair, eczematoid or seborrheic dermatitis, growth retardation, and seizures. Persistent vomiting may occur. The mousy or misty odor of phenylacetic acid can often be detected. Because the disease, if untreated, results in severe mental retardation, any delay in the diagnosis and treatment will worsen the degree of mental retardation.

Treatment consists of **dietary manipulation** in which phenylalanine is reduced in the diet. Dietary reduction should be continued until the child is at least 6 years of age and often longer.

Pregnant women with PKU should be maintained on a low phenylalanine diet to prevent spontaneous abortion, microcephaly, mental retardation, and congenital heart disease in their children.

### Tyrosinemia Type I

Tyrosinemia type I, an autosomal recessive disorder, is due to an enzyme deficiency that results in moderate elevation of serum tyrosine and accumulation of toxic intermediate metabolites. Infants with the acute form of this disease will present with failure to thrive, developmental delay, vomiting, hepatomegaly, jaundice, hypoglycemia, and bleeding secondary to severe liver disease.

Older children with the chronic form of tyrosinemia develop cirrhosis, renal tubular dysfunction (Fanconi syndrome), and vitamin D-resistant rickets.

Dietary therapy may be partially effective; however, liver transplantation may be the only effective form of treatment.

### Homocystinuria

Homocystinuria is an autosomal recessive disorder in which homocysteine, an intermediate metabolite of methionine, accumulates due to a deficiency of the enzyme cystathionine synthase. Affected infants develop failure to thrive and developmental delay. Findings in early childhood include subluxation of the lens and skeletal abnormalities resembling Marfan syndrome. Seizures, mental retardation, psychiatric disorders, and thromboembolisms also occur.

Treatment consists of **dietary restriction of methionine**, supplemental cysteine, and high doses of vitamin B6.

## Maple Syrup Urine Disease

Maple syrup urine disease (**MSUD**) is an autosomal recessive disorder which is caused by a deficiency of the enzyme system involved in the metabolism of the branched-chain amino acids (valine, leucine, and isoleucine). Infants with this disorder rapidly develop poor feeding, lethargy, vomiting, opisthotonos, seizures, and coma. The urine, sweat and cerumen have the distinctive odor of maple syrup. Rapid removal of the toxic amino acids can be achieved by peritoneal dialysis. Subsequent therapy, which should be instituted before 2 weeks of age, involves a diet low in branched-chain amino acids.

## Urea Cycle Defects

Urea cycle defects, which are caused by deficiencies of the five enzymes of the urea cycle, have a prevalence of 1 in 30,000 live births. **Ornithine transcarbamylase (OTC) deficiency,** the most common urea cycle disorder, is an X-linked dominant disorder. Female carriers of OTC deficiency may also have symptoms, depending on the pattern of X-chromosome inactivation. Infants with the disorder present with poor feeding, vomiting, hepatomegaly, lethargy, coma, and seizures. Older children manifest CNS dysfunction of confusion, lethargy, altered behavior, and ataxia. An elevated plasma ammonia level is diagnostic, but hyperammonemia may be found in other inborn errors of metabolism, particularly the **organic acidemias** and **transient hyperammonemia of the newborn.**

# PEROXISOMAL DISORDER

## X-Linked Adrenoleukodystrophy

X-linked adrenoleukodystrophy (ALD) is characterized by the accumulation of very long chain fatty acids due to a degradation defect. ALD causes adrenal dysfunction. CNS involvement occurs in approximately two thirds of affected patients and does not correlate with the biochemical defect. Several forms of this disorder have been described.

The **childhood cerebral form**, which occurs between 4 to 8 years of age, is characterized by hyperactivity, poor school performance, vision and hearing problems, and seizures. Adrenal dysfunction is a less prominent presenting feature, but most children with the disorder will have elevated levels of ACTH; adrenal insufficiency develops later. Computerized tomography (CT) of the brain shows characteristic lesions in the periventricular white matter. These children undergo rapid deterioration in their neurologic status.

# SPHINGOLIPIDOSES

### Tay-Sachs Disease

Tay-Sachs disease, most frequent in children of Ashkenazi Jewish descent, is due to a **deficiency of β-hexosaminidase A**. The disorder affects the CNS; organomegaly is not present. Clinical manifestations that appear during the first year of life include severe hypotonia, blindness, and an exaggerated response to noise. A cherry-red spot can be seen on the macula, a feature also found in Sandhoff disease and Niemann-Pick disease.

### Niemann-Pick Disease

Niemann-Pick disease presents in infants with hepatomegaly and developmental delay. Mental retardation, hypotonia, and vision and hearing problems follow.

### Gaucher Disease

Children with Gaucher disease usually present with splenomegaly due to accumulation of glucocerebroside in the reticuloendothelial system. The accumulation of glucocerebroside in the bone marrow leads to anemia, leukopenia, and thrombocytopenia. Early CNS involvement occurs in infantile Gaucher disease.

### Fabry Disease

Fabry disease, an X-linked recessive disorder, begins in adolescent males with painful crises of the limbs due to accumulation of sphingolipids. Involvement of the skin, cornea, heart, and kidneys develops later.

## Krabbe Disease

Krabbe disease is a progressive degenerative disorder of the white matter in the brain.

## DISORDERS OF CARBOHYDRATE METABOLISM

### Galactosemia

Classic galactosemia, an autosomal recessive inborn error of carbohydrate metabolism, results from a deficiency of the enzyme galactose-1-phosphate uridyltransferase. The absence of this enzyme causes a gradual and toxic accumulation of galactose in all body tissues.

Infants with galactosemia appear normal at birth and only develop symptoms when fed milk that contains galactose (lactose consists of glucose and galactose). Although the onset of symptoms is variable, typically infants present with failure to thrive, vomiting, jaundice, hepatosplenomegaly, hypoglycemia, seizures, and cataracts. Infants with galactosemia are at increased risk of gram-negative sepsis, which may be the presenting clinical picture. Children with untreated galactosemia develop cirrhosis and severe mental retardation.

The disease, which should be considered in any infant with these symptoms, can be diagnosed tentatively by the demonstration of a reducing substance in the urine using the Clinitest technique. The definitive diagnosis is with chromatography or enzyme assay.

The treatment of galactosemia involves the **removal of galactose from the diet**. Lactose-free soy-based formulas are used to replace galactose containing milk-based formulas.

### Hereditary Fructose Intolerance

Hereditary fructose intolerance, an autosomal recessive enzyme deficiency, becomes apparent in infants after they have been exposed to fructose containing food. Signs and symptoms that resemble those of galactosemia include vomiting, hepatomegaly, jaundice, lethargy, and seizures. A reducing substance is also present in the urine when using the Clinitest technique. Elimination of fructose from the diet is required.

# GLYCOGEN STORAGE DISEASES

The glycogen storage diseases are inborn errors of metabolism that cause an abnormal accumulation or structure of glycogen. Numerous enzyme defects have been described and may involve the liver, skeletal muscle, heart, brain, kidneys, intestines, or erythrocytes. The specific organ involvement determines the clinical manifestations of each enzyme defect.

## Glycogen Storage Disease Type Ia

Glycogen storage disease type Ia (**von Gierke disease**) is a deficiency of glucose-6-phosphatase. Affected children have growth failure, hepatomegaly, enlarged kidneys, hypoglycemia, acidosis, and hyperlipidemia.

## Glycogen Storage Disease Type II

Glycogen storage disease type II (**Pompe disease**) is characterized by accumulation of glycogen in all organs, including the heart and skeletal muscle. Affected infants develop severe cardiomyopathy and hypotonia. The classic form of this disease is ultimately fatal, usually within the first 2 years of life.

## Glycogen Storage Disease Type V

Glycogen storage disease type V (**McArdle syndrome**) affects skeletal muscle. Children with this disorder develop severe muscle pains and cramps after exercise.

## Glycogen Storage Disease Type VI

In glycogen storage disease type VI, children develop massive hepatomegaly but are otherwise well.

# MUCOPOLYSACCHARIDOSES

The mucopolysaccharidoses are inborn errors of metabolism due to defects in the metabolism and storage of mucopolysaccharides. The accumulation in specific organs determines the clinical manifestations of the various enzyme defects. Involvement of bones, joints, CNS, heart, liver, spleen, and skin are common.

## Hurler Syndrome

Hurler syndrome (MPS IH) is an enzymatic defect that results in accumulation of mucopolysaccharides in almost all tissues. It is the most severe of these disorders. Affected children develop characteristic, coarse facial features, corneal opacities, hepatosplenomegaly, kyphosis, contractures, and mental retardation. The characteristic radiographic findings include a thick skull, beaked vertebral bodies, and changes in the wrists and hands.

## Scheie Syndrome

Scheie syndrome (MPS IS) is the mildest of the mucopolysaccharidoses and is characterized by corneal opacities, joint contractures, and aortic regurgitation.

## Hunter Syndrome

Hunter syndrome (MPS II) is an X-linked disorder that resembles Hurler syndrome in its clinical manifestations. Affected boys have short stature, coarse facial features, joint stiffness, hepatosplenomegaly, hernias, and mental retardation.

## Sanfilippo Syndrome

Children with Sanfilippo syndrome (MPS III) also have hepatosplenomegaly, joint involvement, mental retardation, and radiographic changes. The disease, however, becomes rapidly progressive in later childhood.

## Morquio Syndrome

Morquio syndrome (MPS IV) does not involve the CNS, but it results in short stature, skeletal changes, corneal opacities, dental abnormalities, and hepatosplenomegaly.

## Maroteaux-Lamy Syndrome

Maroteaux-Lamy syndrome (MPS VI) resembles Hurler syndrome, but children with this syndrome do not develop mental retardation.

### Lesch-Nyhan Syndrome

Lesch-Nyhan syndrome is an X-linked disorder caused by a deficient enzyme in the purine salvage pathway. Affected boys have developmental delays, choreoathetosis, self-destructive behavior (notably biting of the fingers and lips), and elevated serum uric acid levels.

### Orotic Aciduria

Children with orotic aciduria have a defect in the metabolism of orotic acid, which is a metabolite of pyrimidine synthesis. These children develop mental retardation, growth failure, and megaloblastic anemia.

## THYROID DISORDERS

### Congenital Hypothyroidism

Congenital hypothyroidism has an incidence of 1 in 4000 live births; females are more commonly affected than males. Most children with congenital hypothyroidism have congenital structural lesions of the thyroid, either thyroid aplasia or ectopic (lingual) thyroid. Congenital hypothyroidism may also be caused by congenital pituitary lesions, defective synthesis of thyroxine, thyrotropin (thyroid stimulating hormone [TSH]), or thyroxine unresponsiveness and maternal intake of radioiodine during pregnancy.

Although infants with congenital hypothyroidism may be asymptomatic at birth, the disease presents classically with a history of prolonged neonatal jaundice, feeding problems, constipation, and mottling of the extremities. On physical examination, a child with congenital hypothyroidism will have growth failure with the height more seriously affected than weight, developmental delay, general hypotonia, coarse facial features, widely open fontanelles, flattened nasal bridge, protruding tongue, hoarse cry, myxedema, and an umbilical hernia.

The diagnosis is established by measurement of **low levels of T4 and T3** and **elevated levels of TSH**. Newborn screening programs in the United States measure T4 levels with subsequent measurement of TSH when low T4 levels are discovered.

If untreated, these children will become mentally retarded, but early diagnosis and **replacement therapy with thyroid hormone** (L-thyroxine) can do much to prevent the mental retardation and growth failure.

## Lymphocytic (Hashimoto) Thyroiditis

Lymphocytic thyroiditis, or Hashimoto thyroiditis, is the most common cause of hypothyroidism and of a thyroid goiter in children and adolescents. This autoimmune condition is caused by lymphocytic infiltration of the thyroid and the development of antithyroid antibodies. Adolescent girls, who are most commonly affected, present with a **goiter** and the signs and symptoms of hypothyroidism. However, many children with this disease are **euthyroid**. Thyroid replacement hormone is indicated for those children with lymphocytic thyroiditis who have documented hypothyroidism. The condition may spontaneously remit.

## Hyperthyroidism

Hyperthyroidism in children is caused by increased excretion of thyroid hormone due to a diffuse **toxic goiter** (Graves' disease). **Graves' disease** is also an autoimmune condition characterized by infiltration of the thyroid and retro-orbital tissues with lymphocytes and the production of antithyroid antibodies. One type of antibody mimics TSH by binding and activating the TSH receptor, causing a release of thyroid hormone. Although the disease can present at any time during childhood, it usually presents during adolescence and is much more common in girls than in boys.

Children with hyperthyroidism initially present with symptoms of emotional lability, hyperactivity, and a decline in school performance. Weight loss in spite of an increasing appetite is also common. On physical examination tachycardia, fine tremors of the hands, smooth skin, lid lag of the eyes, exophthalmos, lymphadenopathy, and splenomegaly are characteristic. Thyroid enlargement may be present. On laboratory investigation, serum levels of thyroxine (**T4**), triiodothyronine (**T3**), **free T4**, and **free T3 are elevated**. **TSH** levels are **depressed**. Antimicrosomal antibodies can frequently be documented.

Medical therapy for hyperthyroidism involves the use of either of two antithyroid drugs, **propylthiouracil or methimazole**, which block the incorporation of iodide into organic compounds. Propranolol, a β-adrenergic blocker, can be used to manage severe symptoms. For children, medical therapy is preferred to subtotal thyroidectomy, another therapeutic option.

## Hypoparathyroidism

Hypoparathyroidism may occur on an autoimmune or familial basis. **DiGeorge anomaly**, which is caused by developmental defects of the third and fourth pharyngeal pouches, results in aplasia or hypoplasia of the thymus and parathyroid glands and congenital heart disease (coarctation of the aorta and truncus arteriosus).

Children with hypoparathyroidism present with the signs and symptoms of **hypocalcemia**: muscle cramps, tingling of the hands and feet, carpopedal spasms, and seizures. Laboratory evaluation reveals a low serum calcium and phosphorus level. Functional immaturity of the parathyroid glands may be a contributing factor to the hypocalcemia commonly found in premature infants, infants of diabetic mothers, and infants with birth asphyxia.

# ADRENAL DISORDERS

## Adrenocortical Insufficiency

Adrenocortical insufficiency may result from a variety of lesions of the hypothalamus, pituitary gland, or adrenal glands. In infants, the salt-losing form of **congenital adrenal hyperplasia** is the most common cause of adrenocortical insufficiency. **Addison disease** can occur in older children as the result of autoimmune destruction of the adrenals. **Waterhouse-Friderichsen syndrome** is characterized by adrenal hemorrhage during meningococcemia. Children treated with **high doses of corticosteroid** may develop adrenocortical insufficiency, particularly when stressed by infections or surgery. **Adrenal crisis**, heralded by tachypnea, tachycardia, and hypotension, can be fatal if not immediately recognized and treated.

## Congenital Adrenal Hyperplasia

Congenital adrenal hyperplasia, an inborn error of metabolism in the biosynthesis of adrenal corticosteroid, is inherited as an autosomal recessive trait. Although five different enzymatic defects in the synthesis of adrenal corticosteroid have been described, 95% of the cases are caused by a **deficiency in 21-hydroxylase**. The second most frequent cause of the disease, caused by a **deficiency in 11-β hydroxylase**, is especially common in children of North African Jewish ancestry. The 11-β hydroxylase deficiency does not result in salt wasting.

In all forms of the disease, the deficiency in cortisol production causes an **increased secretion of ACTH**, which leads to adrenal hyperplasia and excess production of intermediary metabolites of cortisol.

About three fourths of cases of children with the 21-hydroxylase defect will present with metabolic symptoms of adrenal insufficiency. These "**salt losers**" present within the first few weeks to months of life with failure to thrive, arrhythmias, vomiting, and dehydration, leading to vascular collapse and death. Measurements of serum electrolytes show levels of a low serum sodium and chloride with high serum potassium and blood urea nitrogen. Cortisol levels are low, and levels of the intermediary metabolite 17-hydroxyprogesterone are elevated; the latter is converted to testosterone. Virilization of the genitalia, which will occur in girls, is a clue to the diagnosis. In male infants, however, the genitalia appear normal. Treatment consists of replacement therapy with glucocorticoids and mineralocorticoids.

In **boys**, the **simple virilizing form of 21-hydroxylase deficiency** presents as premature isosexual precocity, usually within the first 6 months of life. Enlargement of the penis, scrotum, and prostate, deepening of the voice, and the appearance of pubic hair in young boys are all clinical signs of the virilization typical of the disease. Bone age is advanced for chronologic age, and the premature closure of the epiphyses results in short stature as adults.

In **girls**, congenital adrenal hyperplasia causes **pseudohermaphroditism**, which is evident at birth. The degree of virilization may vary from mild clitoral hypertrophy and labial fusion to true ambiguous genitalia. All newborns with **ambiguous genitalia** must be carefully investigated immediately to ensure that the appropriate sex is assigned and that therapy is instituted promptly.

## Cushing Syndrome

Cushing syndrome in infants and children is usually due to **adrenocortical tumors** (adenomas or carcinomas), adrenal hyperplasia secondary to pituitary adenomas, or as a result of an autoimmune disease with immunoglobulins activating the ACTH receptor. Chronic administration of corticosteroids can result in a similar clinical picture.

Children with Cushing syndrome are short and obese with a round, flushed face, and a buffalo hump. Signs of virilization, striae and osteoporosis may be present. Hypertension is common. Treatment depends upon the etiology.

# DISORDERS OF THE PITUITARY GLAND

## Hypopituitarism

Hypopituitarism in children can result from cranial defects (anencephaly), **septo-optic dysplasia** (optic nerve hypoplasia and absence of the septum pellucidum), **craniopharyngiomas**, Langerhans' cell histiocytosis, trauma, and cranial radiotherapy. In many children, no etiology can be demonstrated.

Hypopituitarism results in thyroid, adrenal and gonadal dysfunction. **Growth retardation** is a common feature because of growth hormone deficiency. Therapy with recombinant growth hormone restores growth in children with growth hormone deficiency.

Trials of growth hormone therapy have been undertaken in children with other causes of short stature, including those with Turner syndrome and chronic renal failure. Children who received cadaver pituitary extracts, prior to the development of recombinant growth hormone, are at risk for **Creutzfeldt-Jacob disease**, a neurodegenerative disorder.

## Diabetes Insipidus

Diabetes insipidus, which results from deficiency of antidiuretic hormone (arginine vasopressin), presents with symptoms of polyuria and polydipsia. The etiologies of diabetes insipidus are similar to those of hypopituitarism (craniopharyngiomas, Langerhans' cell histiocytosis, and trauma); autoimmune, hereditary, and idiopathic forms also exist. Affected children have excessive urinary output and a low urine specific gravity, which rises to a maximum of 1.010 with water deprivation. Vasopressin levels are low.

Several conditions can mimic diabetes insipidus, including hypercalcemia, potassium deficiency, chronic renal disease, and nephrogenic diabetes insipidus. Treatment consists of intranasal administration of desmopressin (DDAVP).

## Syndrome of Inappropriate Antidiuretic Hormone

Inappropriate secretion of antidiuretic hormone, or **SIADH**, is a syndrome that is often asymptomatic and characterized by low serum sodium levels. Neurologic symptoms of increasing severity occur with worsening hyponatremia. The syndrome is associated with numerous underlying conditions including meningitis, encephalitis, brain tumors, head trauma, pneumonia, and tuberculosis. The diagnosis is confirmed by the demonstration of a less than maximally dilute urine in the face of low serum osmolality. The therapy involves fluid restriction and treatment of the underlying disorder.

# DISORDERS OF PUBERTY

## Precocious Puberty

Precocious puberty may be true precocious puberty, which is always isosexual and gonadotropin-dependent, or precocious pseudopuberty, which can be either isosexual or heterosexual, and is independent of gonadotropin function.

## True Precocious Puberty

True precocious puberty can be due to lesions of the CNS (tumors, meningitis, trauma, hydrocephalus), therapy for other endocrine diseases, or idiopathic. Idiopathic true precocious puberty is more common in girls and begins with breast development followed by pubic hair. Growth is accelerated, and premature closure of the epiphyses results in eventual short stature. Treatment involves the administration of a luteinizing hormone releasing hormone (LHRH) analog to suppress gonadotropin release.

**McCune-Albright syndrome** is more common in girls and is characterized by precocious puberty, abnormal pigmentation of the skin, fibrous dysplasia of the bones and pituitary, thyroid, and adrenal dysfunction. Affected children are prone to repeated fractures and skeletal deformities.

## Precocious Pseudopuberty

Precocious pseudopuberty can be caused by congenital adrenal hyperplasia and other adrenal disorders and by gonadal tumors (ovarian, testicular).

## Testicular Feminization Syndrome

Testicular feminization syndrome is an X-linked recessive disorder of the androgen receptor in which genetic males have the phenotype of a female with a vaginal pouch and no uterus. The testes are intraabdominal or located within the inguinal canal; in fact, the condition is frequently diagnosed when **testes are found in a girl with an inguinal hernia**, as occurs in 1% to 2% of cases. The testes should be removed because of a high risk of the development of malignant seminomas. Adolescents present with primary amenorrhea. Children with testicular feminization syndrome should be raised as girls.

## Breast Masses

Breast masses can occur in infants and adolescents. Newborn infants may develop neonatal breast hypertrophy as a consequence of maternal estrogens. The condition resolves spontaneously. Newborns may also develop breast abscesses. Causes of breast masses in adolescent girls include fibrocystic disease, which varies in size throughout the menstrual cycle, and fibroadenomas, which require resection. Obese adolescent boys are prone to develop gynecomastia.

# DISORDERS OF THE PANCREAS

## Insulin-Dependent Diabetes Mellitus and Diabetic Ketoacidosis

Insulin-dependent diabetes mellitus (**IDDM**, or **type I diabetes**) is a familial, chronic disorder of carbohydrate, protein, and fat metabolism, and it results from an absolute deficiency of endogenous insulin. The metabolic derangements are exacerbated by secretion of the counter-regulatory hormones glucagon, epinephrine, growth hormone, and cortisol.

The most common metabolic or endocrine disorder of children, insulin-dependent diabetes mellitus has a prevalence of 1.9/1000 in school age children. There is strong evidence that IDDM is the result of autoimmune **destruction of pancreatic islet cells**, perhaps triggered by a viral infection in persons with a genetic predisposition, particularly those with certain HLA types. The autoimmune basis is suggested by the presence of anti-islet cell antibodies, lymphocytic infiltration of the pancreas, and association with other autoimmune, endocrine diseases (lymphocytic thyroiditis, Addison disease).

The disease usually presents in the **early school years** or during **adolescence**. Classically, children with diabetes mellitus present with rapid weight loss, fatigue, polyuria, polydipsia, and polyphagia. However, the disease may first manifest with the abrupt onset of diabetic ketoacidosis, triggered by an infection or trauma. The classic laboratory findings of IDDM are **hyperglycemia and glucosuria**.

The **treatment** of diabetes mellitus in children includes the twice daily administration of **insulin**, usually a combination of rapid and intermediate-acting preparations, glucose monitoring, dietary management, and exercise. Continuous monitoring is critical and involves periodic measurement of blood glucose levels and glucosuria. Long-term glycemic control can be monitored by measurement of **glycosylated hemoglobin**, which reflects the average blood glucose concentration for the preceding 2 to 3 months. Social support and health education for the child and parents are equally important in the management of this chronic disease.

Because episodes of hypoglycemia are not infrequent, the child and parents should be taught to recognize the signs and symptoms of hypoglycemia. Most episodes can be managed with a carbohydrate snack. Severe episodes should be treated with the intramuscular administration of glucagon.

The **"honeymoon period"** is the return of residual islet cell function in children with newly diagnosed diabetes mellitus. Recurrent episodes of hypoglycemia signal the "honeymoon period," which usually lasts from several weeks to months, but may last several years. During this period, a temporary reduction in the insulin dosage is required.

The **Somogyi phenomenon** represents early morning hypoglycemia, as a result of excessive administration of insulin, followed by rebound hyperglycemia. In this situation, the dose of insulin should be reduced. The **dawn phenomenon** is a naturally occurring, early morning hyperglycemia, without preceding hypoglycemia. In dealing with the dawn phenomenon, the evening dose of intermediate-acting insulin should be increased or delayed.

Rarely, children may develop antibodies to insulin that cause insulin resistance. A change in the type of insulin preparation (pork, beef, human) may be beneficial.

Long-term **complications** of type I diabetes mellitus include retinopathy, renal disease, atherosclerotic heart disease, and peripheral neuropathy. Considerable scientific data suggest that these complications can be prevented through rigorous insulin therapy with strict control of serum glucose levels.

## Diabetic Ketoacidosis

**Diabetic ketoacidosis** (**DKA**) is an acute, life-threatening complication of insulin-dependent diabetes mellitus, characterized by marked **hyperglycemia**, which causes a profound osmotic diuresis, metabolic acidosis, and ketonemia. The signs and symptoms of DKA include dehydration, vomiting, abdominal pain (which can mimic an acute surgical condition), polyuria, lethargy and coma. The metabolic acidosis induces a compensatory respiratory alkalosis, manifest by **Kussmaul respirations**. The generation of ketone bodies, which produces the characteristic acetone odor of the breath, stimulates vomiting.

Measurement of serum pH, bicarbonate, and $PCO_2$ document the acid-base disturbances of DKA, typically a metabolic acidosis with an elevated anion gap and a compensatory respiratory alkalosis. Measurement of urine or serum ketones can be used to confirm the diagnosis of diabetic ketoacidosis. Hyponatremia, hyperkalemia with a low total body potassium, and azotemia are features of diabetic ketoacidosis.

The **treatment** of diabetic ketoacidosis involves meticulous **fluid and electrolyte replacement** (particularly potassium); intravenous administration of insulin; and glucose administration once the serum glucose level has fallen. In some cases, cautious administration of bicarbonate is warranted.

The complications of diabetic ketoacidosis and its therapy include hypoglycemia, hypokalemia, hypocalcemia, and cerebral edema. Cerebral edema, which can be fatal and occurs several hours after the onset of therapy, is indicated by the onset of headache, altered mental status, vomiting, and bradycardia.

# Chapter 11

# Hematologic and Malignant Disorders

## ANEMIA

Anemia in children results from either decreased production, increased destruction (hemolysis), or increased loss of red blood cells. Decreased production can result from deficiency states (iron, folic acid, vitamin B12), chronic renal disease, infections and inflammation, or genetic defects. Table 11-1 provides the normal hematologic values for children.

**Blackfan-Diamond syndrome**, or congenital pure red cell aplasia, is a rare genetic defect of red cell production that presents in the first few months of life with severe anemia, low reticulocyte count, and congestive heart failure. An examination of the bone marrow shows marked reduction of red cell precursors. Corticosteroid therapy may be effective in stimulating red blood cell production; otherwise, affected children are dependent on frequent blood transfusions. Spontaneous remission may occur.

## IRON DEFICIENCY ANEMIA

Iron deficiency anemia, the most common cause of anemia in children, results from an absolute deficit in the body's iron stores. Factors associated with iron deficiency include lower socioeconomic status, multiple gestational births, iatrogenic blood loss, early introduction of whole cow's milk, and delay in the introduction of iron fortified cereals.

With the advent of the federal Women, Infants, and Children (WIC) program in which eligible poor children can receive nutritional supplements in the form of iron-fortified proprietary formula, the incidence of nutritional iron deficiency anemia in infants and children has decreased substantially in the United States.

## TABLE 11-1. Normal Hematologic Values for Children

| Age | Hb (g/dL) Mean | -2 SD | Hematocrit% Mean | -2 SD | MCV (fL) Mean | -2 SD | MCHC (g/dL RBC) Mean | -2 SD | Reticulocyte (%) | WBC (1000/mm³) Mean | 95% CI | Platelets (1000/mm³) Mean (Range) |
|---|---|---|---|---|---|---|---|---|---|---|---|---|
| Term (cord blood) | 16.5 | 13.5 | 51 | 42 | 108 | 98 | 33.0 | 30.0 | 3.0–7.0 | 18.1 | 9.0–30.0 | 290 |
| 1–3 days | 18.5 | 14.5 | 56 | 45 | 108 | 95 | 33.0 | 29.0 | 1.8–4.6 | 18.9 | 9.4–34.0 | 192 |
| 2 weeks | 16.6 | 13.4 | 53 | 41 | 105 | 88 | 31.4 | 28.1 | | 11.4 | 5.0–20.0 | 252 |
| 1 month | 13.9 | 10.7 | 44 | 33 | 101 | 91 | 31.8 | 28.1 | 0.1–1.7 | 10.8 | 5.0–19.5 | |
| 2 months | 11.2 | 9.4 | 35 | 28 | 95 | 84 | 31.8 | 28.3 | | | | |
| 6 months | 12.6 | 11.1 | 36 | 31 | 76 | 68 | 35.0 | 32.7 | 0.7–2.3 | 11.9 | 6.0–17.5 | |
| 6–24 months | 12.0 | 10.5 | 36 | 33 | 78 | 70 | 33.0 | 30.0 | | 10.6 | 6.0–17.0 | (150–300) |
| 2–6 years | 12.5 | 11.5 | 37 | 34 | 81 | 75 | 34.0 | 31.0 | 0.5–1.0 | 8.5 | 5.0–15.5 | (150–300) |
| 6–12 years | 13.5 | 11.5 | 40 | 35 | 86 | 77 | 34.0 | 31.0 | 0.5–1.0 | 8.1 | 4.5–13.5 | (150–300) |
| 12–18 years (M) | 14.5 | 13.0 | 43 | 36 | 88 | 78 | 34.0 | 31.0 | 0.5–1.0 | 7.8 | 4.5–13.5 | (150–300) |
| 12–18 years (F) | 14.0 | 12.0 | 41 | 37 | 90 | 78 | 34.0 | 31.0 | 0.5–1.0 | 7.8 | 4.5–13.5 | (150–300) |

CI = confidence interval; F = female; Hb = hemoglobin; M = male; MCHC = mean corpuscular hemoglobin concentration; MCV = mean corpuscular volume; RBC = red blood cells; SD = standard deviation; WBC = white blood cells.
Adapted from Oski FH, et al, Principles and Practices of Pediatrics, 2nd ed. Philadelphia: JB Lippincott; 1994, p. 2168.

In full-term infants, iron stores are sufficient for the first 4 months of growth. **Premature infants** have proportionally the same amount of iron per body weight as full-term infants, but they have a higher rate of growth and thus a **greater propensity to develop iron deficiency anemia**. To prevent iron deficiency, full-term infants should receive iron supplementation starting at no later than 4 months of age and continuing to 3 years of age. Because low-birth-weight infants require more iron per kilogram of body weight, supplementation should be started no later than 2 months of age.

Both breast milk and cow's milk contain 0.5 to 1.0 mg of iron per liter. However, about 50% of the iron in breast milk is absorbed when compared with only 10% absorbed from cow's milk. Iron-fortified formulas contain 12 mg of iron per liter; however, only 4% is absorbed. Iron absorption is increased by ascorbic acid and diminished by bran, fiber, phosphates, and the tannins in tea. Whole cow's milk given in the first year of life may cause occult gastrointestinal bleeding and iron deficiency anemia.

Iron requirements **increase** during **adolescence**. This increased requirement, combined with poor dietary intake of iron and the loss of iron through menstruation, can result in significant iron deficiency, especially in adolescent girls.

A child with iron deficiency may have few **symptoms** or may present with increased fatigue, decreased exercise tolerance, anorexia, and increased irritability. On examination, only pallor of the skin and mucous membranes may be evident. Children with severe iron deficiency may present with signs of congestive heart failure. Anemia is only one late manifestation of iron deficiency. The most important abnormality in iron deficient infants is a **decrease in cognitive function**.

The anemia of iron deficiency is the end result of a loss of iron from the bone marrow and serum. The anemia is characterized by a low mean cell volume (MCV), low serum iron level, low serum ferritin, increased serum iron-binding capacity (TIBC) and increased red cell protoporphyrin level (FEP). An increased red cell distribution width (RDW) in conjunction with a low MCV is strong evidence of iron deficiency. The diagnosis is confirmed by a positive response to a therapeutic trial of iron.

Iron deficiency anemia is treated with ferrous sulfate. Dietary counseling and careful follow-up are also important parts of the management of this condition.

## MEGALOBLASTIC ANEMIAS

Megaloblastic anemias in children are due to deficiencies of folic acid and vitamin B12. **Folic acid deficiency** is most common in infants 4 to 7 months of age and is associated with megaloblastic anemia, failure to thrive, irritability, chronic diarrhea, neutropenia, and thrombocytopenia. Folic acid deficiency is also found in children with malabsorption syndromes, those taking some medications such as methotrexate, trimethoprim-sulfamethoxazole, and anticonvulsants, and those fed goat's milk. **Vitamin B12 deficiency** occurs in children with juvenile pernicious anemia (absence of gastric intrinsic factor) or diseases of the terminal ileum such as necrotizing enterocolitis.

## HEMOLYTIC ANEMIAS

Hemolytic anemia occurs when the lifespan of the red blood cell is shortened. These conditions are characterized by anemia, reticulocytosis, increased erythropoiesis in the bone marrow, and elevations of indirect bilirubin. Hemolytic anemia may be caused by hemoglobinopathies, structural abnormalities, enzyme defects, autoimmune antibodies, or traumatic destruction.

# PEDIATRICS

## Sickle Cell Anemia

Sickle cell anemia is a **chronic hemolytic anemia** caused by the presence of a structural substitution of valine for glutamic acid in the sixth position of the beta-globin chain of hemoglobin, resulting in **hemoglobin S**. This single amino acid substitution results in the formation of polymers and aggregates that deprive sickle red cells of their deformability under conditions of low oxygen tension. The disease is transmitted as an autosomal recessive condition.

**Sickle cell anemia**, the **homozygous** condition, is found in about 1 in 600 African Americans in the United States. Sickle cell anemia can be diagnosed through neonatal screening programs and prenatally by using chorionic villus biopsy or amniocentesis, although newborns have hemoglobin F and little sickle hemoglobin. In children with sickle cell anemia, the hemoglobin contains about 90% hemoglobin S and 2% to 10% hemoglobin F. Red blood cells contain no hemoglobin A.

Infants older than 6 months of age frequently present with **dactylitis** (hand and foot syndrome), which causes a painful swelling of the hands and feet. Children with sickle cell anemia present with characteristic signs of chronic hemolytic anemia, including reticulocytosis, intermittent indirect hyperbilirubinemia, and moderate to severe anemia.

Children with sickle cell anemia also have episodes of pain caused by the occlusion of capillaries and small blood vessels by the distorted sickled red blood cells, resulting in microinfarctions. These **painful crises**, which commonly occur in the extremities, head, chest, and back, can be triggered by infections, dehydration, or other illnesses.

Recurrent **splenic infarcts** result in autosplenectomy and functional asplenia. Infarction and infection of the lungs can result in **acute chest syndrome**, which may rapidly progress to respiratory failure. Occasionally a child with sickle cell disease will suffer an **infarction of the brain**, resulting in serious brain damage as a result of occlusion of vessels supplying the central nervous system (CNS). **Priapism** is the result of pooling of blood in the corpora cavernosa.

Children with sickle cell anemia are prone to serious **bacterial infections**, particularly with encapsulated organisms (*Streptococcus pneumoniae* and *Haemophilus influenzae*) and *Salmonella*, because of an impairment in splenic function as well as a deficiency in serum opsonins. The risk of serious bacterial infection is greatest in the first year of life. Osteomyelitis, another relatively common infectious complication, can be difficult to diagnosis in children with sickle cell disease because of the frequency of bone infarction.

Infants and young children with sickle cell disease may develop an acute splenic sequestration in which blood pools acutely in the spleen and occasionally in the liver. Children with **acute splenic sequestration** may rapidly develop vascular shock and require emergency blood transfusions. Children with concomitant glucose-6-phosphate dehydrogenase (**G6PD**) **deficiency** can develop a severe hemolytic crisis. Other complications of sickle cell anemia include gallstones, folic acid deficiency, cardiomegaly, hyposthenuria, and renal papillary necrosis.

These children, as well as those with other chronic hemolytic anemias, when infected with parvovirus B19, may develop an aplastic crisis characterized by the onset of severe anemia associated with low reticulocyte counts. Transfusion with packed red blood cells can be lifesaving in this situation.

The treatment of children with sickle cell anemia involves the management of the acute episodes with antibiotics, hydration, and transfusions as necessary. Most authorities recommend the administration of the pneumococcal vaccine at the appropriate age and daily prophylactic penicillin as methods for the prevention of serious pneumococcal infections in these children.

## Sickle Cell Trait

Sickle cell trait, the **heterozygous** form of the condition, is found in about 8% of the African American population of the United States. Sickle cell trait provides protection against severe forms of malaria. Children with sickle cell trait have between 35% to 45% of total hemoglobin in the form of **hemoglobin S**. This level of hemoglobin S is not sufficient for the development of any physical abnormalities, symptoms, or anemia. However, when children with sickle cell trait undergo general anesthesia, care must be taken to ensure that no periods of hypoxia occur because extreme hypoxia can cause sickling of their red cells and thrombosis can occur.

## Other Sickle Hemoglobinopathies

**Hemoglobin S** can exist in combination with other hemoglobinopathies, including **beta** and **alpha thalassemia**. Children with a combination of hemoglobin S and hemoglobin C (in which lysine replaces glutamic acid at the 6th position on the β chain) usually have milder symptoms than those with sickle cell anemia. **Splenomegaly**, however, is prominent in Hb SC disease and the **retinopathy** is more severe.

Hereditary persistence of fetal hemoglobin is due to an inability to shift from γ chain production to β chain production. Persons who concurrently have sickle cell anemia usually have few or no symptoms because of the protective effect of hemoglobin F.

## Thalassemias

The thalassemias are a group of genetic defects of globin chain synthesis, both beta and alpha, that result in chronic hypochromic anemia. More than 100 different genetic defects have been described, resulting in conditions with variable levels of globin chain synthesis.

***Homozygous beta⁰-thalassemia*** (**Cooley's anemia or thalassemia major**) is a chronic congenital hemolytic anemia characterized by the **complete absence of beta-globin chain production**. Therefore, hemoglobin A, which consists of alpha-globin and beta-globin chains, cannot be synthesized. Other forms of thalassemia, in which there is milder symptomatology and in which the synthesis of the globin chains is not completely suppressed, are labeled with such superscript distinctions as B± thalassemia.

Transmitted as an autosomal recessive trait, children with homozygous beta⁰-thalassemia present in the first year of life with failure to thrive, pallor, jaundice, hepatosplenomegaly, and a typical facies, which develops with time as a result of bone marrow hyperplasia in the skull and face. Red blood cells contain more than 90% hemoglobin F, which consists of alpha and gamma chains.

***Heterozygous defects*** that result in some beta-globin chain production, homozygous beta⁺-thalassemia, or thalassemia intermedia produce clinical syndromes similar to but milder than homozygous beta⁰-thalassemia with mild microcytic anemia. Children with thalassemia trait are often misdiagnosed with iron deficiency anemia. However, children with thalassemia trait have elevated levels of hemoglobin $A_2$, whereas children with iron deficiency anemia have an increased red cell distribution width (RDW).

***Alpha-thalassemia*** is caused by the **absence** or **deficient synthesis of alpha-globin chains**. Since four alpha-globin genes are present, four subtypes have been identified. Persons with deletion of a single alpha-globin gene are usually asymptomatic and are referred to as silent carriers. Deletion of two alpha-globin genes (alpha-thalassemia trait) is characterized by a mild microcytic anemia. Deletion of three alpha-globin genes (hemoglobin H disease) results in a more severe microcytic anemia. Hemoglobin H is a tetramer of beta-globin chains that forms because of the deficiency of alpha-globin chains. **Deletion** of all **four alpha-globin genes** results in the absence of hemoglobin F, A, and $A_2$, all of which require alpha-globin chains. Most of the hemoglobin is in the form of **hemoglobin Bart's**, a tetramer of gamma chains that cannot transport oxygen. These infants present at birth with **hydrops fetalis**.

The only treatment for severe forms of thalassemia is regular and frequent **blood transfusions**. Deferoxamine, an iron chelating agent, is used to prevent or ameliorate the hemosiderosis that is the inevitable complication of transfusion therapy. Deposition of iron in the myocardium and liver can be fatal. Hypersplenism, another complication of thalassemia, frequently requires splenectomy.

## Congenital Spherocytosis

Congenital spherocytosis is a hemolytic anemia caused by a **defect in the cell wall** (spectrin) of **red blood cells**, causing them to be more vulnerable to destruction as they circulate through the spleen. Commonly transmitted as an autosomal dominant trait, spherocytosis may also be transmitted as an autosomal recessive trait or result from a sporadic mutation.

Spherocytosis is variable in its severity, but it may present in the newborn period with prolonged or severe hyperbilirubinemia. Typically, children with this disease have moderate anemia, jaundice, and splenomegaly. Gallstones and aplastic crises, secondary to infection with parvovirus B19, are complications.

On laboratory evaluation, anemia, reticulocytosis, and increased serum unconjugated bilirubin levels are found. Examination of a peripheral blood smear reveals spherocytes that are smaller than normal red cells and lack central pallor. The osmotic fragility test confirms the diagnosis. The basis of this test is that normal biconcave red cells can swell when placed in a hypertonic solution. Spherocytes, however, are at maximum volume for their surface area and thus rupture.

The treatment of this disease involves **splenectomy**. However, delay in surgery is warranted until the child reaches school age to avoid the danger of bacterial sepsis found in asplenic children. Children who have a splenectomy are at increased risk for serious bacterial sepsis, and should receive vaccines that protect against *H. influenzae* type b and pneumococcus. They should also be placed on **prophylactic penicillin**.

## Autoimmune Hemolytic Anemias

Autoimmune hemolytic anemias may be primary (idiopathic) or secondary to other conditions. Diseases that induce hemolytic anemia include systemic lupus erythematosus, lymphoma, human immunodeficiency virus (HIV) infection, and other viral infections. Drugs can induce hemolytic anemia by either altering the red blood cell epitopes (penicillin, cephalosporins) or by forming immune-complexes that attach to the surface of the red cell (quinidine). The combination of autoimmune hemolytic anemia and thrombocytopenia constitutes **Evans syndrome**.

The laboratory hallmark of autoimmune hemolytic anemias is a **positive direct Coombs' test**. Antibodies may be IgG ("warm") or IgM ("cold"). Steroids and blood transfusion are used to treat autoimmune hemolytic anemias. However, finding matching compatible blood may be difficult.

## Glucose 6-Phosphate Dehydrogenase (G6PD) Deficiency

**G6PD deficiency** is a common, highly variable genetic defect that results in hemolytic anemia. Because the gene for G6PD is located on the X chromosome, males are more seriously affected than females. After ingestion of oxidants, particularly drugs, hemolysis results within 2 to 3 days. Drugs with oxidant properties include antimalarials, antipyretics, and sulfonamides. Infections may also induce hemolysis. The diagnosis can be confirmed by measurement of enzyme activity.

### Pyruvate Kinase Deficiency

Pyruvate kinase deficiency is a rare, autosomal recessive defect that results in variable clinical signs and symptoms, including anemia and jaundice. The diagnosis also is made by measurement of enzyme activity.

## PANCYTOPENIA

Pancytopenia, the presence of anemia, thrombocytopenia, and neutropenia, may be genetic or acquired. Acquired pancytopenia may result from exposure to toxins, radiation, or chemotherapeutic drugs. Chloramphenicol induces aplastic pancytopenia in 1 in 24,000 to 60,000 patients. Hepatitis and other viral infections can also cause pancytopenia. Pancytopenia due to infiltration of the bone marrow occurs with neuroblastoma and leukemia.

Symptoms of pancytopenia include bleeding due to thrombocytopenia, infections secondary to neutropenia, and anemia. The **prognosis** for children with severe pancytopenia is **poor**. Attempts at treating children with acquired pancytopenia include the use of bone marrow transplantation, cyclosporin, and antithymocyte globulin.

### Fanconi Pancytopenia

Fanconi pancytopenia is a syndrome of pancytopenia and congenital anomalies, including absent radii and thumbs, hyperpigmentation, microcephaly, short stature, and cardiac and renal anomalies. The onset of the pancytopenia is variable, but presents most often in school-age children. Affected children have a characteristic **red blood cell macrocytosis**, which may precede the onset of the pancytopenia. Abnormalities of the chromosomes are also found. In contrast to children with acquired pancytopenia, children with Fanconi syndrome may respond to treatment with androgens.

# THROMBOCYTOPENIA

## Autoimmune Thrombocytopenia

Autoimmune thrombocytopenic purpura or **idiopathic thrombocytopenic purpura** (**ITP**) usually occurs in children between the ages of 2 to 8 years. The disorder presents several weeks after a minor viral illness, with the abrupt onset of petechiae and/or purpuric skin lesions. Intracranial hemorrhage is a rare but serious complication.

On laboratory evaluation, the total platelet count is low, and the hematocrit and hemoglobin may be low if bleeding is severe. Platelets visible on blood smear are large, reflecting new platelet production. Bone marrow examination reveals a normal or increased number of megakaryocytes; other elements of the bone marrow are normal. The condition remits without any therapy within a few weeks or months in most children. Some authorities suggest the use of corticosteroid or intravenous gamma globulin for the treatment of this disease, particularly if it is severe.

**Thrombocytopenia** can be an early manifestation of leukemia, lymphoma, systemic lupus erythematosus, and HIV infection. Several other disorders of children are associated with thrombocytopenia.

The **thrombocytopenia absent radius (TAR) syndrome** is an inherited disorder of severe thrombocytopenia, aplasia of the radius, and cardiac and renal anomalies.

**Wiskott-Aldrich syndrome**, an X-linked recessive disorder, consists of thrombocytopenia, eczema, and immunologic defects predisposing to infections.

Children with large, cavernous hemangiomas can develop thrombocytopenia, the **Kasabach-Merritt syndrome**. Platelets are trapped and destroyed, and red blood cells are fragmented within the hemangioma.

**Disseminated intravascular coagulation (DIC)** is also associated with thrombocytopenia.

# HEMOPHILIAS

## Hemophilia A

Hemophilia A (**factor VIII deficiency**), a disease transmitted by X-linked recessive inheritance, is the most common hereditary coagulation disorder. In one third of cases of children with hemophilia A, the disease is the result of a new genetic mutation. A variety of genetic mutations cause hemophilia, including deletions, missense mutations, and nonsense mutations.

Children with hemophilia present in early childhood with easy bruising, the formation of large hematomas after trivial trauma, and prolonged bleeding at surgery. Bleeding into joints and muscles can cause serious acute or chronic injury. Intramuscular hematomas can compress nerves and vessels. **Hemarthroses** result in pain and swelling of the affected joint, most commonly the knees, elbows, ankles, shoulders, and hips. Repeated hemorrhage and inflammation lead to chronic joint disease, limitation of motion, and permanent disability. Severe intracranial bleeding, particularly after head trauma, can be fatal.

The clinical severity of this disease varies greatly. Children with severe **hemophilia A** have **no detectable factor VIII**. Children with moderate disease have factor VIII levels that range from 1% to 4% of normal levels; those with mild disease have levels that range from 5% to 25% of normal. These distinctions are important for both prognosis and treatment.

On laboratory evaluation, children with hemophilia A and hemophilia B have a normal platelet count and prothrombin time, but **prolonged activated partial-thromboplastin time** (APTT). Coagulation factor assays are required to differentiate hemophilia A and hemophilia B.

The treatment of hemophilia A involves replacement of the missing clotting factor with fresh frozen plasma, plasma cryoprecipitate, or factor VIII concentrates, which contain increasing concentrations of factor VIII. Factor VIII concentrates are prepared from the pooled plasma from 2000 to 200,000 donors.

In 10% to 20% of children, treatment of hemophilia may be complicated by the development of antibodies to factor VIII (inhibitors). These children do not respond to standard factor VIII replacement therapy.

Recently, factor VIII concentrates have been developed using recombinant DNA technology. These forms of concentrate have the advantage of safety in regard to infectious agents but are more expensive.

## Hemophilia B or Christmas Disease

**Factor IX deficiency**, called hemophilia B or Christmas disease, is also transmitted as an X-linked recessive disorder. Although clinically indistinguishable from hemophilia A, treatment of the two disorders differs. Treatment of children with factor IX deficiency requires replacement therapy with fresh frozen plasma or factor IX concentrate.

With the identification of the HIV, a significant number of children with hemophilia were found to be infected with HIV as a result of contamination of plasma used to prepare the replacement therapy. Other viruses capable of being transmitted through plasma preparations include hepatitis B and hepatitis C. With widespread screening of blood donations for the presence of antibodies to HIV and to viral hepatitis and with new methods of viral inactivation, this problem has largely been solved. However, children with hemophilia represent a significant proportion of the children with HIV disease in the United States.

## Von Willebrand Disease

Von Willebrand disease, classically an autosomal dominant disorder, is caused by a deficiency of functional von Willebrand protein. Affected children present with bleeding of the mucous membranes and prolonged bleeding after trauma or surgery, but spontaneous hemarthroses are uncommon. Because von Willebrand protein transports factor VIII, children with von Willebrand disease have decreased factor VIII activity and a prolonged partial thromboplastin time. Platelet aggregation and adhesiveness are also diminished. Treatment is with fresh frozen plasma or cryoprecipitate.

# MALIGNANT DISORDERS

Malignant disease is the principal medical cause of death, following accidental injury and poisoning, in the 1- to 14-year age group. Leukemia, lymphomas, and brain tumors account for the majority of neoplasms in childhood. Infants and young children develop Wilms' tumor, neuroblastoma, and retinoblastoma. Older children and adolescents are prone to tumors of the bones, ovary, testis, and thyroid gland. Rhabdomyosarcomas and other soft tissue tumors occur throughout childhood.

# LEUKEMIAS

Leukemia is a disease characterized by the proliferation of immature white blood cells, and it is the most common neoplasm of children. Leukemia is classified according to the involved white blood cell line. Acute lymphocytic leukemia (ALL) accounts for approximately 80%, and acute nonlymphocytic leukemia accounts for approximately 15% of leukemia in children. Chronic myelogenous leukemia accounts for the remainder of cases of leukemia in childhood.

## Acute Lymphocytic Leukemia

**ALL** (also termed lymphoblastic) leukemia has a peak incidence in children between the ages of 3 to 6 years. Children with trisomy 21 and immunodeficiencies are at increased risk for the disease. Several different types of analysis are used to classify ALL: cytologic appearance, histochemical stains, presence or absence of specific enzymes, chromosomal translocations, and cell surface antigens, including common ALL antigen (cALLa). Surface antigens are used to identify the leukemic cells as either T-cell or B-cell lineage and their maturational stage. Most children with leukemia have cells that derive from a very early B-cell clone.

Children with acute lymphoblastic leukemia present with a history of irritability, fatigue, fever, easy bruising, bone pain, arthralgia, and weight loss. On physical examination pallor, ecchymoses, petechiae, generalized lymphadenopathy, splenomegaly, hepatomegaly, and bone tenderness may be found.

The diagnosis is made by examination of the blood smear and bone marrow for the presence of typical immature blast cells. The white blood cell count varies; some children with ALL have a markedly **elevated white blood cell count**, and others have leukopenia. Many children with ALL also have anemia and thrombocytopenia. The evaluation of children with ALL should include a chest radiograph to determine the presence of a mediastinal mass common in T-cell leukemia and a lumbar puncture to identify leukemic cells.

Therapy of ALL includes antineoplastic agents, prophylactic treatment of the CNS with either intrathecal chemotherapy or cranial radiation, and several years of maintenance therapy with antineoplastic agents.

Without prophylactic treatment, the **CNS** is a **common site of relapse**. Relapse involving the CNS presents with signs and symptoms of increased intracranial pressure. The **testes** also represent a "sanctuary" or site of relapse. Testicular relapse presents with painless swelling of one or both testes.

A **poorer prognosis** of the disease is associated with **age of less than 2 or more than 10 years**; white blood cell count over 100,000/mm$^3$; the presence of a mediastinal mass; or evidence of CNS involvement.

Children with **null cell ALL**, those without definite markers for either mature T or B cells, have the **best prognosis**. Ninety-five percent of these children will have a period of remission, 75% survive beyond 5 years, and most can be cured. About half of the cases of children with T-cell leukemia are cured; however, almost all of children with mature B-cell leukemia succumb to their disease. Children who fail to respond to intensive chemotherapy may be candidates for bone marrow transplantation.

## Acute Nonlymphocytic Leukemia

Acute nonlymphocytic leukemia (**ANLL**) has numerous subtypes, based on cellular morphology; the vast majority resemble myeloblasts or monoblasts. ANLL presents in children later than ALL. Predisposing conditions include other malignancies and such **chromosomal breakage syndromes** as Fanconi pancytopenia and Bloom syndrome, caused by a genetic mutation in a helicase gene, an enzyme that unwinds paired DNA strands.

The clinical picture of children with ANLL resembles ALL. The diagnosis must be confirmed by examination of the blood smear and bone marrow. The treatment of ANLL resembles that of ALL, with induction, CNS prophylaxis, and maintenance chemotherapy. However, the prognosis of ANLL is not as favorable; only **30% to 40%** of children are **cured**.

# LYMPHOMAS

## Hodgkin's Disease

Hodgkin's disease is characterized histologically by the Reed-Sternberg cell, and has a peak incidence in **adolescence** and **early adulthood** with a second peak **after age 50 years**. Adolescents usually present with an enlarged cervical or supraclavicular lymph node without evidence of inflammation. Other lymph nodes may also be involved; mediastinal lymph node involvement can cause airway compression and cough. Metastatic disease occurs in the lungs, liver, and bone marrow. Both the disease and therapy for the disease can result in impaired cell-mediated immunity and susceptibility to opportunistic infections.

The diagnosis is confirmed by histologic examination of a lymph node biopsy, which is classified into **four histologic subtypes** with **differing prognosis**: nodular sclerosing (the most common subtype in children and adolescents); lymphocyte predominant (best prognosis); mixed cellularity; and lymphocyte depletion (least common and worst prognosis).

Chest radiograph and computerized tomography (CT) scan are required to assess mediastinal and pulmonary involvement. A staging laparotomy, consisting of splenectomy, liver biopsy, and lymph node biopsy, is frequently performed.

The treatment of Hodgkin's disease involves radiotherapy and chemotherapy, depending on the stage of disease.

## Non-Hodgkin's Lymphoma

Non-Hodgkin's lymphoma (**NHL**) refers to a group of lymphomas with different characteristics and cells of origin. Non-Hodgkin's lymphomas are more common in young children than Hodgkin's disease. Such immunocompromised children as those with HIV infection, severe combined immunodeficiency (SCID), X-linked agammaglobulinemia, Wiskott-Aldrich syndrome, and ataxia-telangiectasia are at particularly high risk of NHL.

Children with NHL commonly present with lymphadenopathy of the head or neck. Lymph node enlargement may be extremely rapid, particularly with **Burkitt lymphoma**. Anterior mediastinal involvement helps to distinguish lymphoma from neuroblastoma, which involves the posterior mediastinum. Abdominal lymphomas frequently involve the ileocecum and may cause intestinal obstruction or intussusception. Disseminated disease involves the meninges and bone marrow.

Therapy is primarily with **chemotherapeutic regimens**; surgical excision of abdominal tumors and cranial radiation is useful for some patients.

# TUMORS OF THE CENTRAL NERVOUS SYSTEM

**Brain tumors** are the **most common solid tumors** in children. Because half of all brain tumors in children over 1 year of age are located **infratentorially**, most present with symptoms of **cerebellar dysfunction**. Children with these tumors typically present with nystagmus, ataxia, head tilt, and uncoordinated movements. Signs and symptoms of increased intracranial pressure, such as vomiting and papilledema, result from obstructive hydrocephalus. Papilledema is rare in infants because intracranial pressure is decompressed through the fontanelles. Older children may complain of headache and diplopia. Irritability, lethargy, and failure to thrive occur in children with infratentorial and supratentorial brain tumors. Focal neurologic signs and seizures are more common in children with supratentorial tumors. Brain tumors are diagnosed using CT and magnetic resonance imaging (MRI).

## Medulloblastomas

Medulloblastomas, which account for 20% to 25% of **intracranial** tumors in children, are primitive neuroectodermal tumors that commonly invade the fourth ventricle and cerebellar hemispheres. These tumors are more common in boys than in girls, and they have a peak incidence between the ages of 2 to 6 years. Medulloblastomas **disseminate along the spinal cord**.

The therapy for medulloblastomas involves surgical removal accompanied by radiation therapy, which includes the spinal cord. Adjuvant chemotherapy may be added for children at high risk of recurrence.

## Cerebellar Astrocytomas

Cerebellar astrocytomas are usually low-grade **cystic gliomas** that account for 15% of brain tumors in children. They generally occur in children between the ages of 6 to 9 years and are rather **slow-growing malignancies**. The signs and symptoms include the appearance of a unilateral ataxia, accompanied by a tilting of the head toward the side of the tumor. Cerebellar astrocytomas may also cause obstructive hydrocephalus. Prompt surgical removal results in long-term survival in about 90% of children. Radiotherapy and chemotherapy are used in children with incompletely removed cerebellar astrocytomas.

## Brain Stem Gliomas

Brain stem gliomas constitute about 10% of brain tumors in children. These tumors invade surrounding tissue, resulting in cranial nerve palsies and upper motor neuron signs. Because most of these gliomas cannot be surgically resected, *radiotherapy* is the treatment of choice. However, the prognosis is poor, with a median survival of less than 1 year after diagnosis.

## Ependymomas

Ependymomas constitute 5% to 10% of brain tumors in children. Because they arise within the fourth ventricle, the presenting clinical picture is of **obstructive hydrocephalus** and **increased intracranial pressure**. Herniation of the cerebellar tonsils may result in nuchal rigidity and torticollis; lumbar puncture may be fatal. Treatment consists of surgical excision and radiotherapy.

## Supratentorial Astrocytomas

Supratentorial astrocytomas and gliomas can occur in the cerebral hemispheres in children. The prognosis for children with supratentorial astrocytomas is less favorable than those with infratentorial tumors.

## Craniopharyngiomas

Craniopharyngiomas, which account for approximately 5% to 10% of pediatric brain tumors, cause **pituitary and hypothalamic dysfunction**, especially short stature and symptoms of diabetes insipidus. Invasive disease can cause **visual disturbances**, including visual field defects due to compression of the optic chiasm as well as hydrocephalus. The majority are calcified and can be seen on skull radiographs. Treatment is surgical excision.

## Diencephalic Syndrome

The diencephalic syndrome, which is characterized by anorexia and wasting but normal linear growth, is associated with optic nerve gliomas.

## Parinaud Syndrome

Parinaud syndrome, paralysis of upward gaze and loss of the pupillary reflex, is associated with tumors of the pineal gland that compress the quadrigeminal plate.

# NEUROBLASTOMA

**Neuroblastoma** is a malignancy of the sympathetic nervous system. It may appear anywhere this tissue is found, but it most often arises from the adrenal glands or from the thoracic or abdominal sympathetic chains. Neuroblastoma is a tumor of childhood; 75% of children have been identified by the age of 5 years, with a median age at diagnosis of 2 years. An unusual feature of neuroblastoma is a **high rate of spontaneous regression in early infancy**.

The presenting symptoms depend on the location of the tumor. Because the tumor commonly arises in the abdomen, the **usual presenting sign** is a **firm, nontender abdominal mass**. Thoracic neuroblastomas usually occur in the posterior mediastinum. Neuroblastomas that arise from the sympathetic chain may extend into the spinal canal and compress the spinal cord ("dumbbell" tumors). Disseminated neuroblastoma involves the liver, bones, and dura.

Occasionally, neuroblastoma presents with **unilateral proptosis**, periorbital swelling, and ecchymoses caused by metastasis of the tumor to the eye. Symptoms of **diarrhea, sweating**, and flushing are due to excretion of vasoactive substances by the tumor. Neuroblastoma may be associated with **opsoclonus-myoclonus**, a condition of ataxia, myoclonic jerks, and jerking eye movements.

The **diagnosis** of neuroblastoma is assisted by computerized tomography. The tumor commonly contains areas of calcification, hemorrhage, and necrosis. Bone scan and nuclear medicine scans may also be useful in assessing the primary tumor and extent of metastatic disease. Because these tumors produce elevated levels of catecholamines, measurement of catecholamine metabolites in the urine, including vanillylmandelic acid (VMA) and homovanillic acid

(HVA), is used as an adjunct to the diagnosis. The definitive diagnosis is made by surgical biopsy.

**Treatment** of neuroblastoma includes surgical resection, chemotherapy, and irradiation. The prognosis for children with neuroblastoma is worse for older children and those with metastatic disease. An increased number of copies of the oncogene *N-myc*, are associated with poor prognosis.

# WILMS' TUMOR

Wilms' tumor, or **nephroblastoma**, occurs in early childhood, with a median age at presentation of 3 years of life. This tumor is usually **unilateral**, but bilateral Wilms' tumor occurs in 10% to 15% of patients. Wilms' tumor must be distinguished from neuroblastoma in the young child with an abdominal mass.

Children with the familial form of Wilms' tumor, which is more commonly bilateral, are also at higher risk of associated congenital anomalies, including genitourinary anomalies, hemihypertrophy, and aniridia. The hemihypertrophy is not always apparent at the time of diagnosis and may become manifest during adolescence.

Children with Wilms' tumor typically present with an **asymptomatic abdominal mass** that does not cross the midline. Hypertension usually due to compression of the renal artery is present in 30% to 60% of patients. Hematuria may also be present. Metastases commonly occur to the lung, liver, and adjacent lymph nodes.

The diagnosis is made by abdominal CT scan, which demonstrates an intrarenal mass. Therapy includes surgical removal of the involved kidney with the addition of chemotherapy and radiation therapy, depending on the stage of disease.

# RHABDOMYOSARCOMA

Rhabdomyosarcoma is a **soft tissue sarcoma of skeletal muscle**, and is the most common soft tissue sarcoma of childhood. It occurs in young children in the head, bladder, prostate, and vagina. In adolescents, the tumor is found in the genitourinary tract.

## Sarcoma Botryoides

Sarcoma botryoides is a specific subtype of rhabdomyosarcoma in which the tumor extends into a body cavity such as the vagina, bladder, or nasopharynx. Children frequently present with a mass; children with metastatic disease may have bone pain or respiratory symptoms secondary to bone or pulmonary metastases. Treatment consists of surgical resection and chemotherapy.

# BONE TUMORS

Bone tumors are more common in adolescents than in younger children. **Osteogenic sarcoma**, the most common malignant bone tumor of children, occurs at the **metaphyses of long bones** during the period of accelerated growth. The distal femur, proximal humerus, and proximal tibia are the common sites. Children present with pain and a mass at the site of the tumor. Metastatic disease involves the lungs.

The typical radiographic appearance is of a destructive mass breaking through the bony cortex, with marked periosteal reaction and calcification creating a "sunburst" pattern.

Treatment includes extensive local excision or amputation of the affected limb and intensive chemotherapy with multiple drugs.

### Ewing's Sarcoma

Ewing's sarcoma, less common than osteogenic sarcoma and extremely rare in black children, also most commonly involves **long bones**, particularly the femur. However, Ewing's sarcoma may also involve **flat bones** such as the pelvis. The clinical picture may mimic osteomyelitis. This tumor usually metastasizes to the lungs and other bones. Combination radiotherapy and chemotherapy is the treatment of Ewing's sarcoma.

# RETINOBLASTOMA

Although retinoblastoma is rare, it is the most common **malignant tumor of the eye** in children. In about one third of children with retinoblastoma, both eyes are involved. Children with bilateral retinoblastoma usually present in the first year of life; children with unilateral retinoblastoma present at about 2 years of age. Bilateral retinoblastoma has a genetic predisposition associated with a retinoblastoma gene located on the long arm of **chromosome 13**. This genetic defect also predisposes to osteogenic sarcoma in later childhood and other malignancies in adulthood.

Retinoblastoma usually presents with **leukokoria**, a whitish reflex in the pupil due to growth of the tumor from the retina. More advanced disease presents with pain and loss of vision. Unilateral disease is treated with enucleation of the eye. Radiotherapy is the treatment of choice for bilateral retinoblastoma, although unilateral enucleation is sometimes warranted. Chemotherapy may be useful for metastatic disease.

# HISTIOCYTOSES

**Langerhans' cell histiocytosis**, formerly called histiocytosis X, is a term used to describe a group of relatively rare diseases characterized by the clonal proliferation of Langerhans' cells at one or more sites in the body. Langerhans' cell histiocytoses form a subgroup of **histiocytosis syndromes**, three classes of which have been described. The majority are not malignant.

**Class I histiocytoses** consists of Langerhans' cell histiocytoses and the conditions previously called eosinophilic granuloma, Hand-Schüller-Christian disease and Letterer-Siwe disease. **Cystic bone lesions** are common, most frequently involving the skull. Other manifestations, depending on the severity of disease, include fever, failure to thrive, pituitary dysfunction, seborrheic dermatitis, exophthalmos, lymphadenopathy, hepatosplenomegaly, and bone marrow suppression, resulting in anemia and thrombocytopenia. The diagnosis is confirmed by biopsy.

Isolated bone lesions can be excised. Steroids, chemotherapy, and irradiation are used in the treatment of the progressive forms of the disease.

**Class II histiocytoses** consist of erythrophagocytic and hemophagocytic syndromes. True malignancies comprise *class III histiocytoses*, including specific types of leukemia and lymphoma.

# Chapter 12

# Disorders of the Central Nervous System

Almost any serious disease or condition has the potential for damage to the central nervous system (CNS). Birth asphyxia, inborn errors of metabolism, genetic disorders, meningitis and encephalitis, trauma, and chronic lead intoxication or other environmental agents are among the common causes of serious neurologic disorders in childhood.

## CONGENITAL MALFORMATIONS OF THE CENTRAL NERVOUS SYSTEM

### Neural Tube Defects

Neural tube defects are the most common congenital defects of the CNS. The neural tube normally closes between 3 to 4 weeks of embryonic life. Failure of closure of the neural tube causes a spectrum of defects. Some evidence suggests that **folic acid supplementation** for pregnant women, begun before conception, will reduce the risk of this lesion in their newborns. Because the neural tube closes before most pregnancies are recognized, women of childbearing age should take daily folic acid supplementation prophylactically. Many neural tube defects can be detected prenatally by detection of an elevated alpha-fetoprotein level.

The most benign form of neural tube defect is **spina bifida occulta**. Usually asymptomatic, the condition can be recognized by hyperpigmentation, hair, or a dermal sinus in the midline of the lower lumbar region. A cleft in the posterior vertebral arches and laminae of L5 and S1 is evident on radiographs of the lower spine.

### Myelomeningoceles

Myelomeningoceles, the most severe neural tube defects involving the spine, are relatively common (1 in 1000 live births). In this anomaly, usually but not always located in the lumbosacral region, both the spinal cord and the meninges herniate through the bony defect in the spine causing severe neurologic deficits. Paralysis of the legs, deformities of the hips and feet, bladder and bowel dysfunction, perineal anesthesia, and obstructive hydrocephalus (Chiari malformation) are common. An associated leakage of cerebrospinal fluid (CSF) increases the risk of meningitis. When only the meninges herniate through the spine, the condition is called a **meningocele**. Treatment consists of surgical correction, intermittent bladder catheterization, intensive physiotherapy, and social support.

### Encephalocele

An encephalocele is a severe form of neural tube defect involving the skull, with protrusion of the brain through a midline defect, which may be located in the occipital or frontal region.

### Anencephaly

Anencephaly is a condition in which most of the brain, including the cerebral cortex and cerebellum, is missing. The skull is markedly abnormal. Infants with this condition die soon after birth.

### Craniosynostosis

Craniosynostosis is a condition of **premature closure of the cranial sutures**. Most affected infants present at birth with an abnormal skull, the shape of which depends on which sutures fused prematurely. The sagittal suture is most commonly involved. **Hydrocephalus** can result when several sutures close prematurely.

Children with **Crouzon syndrome**, which is inherited as an autosomal dominant trait, usually have brachycephaly and proptosis.

**Apert syndrome** is characterized by craniosynostosis, asymmetric facies, syndactyly and fusion of the bones of the hands, feet, and cervical spine.

**Carpenter syndrome** is characterized by craniosynostosis with an unusually shaped head, syndactyly, and mental retardation.

## NEUROCUTANEOUS SYNDROMES

### Neurofibromatosis

Neurofibromatosis, or **von Recklinghausen disease**, is an autosomal dominant disorder with two distinct forms (types 1 and 2). **Neurofibromatosis type 1, which accounts for 90% of all cases, is caused by a gene located on **chromosome 17**; about half of all cases result from spontaneous mutations. The clinical manifestations of neurofibromatosis type 1 include café-au-lait spots, axillary or inguinal freckling, neurofibromas, Lisch nodules (hamartomas of the iris), optic gliomas, and kyphoscoliosis. Seizures, learning disorders, and malignancies are also common.

Children with **neurofibromatosis type 2** characteristically develop **bilateral acoustic neuromas**. Other clinical manifestations include cataracts and brain tumors. Café-au-lait spots and neurofibromas frequently are absent.

## Tuberous Sclerosis

Tuberous sclerosis, also an autosomal dominant genetic disorder with a spontaneous mutation rate of 50%, is characterized by **calcified periventricular tubers of the cerebral cortex**. The signs of tuberous sclerosis include skin manifestations such as hypopigmented "ash leaf" lesions, which are more apparent when visualized with a Wood's ultraviolet lamp, sebaceous adenomas around the nose, and a shagreen patch in the lumbosacral area. Infantile spasms, seizures, and mental retardation are common. Obstructive hydrocephalus may result from compression on the ventricular system. Other clinical manifestations include cardiac rhabdomyosarcomas, retinal lesions, and renal disease.

## Sturge-Weber Disease

Sturge-Weber disease consists of a unilateral, facial nevus (port-wine stain), seizures, and hemiparesis. Computerized tomography (CT) of the brain typically shows unilateral intracranial calcification and cortical atrophy. Children with this condition often also have mental retardation.

## Von Hippel-Lindau Disease

Children with von Hippel-Lindau disease develop cerebellar hemangioblastomas and retinal angiomata; the spinal cord, kidneys, and pancreas are also frequently involved.

# SEIZURE DISORDERS

Seizures are common neurologic problems of children and are classified as partial or generalized (Table 12-1). Recurrent seizures,

**TABLE 12-1.**
**Classification of Seizures**

**Partial seizures**
Simple partial (consciousness preserved)
    Motor signs
    Sensory symptoms
    Autonomic signs or symptoms
    Psychic symptoms
Complex partial (consciousness impaired)
    Simple partial onset followed by impaired consciousness
    Impaired consciousness at onset
Partial seizures with secondary generalization
**Generalized-onset seizures**
Tonic-clonic seizures
Tonic seizures
Absence seizures
Atypical absence seizures
Atonic seizures
Infantile spasms

*Adapted from Scheuer ML, Pedley TA. The evaluation and treatment of seizures. N Engl J Med 1990;323:1469.*

unrelated to fever, are termed **epilepsy**. The greatest risk of recurrence is in the first year after the initial seizure, but many children with a single afebrile seizure will not have a recurrence. The classification of the type of seizure is assisted by the electroencephalogram (EEG). Neuroimaging (CT or magnetic resonance imaging [MRI]) is usually reserved for children with focal findings on neurologic examination or EEG.

## Partial Seizures

Partial seizures are common in children. In contrast to adults, most children with focal seizures do not have an identifiable local lesion. **Simple partial seizures** consist of short episodes (10 to 20 seconds) of clonic or tonic movements of the face, neck, and extremities, without impairment of consciousness. Simple partial seizures may be confused with tics.

## Complex Partial Seizures

Complex partial seizures, manifest by unresponsiveness and staring for 1 to 2 minutes, are commonly associated with an aura. Such automatisms as lip smacking, chewing, swallowing movements, or purposeful gestures in older children are frequent. The characteristic EEG shows temporal lobe sharp waves and focal spikes. Precipitating lesions of the temporal lobe include mesial temporal sclerosis, postencephalitic gliosis, hamartomas, and gliomas. Complex partial seizures may be followed by generalized seizures.

## Generalized Seizures

Generalized seizures include absence, tonic-clonic, atonic, myoclonic seizures, and infantile spasms. Generalized tonic-clonic seizures, common in children, are associated with bladder incontinence and tongue biting. They are usually followed by a postictal state of lethargy and drowsiness that lasts several hours.

## Absence Seizures

Absence seizures are found in older children and are brief (less than 30 seconds) episodes of staring and loss of motor function; postural tone remains. There is no aura or postictal state. Absence seizures can be induced by hyperventilation. The EEG pattern is typical. Absence seizures can be confused with complex partial seizures.

## Infantile Spasms

Infantile spasms classically present in early infancy as episodes in which the infant's **head suddenly drops to the chest**, the **thighs flex** on the abdomen, and the **arms adduct** and **flex** on the chest. **Extensor spasms**, rather than flexor spasms, also occur; the majority of infants present with a mixture of types. The individual episodes are brief, but they may be extremely frequent, with another following in rapid succession. The EEG shows a characteristically disorganized pattern termed **hypsarrhythmia**.

Most infants with infantile spasms have suffered perinatal or subsequent damage to the CNS, including hypoxic-ischemic encephalopathy. Congenital infections, metabolic errors, neurocutaneous syndromes, and trauma are also associated with infantile spasms. Infants with underlying CNS lesions are likely to be mentally retarded. "Cryptogenic" infantile spasms are defined as those without associated underlying CNS lesions. The treatment of infantile spasms is with adrenocorticotropic hormone (ACTH).

## Partial Epilepsy

**Benign partial epilepsy with centrotemporal spikes** is a common partial epilepsy of children with a good prognosis. The partial motor seizures, which commonly occur during sleep, frequently involve the face and neck. The EEG pattern is diagnostic. The seizures disappear during adolescence.

## Myoclonic Seizures and Epilepsy Syndromes

**Myoclonic epilepsy of childhood** begins in infancy or early childhood in a child who is otherwise healthy and who has no previous evidence of neurologic disease. A family history of epilepsy is common. Myoclonic seizures can occur several times a day and can also be accompanied by tonic-clonic seizures. Most children with myoclonic epilepsy will have a spontaneous remission after several years.

Children with **Lennox-Gastaut syndrome** have refractory myoclonic and tonic-clonic seizures, developmental delay, and interictal slow spike waves on EEG.

**Juvenile myoclonic epilepsy** begins in adolescence with early morning myoclonic seizures.

## Febrile Seizures

Febrile seizures, the most common cause of seizures in children, occur in 3% to 4% of all children. Febrile seizures are generalized tonic-clonic seizures that occur commonly in infants between the ages of 9 months and 5 years, with a peak incidence at 18 months. A family history of febrile seizures is common. These episodes are usually of short duration and often occur in the face of a rapid rise in body temperature. Febrile seizures rarely last more than 15 minutes.

The physician's first **priority** should be in the diagnosis of the cause of the fever. Because meningitis can present with seizures and fever, many physicians elect to perform a lumbar puncture in young children with a first febrile seizure to exclude this possibility.

Many children with a single febrile seizure never have more than one seizure, but about one third have recurrent febrile seizures. The risk factors for recurrent febrile seizures include age less than 18 months, family history of febrile seizures, shorter duration of fever before the first seizure, and lower temperature (less than 101°F) associated with the first seizure. One half of febrile seizures recur within the first 6 months of life; most recurrences occur within 2 years.

Approximately 2% to 3% of children with febrile seizures develop **nonfebrile seizures** or **idiopathic epilepsy** later in childhood. Children with a family history of seizures, neurologic abnormalities, focal seizures, repeated seizures within the same febrile episode, or those with a febrile seizure of prolonged duration (greater than 15 minutes) are more likely to develop afebrile seizures. The risk increases to almost 10% when several risk factors are present.

Only rarely do children with febrile seizures require anticonvulsant therapy. The use of antipyretics during febrile illnesses may reduce the risk of recurrence.

## MOVEMENT DISORDERS

Tics are repetitive, stereotyped movements that are more common in boys than in girls; they often occur during times of stress. Tics do not occur during sleep. Eye and facial muscles are frequently involved. Transient tic disorder, which persists for weeks to months, does not require therapy.

**Gilles de la Tourette syndrome** is a chronic tic disorder that begins in childhood. In addition to tics of the eyes, face, neck, and shoulders, children with this syndrome frequently have uncontrollable vocalizations, which may consist of coughing or sniffling sounds, but may also take the form of words. Drug therapy, including haloperidol, is of benefit to some children.

The most common cause of **chorea** in children is **Sydenham chorea**, a manifestation of rheumatic fever. Sydenham chorea is associated with hypotonia and emotional lability.

**Dystonias** are slow twisting movements of the trunk and extremities. Dystonias of childhood include **dystonia musculorum deformans** and **Wilson's disease**. Wilson's disease is an inborn error of copper metabolism associated with cirrhosis. **Acute dystonic reactions** in children frequently follow phenothiazine ingestion. The dystonia rapidly resolves with the administration of diphenhydramine intravenously.

**Ataxia** is associated with disease of the cerebellum. **Acute cerebellar ataxia** frequently follows a viral infection, typically varicella, and is thought to be due to a postinfectious autoimmune response involving the cerebellum.

Such degenerative neurologic conditions as **ataxia-telangiectasia** and **Friedreich's ataxia** are also associated with ataxia.

## INFECTIONS OF THE CENTRAL NERVOUS SYSTEM

### Meningitis

Meningitis, **inflammation of the meninges**, is usually of infectious etiology. **Bacterial** meningitis is one of the more common serious infections of children. Risk factors for bacterial meningitis include young age (less than 1 year); exposure to carriers of pathogenic bacteria (day-care centers); communicating defects with the CNS (basilar skull fracture, myelomeningocele); and immunodeficiencies, including complement deficiencies, splenic dysfunction (sickle cell anemia), and the inability to produce an antibody response to encapsulated bacteria (infants).

In the newborn period, **bacterial meningitis** is commonly caused by group B beta-hemolytic streptococcus and *Escherichia coli* or other gram-negative organisms that colonize in the maternal genitourinary tract. *Streptococcus pneumoniae, Haemophilus influenzae* type b, and *Neisseria meningitides* are the agents responsible for 95% of bacterial meningitis in children over the age of 2 months.

*Haemophilus influenzae* type b infection is more common between the ages of 2 months to 2 years. The incidence of *H. influenzae* type b meningitis, as well as other forms of infections with this organism, has declined substantially with the routine use of the conjugate *H. influenzae* type b vaccine.

In the United States, most meningococcal disease is due to group B. Epidemic meningococcal infections in other parts of the world are usually due to groups A and C.

The pathogenesis of meningitis involves the **nasopharyngeal colonization** with pathogenic bacteria following exposure to respiratory secretions from a carrier. Pathogenic bacteria invade the blood stream, causing bacteremia (the etiologic agent may be cultured from the blood in a majority of children with meningitis). Through this bacteremia, the organisms gain access to the CSF, which has minimal immunologic defenses.

The bacterial cell wall components stimulate an inflammatory response partially responsible for the long-term complications of bacterial meningitis. Because bacterial lysis following antibiotic therapy magnifies this inflammatory response, early treatment with corticosteroids, prior to or coincident with the first administration of antibiotics, may reduce the inflammatory response and minimize sequelae.

The **clinical presentation** of meningitis **varies with the age of the child**. The classic signs and symptoms of meningitis include fever, irritability, lethargy, headache, vomiting, seizures, and nuchal rigidity, with positive Kernig and Brudzinski signs. Petechiae and purpura may be present, but are conspicuous in children with meningitis and overwhelming sepsis, especially in meningococcemia. Infants with meningitis commonly do not exhibit nuchal rigidity. Fever, irritability, lethargy, and bulging of the anterior fontanelle may be the only signs of meningitis.

The **diagnosis** is made by examination of **CSF**. The spinal fluid of a child with bacterial meningitis contains white blood cells, predominantly neutrophils, a decreased glucose level, and an elevated protein level. A very low spinal fluid sugar or a very elevated protein are poor prognostic signs. Gram stain of the fluid may reveal the causative organism. Culture of the spinal fluid may permit the diagnosis of the specific agent.

Because three organisms account for most bacterial meningitis - in children, a regimen of antibiotics with activity against these pathogens is usually instituted until a definitive bacteriologic diagnosis can be made.

The **short-term complications** of bacterial meningitis include subdural effusions, especially in children with *H. influenzae* type b meningitis, the syndrome of inappropriate antidiuretic hormone (SIADH), and an immune mediated arthritis or pericarditis. Subdural effusions are associated with persistent fever.

The **long-term sequelae** of meningitis include hydrocephalus, hearing loss, seizures, speech or developmental delay, and mental retardation. Sensorineural hearing loss is more common in children with pneumococcal meningitis. As many as 10% to 20% of children with meningitis have some neurodevelopmental sequelae.

**Chemoprophylaxis** of the index case and close contacts contains the spread of bacterial meningitis. If there is a child less than the age of 4 years in the home, all household contacts of children with *H. influenzae* type b meningitis should receive **rifampin prophylaxis**. All close contacts of children with meningococcal meningitis should also receive chemoprophylaxis.

**Tuberculosis** and **Lyme disease** are other nonviral causes of meningitis in children.

## Aseptic Meningitis

Aseptic meningitis is characterized by CSF pleocytosis without a positive Gram stain or bacterial culture. It is commonly caused by **viral infection** of the meninges, especially the enteroviruses. In the United States, epidemics occur in the summer and fall.

The clinical picture resembles that of bacterial meningitis, although signs of severe toxicity and neurologic deficits are uncommon. Viral meningitis must be distinguished from partially treated bacterial meningitis. Other signs of enteroviral infection, including rashes, may be present. The pleocytosis may initially show a predominance of neutrophils, but with time lymphocytes predominate. No specific therapy is available for viral meningitis. Hearing loss, especially in children with mumps, represents a complication of viral meningitis.

## Encephalitis

Encephalitis, **inflammation of the brain**, is frequently caused by such viral agents as arboviruses, enteroviruses, and herpes simplex viruses. Herpes encephalitis occurs in newborn infants. The measles and mumps viruses can also cause encephalitis.

## Reye's Syndrome

Reye's syndrome, which is characterized at the cellular level by **mitochondrial dysfunction**, follows apparent recovery from a viral illness, especially influenza and varicella. Reye's syndrome begins with the acute onset of vomiting and mental status changes. The disease process can progress rapidly to include seizures, coma, and fatty degeneration of the liver. Serum levels of ammonia and liver and muscle enzymes are elevated. Treatment is supportive, and includes glucose administration and careful management of increased intracranial pressure.

Since a strong association between Reye's syndrome and **aspirin** use in children with influenza and varicella has been suggested, the incidence of Reye's syndrome has decreased markedly with the reduced use of aspirin in children with febrile illnesses.

# CENTRAL NERVOUS SYSTEM TRAUMA

Although **head injuries** are common in children, they generally are mild and require no treatment. But head injuries are also a major cause of hospitalization, acquired brain damage, and death. Frequent causes of head injuries in children are motor vehicle accidents, falls, and child abuse.

**Concussions** are posttraumatic episodes of transient loss of consciousness, with variable degrees of retrograde and posttraumatic amnesia. Although skull fractures are frequent in children with moderate and severe head trauma, the presence or absence of a skull fracture cannot be used to gauge the degree of underlying injury. Indications for skull radiographs and computerized tomography in children with mild to moderate head trauma remain controversial.

More serious complications of head injury include subdural hematomas, epidural hematomas, cerebral contusions, intracerebral hemorrhages, and cerebral edema.

Children more than 2 years of age have a better prognosis than adults following comparable head injury. The duration of coma is the best predictor of outcome; children with coma for less than 2 weeks have the best prognosis. Seizures, headaches, cognitive disorders, and behavioral disturbances are late complications of head trauma in children.

# NEUROMUSCULAR DISORDERS

## Muscular Dystrophies

Muscular dystrophies are genetic **progressive myopathies**, characterized by muscle degeneration. **Duchenne muscular dystrophy**, an X-linked recessive disorder, is the most common hereditary neuromuscular disease, affecting 1 per 3600 male infants. The genetic defect involves deletion in the gene for dystrophin, a sarcolemmal membrane protein. Approximately one third of cases are due to spontaneous mutations. Boys with Duchenne muscular dystrophy often appear normal in the first 2 years of life or may show mild gross motor delay.

**Gower's sign**, the use of the hands to push up on the legs to achieve an upright posture, is usually evident at 3 to 5 years of age. Most boys lose the ability to walk by 10 to 12 years of age. Progressive weakness eventually affects respiratory and pharyngeal muscles. Other clinical features are pseudohypertrophy of the calf muscles, contractures, scoliosis, cardiomyopathy, and mental retardation. Serum creatinine kinase levels are markedly elevated in those with the disease and are often also elevated in asymptomatic female carriers. Biopsy of a muscle is diagnostic. The diagnosis can also be confirmed by molecular analysis of the dystrophin gene. Treatment is supportive; death usually occurs during adolescence.

**Becker muscular dystrophy** is a similar but less rapidly progressive form of the disease.

**Myotonic dystrophy** is an autosomal dominant disorder, with protean manifestations due to repeated sequences of the trinucleotide CTG within the gene located on chromosome 19. Infants present with hypotonia and characteristic facies. Wasting begins in the distal muscles of the hands, forearms, and legs, and progresses to involve proximal musculature, an unusual pattern of progression for myopathies and more typical of neuropathies. Myotonia, the slow relaxation of muscles following contraction, becomes apparent later in childhood and is evident when grasping the hand. Other clinical findings include dysarthria, dysphagia, constipation, cataracts, heart block, arrhythmias, and mental retardation.

**Endocrinopathies are common**, including diabetes mellitus, hypothyroidism, adrenal insufficiency, and delayed puberty. Children with myotonic dystrophy also have immunodeficiencies, particularly hypogammaglobulinemia. A small percentage of infants born to women with myotonic dystrophy present with severe hypotonia, inability to feed, respiratory distress, and contractures; most of these children die in infancy. The diagnosis of myotonic dystrophy is made by the typical clinical findings, electromyography and muscle biopsy.

## Spinal Muscular Atrophies

The spinal muscular atrophies (SMA), degenerative diseases of motor neurons are also due to trinucleotide repeats, have several forms.

In **Werdnig-Hoffmann disease** (SMA type 1), the most severe form, infants present with severe hypotonia, weakness, poor feeding, muscle wasting, lack of deep tendon reflexes, and respiratory distress. The tongue, face, and jaw are involved, but extraocular muscles spared. Fasciculation, a sign of muscle denervation, is best observed in the tongue, but may be observed in other muscle groups. Most affected children die in early infancy.

In **Kugelberg-Welander disease** (SMA type 3), the mildest form of these atrophies, children typically develop proximal muscle weakness after infancy.

## Polyneuropathy

### Guillain-Barré Syndrome

Guillain-Barré syndrome is a **demyelinating polyneuropathy** that begins with paresthesias of the toes and fingers and progresses to a symmetric, ascending paralysis. Paralysis begins in the legs and is associated with cramping pain and diminished deep tendon reflexes. Examination of the CSF shows an elevated protein level but few or no cells. Nerve conduction studies demonstrate demyelination. The disease process worsens over several weeks, plateaus, and then slowly remits. Most patients have minor, residual neurologic problems.

The condition, which is often milder in children than in adults, frequently follows viral infection, including cytomegalovirus (CMV) and Epstein-Barr virus (EBV), or infection with *Mycoplasma pneumoniae* or *Campylobacter jejuni*.

Supportive care, including mechanical ventilation and intensive care when necessary, is critical. Specific therapies include gamma globulin infusions and plasma exchange; corticosteroids have been shown to be of no benefit.

## Poliomyelitis

Poliomyelitis remains a significant cause of childhood paralysis in Africa and Asia, despite successful attempts to eradicate polio in North and South America. Poliomyelitis follows infection with one of three antigenic types of poliovirus of the genus *Enterovirus*. Humans are the only reservoir of poliovirus, which is transmitted by oral-fecal or respiratory routes.

Most infected children are asymptomatic; however, some develop a minor illness characterized by fever, malaise, headache and sore throat.

**Paralytic poliomyelitis**, which is relatively rare compared with the frequency of poliovirus infection, often presents with the onset of constitutional symptoms, followed in several days with the appearance of severe headache, nuchal rigidity, back and limb pain, and flaccid paralysis. The paralysis characteristically involves the legs, and is asymmetric. Cranial nerve palsies and respiratory failure can occur.

## Charcot-Marie-Tooth Disease

Charcot-Marie-Tooth disease, or peroneal muscular atrophy, is an autosomal dominant disorder and the most common genetic neuropathy. The peroneal and tibial nerves are most severely affected, but the disease process may also involve the forearms and hands. The disease typically presents in late childhood or adolescence with a clumsy gait, bilateral foot drop, and muscle wasting of the anterior lower legs. Sensory loss and autonomic dysfunction may accompany the motor disturbances.

## Familial Dysautonomia

Familial dysautonomia, or **Riley-Day syndrome**, is an autosomal recessive trait of those of eastern European Jewish descent, and is characterized by a reduction in the number of specific nerve fibers, particularly those involved with pain, temperature, and taste sensation, and autonomic function. Children with this condition present with poor feeding, delayed motor and intellectual development, seizures, vomiting, sweating, flushing, and breath holding. Because of insensitivity to pain, children with familial dysautonomia are prone to injuries. Autonomic crises occur with persistent vomiting, irritability, sweating, flushing, and hypertension. The disease is usually fatal by early childhood.

## Botulism

Botulism is caused by the ingestion of the toxin of *Clostridium botulinum*, often from **contaminated honey**. Infants develop symptoms within hours after ingestion, including vomiting, diarrhea, cranial nerve palsies, hypotonia, and respiratory distress.

## Myasthenia Gravis

Myasthenia gravis occurs in infants and children, who typically present with poor feeding, ptosis, and weakness of the extraocular muscles. Infants of women with myasthenia gravis may have **transient neonatal myasthenia gravis**, which presents with respiratory distress, poor feeding, and hypotonia. Symptoms of this syndrome resolve when the acetylcholine receptor-binding antibodies derived from the mother are cleared.

# Chapter 13

# Cardiovascular Disorders

## CONGENITAL HEART DISEASE

With the marked reduction in the incidence of rheumatic fever in the United States, congenital heart disease has become the most common serious cardiac problem in children. Congenital cardiac lesions are associated with a variety of chromosomal abnormalities, genetic conditions, maternal diseases, and congenital infections (Table 13-1). Congenital heart disease is classified as cyanotic or acyanotic. Cyanosis, best seen in the nail beds, lips, and mucous membranes, is due to the shunting of deoxygenated blood from the right side of the heart to the systemic circulation.

### Cyanotic Congenital Heart Disease

*Tetralogy of Fallot*

Tetralogy of Fallot is a common type of **cyanotic congenital heart disease**, which consists of pulmonary valve and infundibular stenosis (in severe cases, pulmonary valve atresia); a ventricular septal defect (**VSD**); dextroposition of the aorta that overrides the septal defect; and right ventricular hypertrophy. Venous blood returning to the right heart cannot exit into the pulmonary artery and instead is shunted to the left ventricle through the ventricular septal defect. Collateral flow to the pulmonary arteries may occur through bronchial vessels and a patent ductus arteriosus.

Most children with tetralogy of Fallot are not cyanotic at birth but present in the **first few weeks or months of life** with failure to thrive, tachypnea, and cyanosis with feeding. With only moderate obstruction to the right ventricular outflow tract, shunting across the VSD may be minimal, resulting in minimal cyanosis ("pink" tetralogy of Fallot). The shape of the heart on chest radiograph resembles a boot, with a narrow base due to the small pulmonary artery and a rounded apex due to right ventricular hypertrophy.

### TABLE 13-1. Congenital Heart Disease in Children

**Chromosomal disorders**

| | |
|---|---|
| Trisomy 21 | Endocardial cushion defects, VSD |
| Trisomies 18 and 13 | VSD, ASD, PDA |
| 5p deletion (cri du chat syndrome) | VSD, PDA, ASD |
| Turner syndrome | Bicuspid aortic valve, aortic stenosis, coarctation of the aorta |

**Syndrome complexes**

| | |
|---|---|
| DiGeorge anomaly | Interrupted aortic arch, truncus arteriosis, VSD |
| Alagille syndrome | Peripheral pulmonic stenosis |
| CHARGE association | VSD, ASD, PDA, tetralogy of Fallot |
| VATER association | VSD, tetralogy of Fallot, ASD |
| Williams syndrome | Supravalvular aortic stenosis |

**Fetal exposures**

| | |
|---|---|
| Congenital rubella | PDA, VSD, ASD, peripheral pulmonic stenosis |
| Maternal diabetes | VSD, septal hypertrophy |
| Maternal SLE | Congenital heart block |
| Fetal alcohol syndrome | ASD, VSD |

ASD = atrial septal defect; PDA = patent ductus arteriosis; SLE = systemic lupus erythematosus; VSD = ventricular septal defect; CHARGE syndrome = coloboma, heart, atresia choanae, retardation, genital and ear anomalies; VATER syndrome = vertebral, anal, tracheoesophageal, radial and renal anomalies.
Adapted from Nelson Textbook of Pediatrics, 14th ed. Philadelphia: WB Saunders, p. 1148.

"Blue spells," or **paroxysmal hypercyanotic attacks**, which are due to reduced pulmonary blood flow, increased right-to-left shunting, worsening hypoxia, and acidosis, can occur in young children. These spells, which last minutes to hours, are characterized by increasing cyanosis, tachypnea, and possible syncope. Placing the child in a knee-chest position and administering oxygen and morphine assist in alleviating the attack.

Treatment of children with tetralogy of Fallot depends on the severity of the lesion. Neonates with severe right outflow tract obstruction and hypoxemia benefit from the administration of **prostaglandin E**, which keeps the ductus arteriosus open, allowing some blood flow to the pulmonary arteries. Once stabilized, infants with severe tetralogy of Fallot may undergo palliative surgery through the placement of a **shunt**, which directs systemic blood into the pulmonary arteries. When the child is older, definitive surgery is required.

## Transposition of the Great Vessels

In transposition of the great vessels, the aorta arises from the right ventricle and the pulmonary artery from the left ventricle, creating two parallel circuits. Oxygenated blood enters the systemic circulation through a patent foramen ovale, and in some children through a VSD or patent ductus arteriosus. Neonates who have an intact ventricular septum are cyanotic shortly after birth and die without prompt diagnosis and treatment.

As is seen in children with severe tetralogy of Fallot, improved arterial oxygenation can be achieved by **maintaining an open ductus arteriosus** with **prostaglandin E**. A balloon atrial septostomy (Rashkind procedure), which creates an atrial septal defect during cardiac catheterization, allows for greater mixing of blood at the atrial level and improved systemic oxygenation. Surgical correction is achieved by an arterial switch (Jatene) procedure performed in the first 2 weeks of life. Children with transposition of the great vessels and a large VSD often present with congestive heart failure and minimal cyanosis, and are at risk of developing severe pulmonary hypertension.

## Truncus Arteriosus

Truncus arteriosus is characterized by a single vessel arising from the ventricles that communicate through a VSD. Blood pumped through this single vessel supplies both the pulmonary and systemic circulations. Infants present with congestive heart failure; older children develop pulmonary hypertension and **cyanosis**.

## Eisenmenger Syndrome

Eisenmenger syndrome is characterized by **right-to-left shunting of blood** through a VSD as a consequence of pulmonary arterial pressures higher than systemic pressures. A loud, single second heart sound is suggestive of pulmonary hypertension.

## Hypoplastic Left Heart Syndrome

Infants with the **hypoplastic left heart syndrome** have a small nonfunctional left ventricle and a high mortality rate.

## Ebstein Anomaly

Ebstein anomaly is the abnormal downward displacement of the tricuspid valve within the right ventricle, resulting in a large right atrium and a small, poorly functioning right ventricle. **Cyanosis** results from right to left shunting through a patent foramen ovale.

Children with severe cyanotic congenital heart disease develop **polycythemia** in response to prolonged hypoxemia. The polycythemia places these children at risk for cerebral thromboses and ischemia. Because of the right-to-left shunt, children with cyanotic congenital heart disease are at risk of brain abscesses, which otherwise are rare in children.

## Acyanotic Congenital Heart Disease

### Ventricular Septal Defect

Ventricular septal defect (**VSD**) is the **most common** congenital cardiac lesion, and it accounts for approximately one fourth of all cases of congenital heart disease. These defects may be single or multiple and may occur in isolation or with other cardiac lesions, notably with tetralogy of Fallot and atrioventricular septal defects. They are characterized by their position and type (**membranous or muscular**). The severity of symptoms varies with the size of the defect.

A VSD may not be apparent immediately after birth because the relatively high pulmonary vascular resistance diminishes the left-to-right shunt. With the drop in pulmonary vascular resistance at several weeks of age, the murmur becomes apparent and signs and symptoms develop. Small defects are asymptomatic, but large left-to-right shunts result in left atrial and ventricular enlargement, congestive heart failure, and pulmonary hypertension.

Signs and symptoms of **heart failure** include failure to thrive, poor feeding, respiratory distress, and sweating. The murmur of ventricular septal defects is typically a **loud, systolic murmur**, heard best along the left sternal border and often associated with a thrill. The diagnosis is confirmed by echocardiography. One third to one half of cases of small ventricular septal defects close in the first year of life. Large defects, which lead to pulmonary hypertension and Eisenmenger syndrome, should be closed surgically.

The risk of endocarditis is minimal, but children with VSDs should maintain good dental hygiene and should receive prophylactic antibiotics for invasive procedures (Table 13-2).

### Atrial Septal Defects

Atrial septal defects (**ASD**) include defects in the ostium secundum and ostium primum. **Ostium secundum defects**, at the fossa ovalis, cause shunting of blood from the **left atrium to the right atrium**, which increases as right ventricular pressures diminish during infancy. Because most infants and many children with ostium secundum defects are asymptomatic, the diagnosis is usually made on routine examination. Increased blood flow across the right ventricular outflow tract generates an ejection systolic murmur best heard at the left upper sternal border. The **second heart sound is widely split** and fixed in both inspiration and expiration.

Right ventricular conduction delay on electrocardiogram (ECG) is characteristic. The diagnosis is confirmed by echocardiography. Complications occur in adults and are related to pulmonary hypertension and atrial dilatation, including atrial arrhythmias, valvular

### TABLE 13-2.
### Recommendations for Bacterial Endocarditis Prophylaxis

**Prophylaxis recommended for the following cardiac conditions:**
- Prosthetic heart valves
- Previous bacterial endocarditis
- Most congenital cardiac defects (see below)
- Valvular disease from rheumatic fever
- Hypertrophic cardiomyopathy
- Mitral valve prolapse with valvular regurgitation

**NOT RECOMMENDED for the following cardiac conditions:**
- Functional heart murmurs
- Isolated ostium secundum atrial septal defects
- Surgical repair without residua of ostium secundum atrial septal defect, ventricular septal defect, patent ductus arteriosis
- Previous Kawasaki disease or rheumatic fever without valvular dysfunction
- Mitral valve prolapse without valvular regurgitation

**Prophylaxis recommended for the following dental or surgical procedures:**
- Dental procedures that induce gingival or mucosal bleeding, including professional cleaning
- Surgical operations that involve intestinal or respiratory mucosa
- Tonsillectomy or adenoidectomy
- Incision and drainage of infected tissue
- Urethral catheterization if urinary tract infection is present

**NOT RECOMMENDED for the following dental or surgical procedures:**
- Dental procedures not likely to induce gingival bleeding, such as dental fillings above the gum line
- Endotracheal intubation
- Bronchoscopy with a flexible bronchoscope
- Tympanostomy tube insertion
- Endoscopy
- Cardiac catheterization

incompetence, and congestive heart failure. The treatment is **surgical correction during childhood**.

**Ostium primum defects**, at the lower atrial septum, are associated with defects of the mitral and tricuspid valves. As with ostium secundum defects, there is **left-to-right intra-atrial** shunting, which is complicated by **mitral insufficiency**. With mild to moderate shunts, most children are asymptomatic. A pansystolic mitral insufficiency murmur distinguishes ostium primum defects from ostium secundum defects. Larger shunts and more severe mitral insufficiency leads to congestive heart failure and recurrent pneumonias. Treatment is surgical correction of the cleft mitral valve and patching of the atrial defect.

Ostium primum defects form part of **atrioventricular septal defects**, also called endocardial cushion defects, which are common in children with trisomy 21. These children present with failure to thrive, congestive heart failure, and recurrent pneumonias. The characteristic ECG includes a superior QRS axis. Because pulmonary hypertension can develop, some children undergo pulmonary artery banding as a palliative procedure. Surgical correction is the treatment.

### Coarctation of the Aorta

Coarctation of the aorta most commonly occurs just below the origin of the left subclavian artery at the site of the **ductus arteriosus**. It is twice as common in boys, is frequently associated with a bicuspid aortic valve, and is a common cardiac anomaly seen in children with Turner syndrome. In infancy, coarctation occurs in conjunction with other congenital cardiac defects such as patent ductus arteriosus and ventricular septal defects.

The clinical picture depends on the coexisting anomalies, but **congestive heart failure** is frequent. Most children diagnosed with coarctation after infancy are asymptomatic. The classic clinical signs of coarctation are systolic hypertension in the upper extremities and weak or absent pulses and lowered blood pressure in lower extremities. In children, normal blood pressure in the legs is 10 to 20 mm Hg higher than pressure in the arms. A **systolic murmur** is frequently audible. Enlarged collateral blood vessels may produce notching of the inferior border of the ribs that is visible on chest radiograph.

Untreated complications of hypertension ensue, including congestive heart failure, coronary artery disease, and intracranial hemorrhage. Treatment is surgical excision of the coarctation with anastomosis.

### Congenital Aortic Stenosis

Congenital aortic stenosis, which is more common in boys than in girls, may be valvular, subvalvular, or supravalvular. Most children are asymptomatic and are found to have a murmur on physical examination. Infants with critical aortic stenosis have **congestive heart failure and low cardiac output**. Children with **Williams syndrome** have supravalvular aortic stenosis, elfin facies, mental retardation, and hypercalcemia.

### Pulmonary Valve Stenosis

Pulmonary valve stenosis, with intact ventricular septum, is also commonly asymptomatic. Infants with critical pulmonary valve stenosis have signs of right ventricular failure and cyanosis caused by shunting through the foramen ovale.

### Anomalous Origin of the Left Coronary Artery

Anomalous origin of the left coronary artery from the pulmonary artery results in decreased perfusion pressure of the left ventricle and myocardial infarction. Recurrent myocardial infarction leads to fibrosis, myocardial dysfunction, and congestive heart failure. Infants may develop angina, manifested by irritability, dyspnea, and sweating. Most affected children die in infancy.

# ARRHYTHMIAS

## Supraventricular Tachycardia

Supraventricular tachycardia (**SVT**), also called paroxysmal atrial tachycardia (PAT), is due to reentry of electrical impulses conducted from the ventricle back to the atrium and again cycling back to the ventricle. On ECG, the heart rate varies between 200 to 300 beats per minute, the QRS complex is usually narrow, and the P waves are abnormal. Normal P waves are upright in leads I, II, and $aV_F$. If prolonged, congestive heart failure may ensue. Modes of treatment include vagal stimulation, digoxin, adenosine, verapamil, and in emergencies synchronized cardioversion.

Most children with SVT have no underlying heart disease, although some have **Wolfe-Parkinson-White syndrome**, characterized by a short PR interval, delta waves, and a wide QRS complex (when the SVT has resolved) on ECG.

SVT must be distinguished from sinus tachycardia, atrial flutter, atrial fibrillation, and ventricular tachycardia. Careful analysis of the cardiac rate, P waves, and QRS complex most often allows for distinction of the various forms of tachycardia.

## Congenital Heart Block

Congenital heart block, a cause of bradycardia, occurs in infants born to mothers with systemic lupus erythematosus (SLE), in whom maternal antibodies damage the infant's conduction system.

# VASCULITIS

## Kawasaki Disease

Kawasaki disease, or **mucocutaneous lymph node syndrome**, is a generalized vasculitis of unknown etiology found in children under the age of 5 years. The disease presents with the abrupt onset of high fever, persisting for weeks, and a variety of signs and symptoms that vary with the stage of disease: lymphadenopathy, conjunctivitis, fissured lips, strawberry tongue, erythematous rash, edema of the hands and feet, and desquamation of the skin. The lymphadenopathy is often of a single, cervical node. The conjunctivitis consists of bilateral conjunctival infection without discharge. The rash varies in form and may be transient. Early desquamation involves the perineal region; late desquamation involves the fingers and toes. Other signs and symptoms include marked irritability, diarrhea, vomiting, myocarditis, symmetric arthritis, hydrops of the gallbladder, sterile pyuria, and iridocyclitis. Characteristic laboratory findings include an **elevated erythrocyte sedimentation rate** and the later development of **thrombocytosis**.

A significant percentage of children develop arteritis of the coronary arteries, which may evolve into coronary aneurysms with subsequent thrombosis and myocardial ischemia and infarction. **Aneurysms** of other vessels can occur as well, and a palpable aneurysm of the axillary artery may be found on physical examination.

The diagnosis is made on clinical criteria. Atypical or incomplete cases of Kawasaki disease can occur, particularly in infants less than 1 year of age. These children are found to have coronary aneurysms without an antecedent history of obvious Kawasaki disease, and have a high rate of complications.

Therapy includes the use of intravenous **gamma globulin** and **salicylate** during the acute phase of the disease. Treatment results in the amelioration of symptoms and, if initiated early in the course of disease, in the prevention of coronary artery aneurysms. Children with Kawasaki disease should be followed up with echocardiograms to detect changes in coronary artery involvement.

## Henoch-Schönlein Purpura

Henoch-Schönlein purpura (HSP) or anaphylactoid purpura is a vasculitis involving small blood vessels. The cause is unknown, but Henoch-Schönlein purpura commonly follows an upper respiratory tract infection or exposure to a drug or allergen. The disease usually occurs in children between the ages of 2 to 8 years and is more common in boys than in girls.

The condition affects the skin, kidneys, joints, and gastrointestinal tract. Children with Henoch-Schönlein purpura present with nonthrombocytopenic purpura, which has a distinctive peripheral distribution over the posterior legs and buttocks. Edema of the scalp, eyelids, hands, and feet may be present. These children may also have colicky abdominal pain, accompanied by gross or occult gastrointestinal bleeding. Occasionally, they develop an acute intussusception secondary to edema and hemorrhage in the intestinal wall. Microscopic hematuria and other signs of glomerulonephritis, as well as arthritis of the large joints and especially the knees and ankles, may also be present. Rarely, seizures and other evidence of central nervous system involvement occur.

The **prognosis** of Henoch-Schönlein purpura is **excellent**. Most children recover within a few weeks or months. However, those with signs of renal involvement may develop chronic renal disease. The treatment of this condition is symptomatic and supportive. Children with severe forms of acute disease, such as gastrointestinal hemorrhage, may benefit from corticosteroid therapy.

# Chapter 14

# Disorders of the Gastrointestinal System

## ESOPHAGEAL FOREIGN BODIES

**Esophageal foreign bodies** commonly lodge in one of three anatomic areas where the esophagus narrows. Children with esophageal foreign bodies present with cough, drooling, and choking. If the foreign body is not detected early, an inflammatory reaction can cause esophageal obstruction and, rarely, compress the airway.

Foreign bodies that require careful medical attention are batteries and sharp objects, such as needles and open safety pins. Coins in the esophagus are almost always seen on edge in a lateral radiograph; when seen on edge in an anterior-posterior radiograph, they are more likely to be in the trachea because of its "U-shaped" cartilaginous structure. Many foreign bodies will safely pass within 24 hours. Objects trapped in the esophagus should be removed by esophagoscopy. It is not necessary to follow the expulsion of most foreign bodies with frequent serial radiographs. Most objects that enter the stomach safely pass through the gastrointestinal tract.

## GASTROESOPHAGEAL REFLUX

**Gastroesophageal reflux** is common in infants and usually is benign and resolves spontaneously as the child grows. Therapies for mild reflux in infants include upright posture during feeding, thickening milk with cereals, and frequent burping.

The few infants and young children with severe reflux may develop failure to thrive and have recurrent episodes of aspiration pneumonia. **Chronic esophagitis** results in blood loss and iron deficiency anemia.

Radiographic examination with a barium swallow can demonstrate anatomic abnormalities such as a **hiatal hernia**. Because reflux is episodic, continuous monitoring of esophageal pH is useful in some cases. The pharmacologic agents metoclopramide and cisapride may be of some benefit in moderate to severe reflux. In severe instances of infants with recurrent aspiration pneumonia, surgical correction may be required.

# PYLORIC STENOSIS

**Pyloric stenosis**, which is due to hypertrophy of the pyloric sphincter and stomach antrum, causes **partial obstruction of the stomach**. Pyloric stenosis is more common in males than females and tends to be familial. The condition presents in the second or third week of life with projectile nonbilious vomiting, failure to thrive, and dehydration. After vomiting, the infant appears hungry and is anxious to feed again.

On examination, a small hard mass may be palpated about midway between the umbilicus and the costal margin at the lateral border of the right rectus muscle. The mass is most easily palpated after vomiting. Peristaltic waves, which begin at the left costal margin and pass toward the midepigastric region, may also be observed.

On ultrasonography, a "doughnut" or "target" sign is seen, which confirms the diagnosis. Because of the protracted vomiting, hypochloremic alkalosis and hypokalemia are frequently present.

The prognosis for children with pyloric stenosis is excellent following surgical **pyloromyotomy**. However, surgery should be delayed until fluid and electrolyte disturbances have been corrected.

# MECKEL'S DIVERTICULUM

**Meckel's diverticulum**, a remnant of the vitelline duct, is a several centimeter diverticulum of the ileum that occurs in 2% to 3% of people. Some Meckel's diverticula contain ectopic gastric or pancreatic mucosa and present with acute, painless, **rectal bleeding** caused by erosion of the mucosa of the diverticulum. Rectal bleeding is the most common complication of a Meckel's diverticulum.

A $^{99m}$technetium scan identifies ectopic gastric mucosa within the diverticulum. If the diverticulum retains its connection with the umbilicus, children may present with acute intestinal obstruction or volvulus. If the diverticulum is in the form of a vermiform appendage to the small intestine, children may present with symptoms that are identical to acute appendicitis. For that reason, a Meckel's diverticulum is always considered during surgery for appendicitis. Other complications include intussusception and herniation (Littre hernia). The treatment for these conditions involves surgical removal of the diverticulum. When the vitelline duct remains patent, an **omphalomesenteric duct** results, connecting the umbilicus with the intestine.

## MALROTATION

**Malrotation** is the incomplete rotation of small and large intestine during fetal development. Malrotation creates conditions for both obstruction and volvulus. With the cecum displaced from its normal position in the right lower quadrant, bands anchoring it can obstruct the duodenum. In addition, the small intestine is then suspended by a narrow pedicle and is prone to volvulus.

Malrotation may present with symptoms of acute or intermittent gastrointestinal obstruction, including **abdominal pain** and **bilious vomiting**. Intestinal volvulus is a surgical emergency because gangrene rapidly ensues. The diagnosis of malrotation and volvulus is made by radiographic examination of the abdomen in which the normal colonic gas pattern is misplaced. Barium enema confirms the abnormally positioned cecum. Upper gastrointestinal radiographic studies show the ligament of Treitz displaced to the right.

## INTUSSUSCEPTION

**Intussusception** is a condition in which one portion of the intestine telescopes or invaginates into another, most commonly the distal ileum into the proximal colon. Intussusception is found most often in boys and in children under the age of 3 years. In less than 10% of cases an identifiable cause such as Meckel's diverticulum, polyp, or Henoch-Schönlein purpura is found.

Typically, children with intussusception present with the abrupt onset of cramping abdominal pain, vomiting, and blood and mucus in the stool ("currant jelly stools"). Irritability and lethargy may be the only prominent symptoms in some children. A tender, sausage-shaped mass can be palpated, most often in the right upper quadrant.

Intussusception can be reduced using the hydrostatic pressure of barium introduced into the rectum and colon, a procedure that is both diagnostic and therapeutic. After barium enema, a coiled-spring appearance of the involved intestine is the characteristic appearance. However, if this maneuver is not successful, or if there is prolonged intussusception or evidence of intestinal perforation, immediate surgery is required. **Untreated intussusception is fatal**.

## ACUTE APPENDICITIS

**Acute appendicitis,** the most common condition requiring abdominal surgery in children, is caused by obstruction of the lumen from a fecalith or calculi or by edema from a bacterial or viral infection. This obstruction causes inflammation, ischemia, and necrosis of the appendix. Appendicitis rarely occurs in a child less than 2 years of age, but when it occurs, the diagnosis is frequently missed until the appendix has ruptured and classic signs of generalized peritonitis have developed.

Children usually present with cramping, **periumbilical pain**, which with time localizes to the site of the appendix, usually the right lower quadrant. If the appendix is not located in the right lower quadrant, the diagnosis is more difficult. Peritoneal pain typically is worse with movement. Other signs and symptoms of appendicitis include fever, anorexia, and vomiting. **Diarrhea** may be present as a result from irritation of the colon by the inflamed appendix. **Pyuria** can be caused by irritation of the bladder from inflammation. Leukocytosis is characteristic but not diagnostic of appendicitis.

The treatment is emergency appendectomy with preoperative antibiotic therapy. In girls, peritonitis from a ruptured appendix can cause inflammatory obstruction of the fallopian tubes and infertility.

## ACUTE GASTROENTERITIS

**Acute gastroenteritis** is one of the most frequent causes of death in children in underdeveloped countries. With the improvement in sanitation and nutrition in the industrialized countries, the mortality rate from gastroenteritis has been reduced markedly. Most children can be managed at home with careful monitoring of fluid intake and of losses due to diarrhea and vomiting. Children with **significant dehydration** require hospitalization and supervised oral rehydration or parenteral administration of fluids.

Acute gastroenteritis may be due to viral, bacterial, or parasitic infection.

### Viral Gastroenteritis

In the United States, viruses cause 30% to 40% of all cases of infectious diarrhea; in 40% of episodes of acute gastroenteritis, the cause is unknown. Five categories of viral gastroenteritis have been identified: rotavirus, enteric adenovirus, calicivirus, astrovirus, and Norwalk virus. **Rotavirus** (specifically group A) is the major cause of

**severe diarrhea** in infants and young children. In the United States, the peak incidence of rotavirus infection occurs between 3 to 15 months of age and during the winter months. Infants less than 3 months of age are most likely protected by passively acquired maternal antibodies.

Infected children present with fever, vomiting, watery diarrhea, and dehydration. Bloody mucoid diarrhea is not a feature of rotavirus infection. Detection of rotaviral antigens in the stool can be used to confirm the diagnosis. Treatment is with oral or parenteral rehydration solutions.

Enteric **adenoviruses** are probably the second most common viral cause of acute gastroenteritis in children. Caliciviruses and astroviruses have been documented to cause outbreaks of diarrhea in children. Norwalk viruses are more commonly associated with epidemics of acute gastroenteritis in adults and older children.

## Bacterial Gastroenteritis

Bacterial causes of acute gastroenteritis are numerous. The most common etiologic agents in children are *Campylobacter jejuni*, *Salmonella enteritidis*, *Shigella* species, pathogenic *Escherichia coli* and *Yersinia enterocolitica*. Children with bacterial (unlike viral) gastroenteritis are more likely to present with high fever, abdominal pain, tenesmus, and the presence of blood, mucus, and leukocytes in the stool. The etiologic agent can be identified by stool culture, although the diagnosis of pathogenic *E. coli* requires special laboratory tests.

Many authorities recommend **antibiotics** for children with gastroenteritis caused by *Shigella* and *Campylobacter*. Children with nontyphoidal salmonella gastroenteritis do not require antibiotics; however, **infants less than 3 months of age** and immunocompromised children should be treated with **antibiotics** because of the risk of disseminated infection.

*Giardia lamblia* is the most common parasitic cause of diarrhea in children in the United States. Outbreaks are not infrequent in day-care centers. Cryptosporidium can also cause outbreaks of gastroenteritis in day-care centers and in human immunodeficiency virus (HIV)-infected children.

# ENZYME DEFICIENCIES

**Disaccharidase deficiencies,** the brush border enzymes that hydrolyze sugars, are most common following gastrointestinal infections. The accumulation of intestinal sugar results in a watery, osmotic diarrhea and bacterial production of organic acids, which lower the stool pH (pH less than 6.0) and cause excoriation of the buttocks. Although **lactase deficiency** is a common transient abnormality of the brush border following acute gastroenteritis, most children with gastroenteritis do not require a lactose-free formula. Because lactose is a reducing sugar, its presence in the stool may be detected by the Clinitest method.

Congenital **lactase deficiency** is extremely rare, despite the widespread use of lactose-free formulas. The development of lactase deficiency is common in adults, particularly in people of African descent.

# FOOD ALLERGIES

**Cow's milk protein allergy** is a rare, usually transitory, allergic response to cow's milk. Gastrointestinal, respiratory, and dermatologic symptoms have been attributed to cow's milk allergy. Classic gastrointestinal symptoms are diarrhea, protein-losing enteropathy, and intestinal blood loss. Symptoms resolve when cow's milk is removed from the diet; however, a causal relationship is often difficult to prove. Children intolerant of cow's milk protein are frequently also intolerant of soy protein.

**Celiac disease**, or gluten sensitive enteropathy, is an immune-mediated, intestinal **intolerance of gliadin**, found in the cereals wheat, rye, and barley. Affected children usually present with failure to thrive, irritability, diarrhea, and vomiting, but the clinical picture is variable. The diagnosis is made by upper small intestinal biopsy and a trial of a gluten free diet. Therapy involves the dietary restriction of gluten containing cereals.

# CROHN'S DISEASE

**Crohn's disease**, or regional enteritis, begins in late childhood and adolescence in 25% to 40% of affected persons. This chronic segmental, inflammatory process may involve **any portion of the gastrointestinal tract** from mouth to anus, with the distal ileum and colon most frequently involved. Children or adolescents with Crohn's disease present with cramping, abdominal pain, diarrhea, and poor growth as well as fever, malaise, and perianal disease. Extraintestinal disease, especially arthritis, is common and may be the presenting illness. The disease follows a course of exacerbations and remissions.

Contrast studies of the gastrointestinal tract demonstrate a classic "cobblestone" appearance of the mucosa, skip lesions, and enteric fistulas. Biopsy of colonic mucosa reveals granulomas. Treatment involves steroid therapy, occasional bowel rest, and intensive support of the child and family.

## ULCERATIVE COLITIS

Approximately 20% of patients with **ulcerative colitis** have the onset of disease in childhood and adolescence. When the disease begins in childhood, it tends to be extensive and severe. The disease process is **restricted to the mucosa**, in contrast to Crohn's disease, which involves the entire intestinal wall, and begins in the rectum and extends proximally. The **entire colon** can be involved. Affected children present with cramping, lower abdominal pain and bloody diarrhea. **Arthritis** may be present in a small proportion of children. The diagnosis is confirmed by colonoscopy.

Toxic megacolon is a serious complication that can lead to perforation and sepsis. Patients with ulcerative colitis are at high risk of subsequent carcinoma of the colon. Therapy is with sulfasalazine, corticosteroids, and for severe disease, surgical resection.

## INDIRECT INGUINAL HERNIAS

**Indirect inguinal hernias** occur in 1% to 3% of children, with 90% occurring in boys. Girls with an inguinal hernia should be suspected of having testicular feminization syndrome, which is found in approximately 1% to 2% of girls with inguinal hernias. Indirect inguinal hernias result from a failure of the proximal part of the processus vaginalis to close in late fetal life. Thus, premature infants are at high risk. In boys, the hernial sac may extend to the tunica vaginalis, the remainder of the processus vaginalis covering the testicle.

Children present with inguinal swelling due to the movement of small intestine into the hernial sac. The swelling may increase in size with increased abdominal pressure, such as crying or coughing, and may resolve when the child relaxes. In girls, the ovary is likely to herniate into the inguinal canal. The treatment is herniorrhaphy. Emergency herniorrhaphy should be performed when the hernia cannot be reduced, an **incarcerated hernia**. However, with time, an experienced physician can reduce most hernias. An incarcerated hernia, although uncommon, can cause venous infarction of the testicle and intestinal obstruction, and is most frequent in the first year of life.

# Chapter 15

# Genitourinary and Renal Disorders

## GENITOURINARY DISORDERS

### Congenital Anomalies

*Phimosis*

The penile foreskin is normally adherent to the glans penis until the age of 3 years. Phimosis is a condition in which the foreskin is adherent after age three. Phimosis may require circumcision, but mild degrees can often be managed with periodic, gentle retraction and patient education on proper hygiene. Good hygiene reduces the risk of inflammatory phimosis. Paraphimosis occurs when the foreskin becomes retracted beyond the coronal sulcus and cannot be reduced.

*Hypospadias*

Hypospadias is a relatively common spectrum of congenital anomalies of the position of the urethral meatus ranging from mild malposition, in which the urethral meatus opens on the ventral surface of the glans, to meatal positions on the penile shaft, penoscrotal junction, or perineum. More severe forms are associated with **chordee**, ventral curvature of the penis. Inguinal hernias and undescended testes are associated with hypospadias. Because the foreskin is crucial for repair, boys with hypospadias should not undergo routine circumcision.

*Hydroceles*

Hydroceles are collections of fluid within the tunica vaginalis which are relatively common in infants, particularly premature infants, and generally resolve spontaneously. Hydroceles are also found in boys with indirect inguinal hernias. In this instance, the size of the hydrocele changes because of the direct connection with the peritoneal cavity.

## PEDIATRICS

### *Undescended Testes*

Undescended testes, especially common in premature infants, is caused by a halt in the normal embryonic migration of the testis into the scrotum, which takes place during the seventh month of gestation. The processus vaginalis is patent, and an indirect inguinal hernia coexists. When the testicle is diverted, usually lateral to the external inguinal canal, **ectopic testes** result. In both cases, testes cannot not be palpated within the scrotum. Cryptorchidism is bilateral in one third of cases of boys with cryptorchidism. The complications of this condition include **testicular malignancy** (seminoma), **infertility**, and **incarceration of the associated inguinal hernia**. Early surgical correction, orchiopexy, reduces the risk of infertility.

Many boys have **retractile testes**, which at times can be brought into the scrotal sac but at other times lodge between the inguinal ring and the scrotum. Retractile testes do not require surgical correction.

### *Testicular Torsion*

Testicular torsion results from an inadequate fixation of the testicle by the tunica vaginalis, which allows the testicle to rotate and occlude its vascular supply. Boys with testicular torsion present with the acute onset of pain and swelling of the involved testicle. Doppler studies and nuclear medicine scans can assist with the diagnosis; however, **surgical exploration should not be delayed more than 6 hours**. The defect is often bilateral, and the contralateral testicle should be repaired at the time of surgery.

**Torsion of the testicular appendix**, which may cause localized tenderness and a "blue dot" sign at the site of the testicular appendix, may be confused with testicular torsion.

### *Vesicoureteral Reflux*

**Primary vesicoureteral reflux** results from **valvular incompetence** at the ureterovesical junction due to a shortened segment of ureter within the bladder wall, the segment that normally closes as a result of bladder muscle contraction during voiding. This valvular incompetence exposes the kidney to bacteria and high pressure. Vesicoureteral reflux is often associated with other genitourinary anomalies.

In anomalous double collecting systems, the reflux usually occurs in the lower ureter. Secondary vesicoureteral reflux may also be found with bladder dysfunction or infection. Vesicoureteral reflux is frequently diagnosed by voiding cystourethrogram in children with a urinary tract infection. Mild vesicoureteral reflux resolves without treatment; however, urinary tract infection must be prevented with prophylactic antibiotics.

Significant reflux results in dilatation of the ureters and renal pelvis and, when associated with infection, with renal scarring and **reflux nephropathy**. Reflux nephropathy is a major cause of hypertension and chronic renal failure in children and adolescents. Renal scarring can be diagnosed by nuclear medicine scan; small kidneys can be documented on ultrasonography. Severe grades of vesicoureteral reflux require surgical reimplantation of the ureters.

### *Urinary Tract Obstruction*

Urinary tract obstruction in infants and children is usually due to congenital anomalies of the genitourinary tract. Obstruction can occur anywhere from the renal pelvis to the urethra and is characterized by dilatation of the collecting system proximal to the site of obstruction. In girls, the most common site of obstruction is at the ureteropelvic junction (renal pelvis). The vesicoureteral junction is another common site of obstruction.

Urinary tract obstruction, particularly when unilateral, is frequently asymptomatic, or a urinary tract infection may be the first manifestation of obstruction. In the neonate severe, bilateral intrauterine obstruction causes oligohydramnios, pulmonary hypoplasia, and Potter syndrome. An abdominal mass in a newborn is frequently caused by a hydronephrotic kidney. Older children with hydronephrosis may present with flank pain or hematuria.

### *Posterior Urethral Valves*

In boys, **posterior urethral valves**, membranes that obstruct the posterior urethra, are the most common cause of obstruction. Posterior urethral valves are associated with vesicoureteral reflux and reflux nephropathy.

Infant boys with posterior urethral valves may present with a weak urinary stream and distended bladder. Older boys with posterior urethral valves present with urinary tract infection and daytime enuresis. The resulting dilatation of the ureters mimics radiographically severe forms of vesicoureteral reflux; the two are distinguished by voiding cystourethrography.

### *Chronic Obstruction*

Chronic obstruction results in **renal failure and obstructive uropathy**. Because of tubular dysfunction, children with renal failure secondary to obstructive uropathy frequently have polyuria rather than oliguria. Other nonspecific signs of renal failure in an infant or young child include failure to thrive and vomiting.

Severe urethral obstruction can result in **prune-belly syndrome** (Eagle-Barrett syndrome), characterized by genitourinary abnormalities (hydronephrosis, renal dysplasia, and patent urachus), deficient abdominal muscles, and undescended testes. Many affected infants are stillborn or die in early infancy.

## Urinary Tract Infection

Urinary tract infection in infants is more common in boys and is due to preceding bacteremia. After infancy, urinary tract infection is more common in girls and results from ascending infection. Colonic bacteria, especially *Escherichia coli*, are the most common infecting organisms. Predisposing factors include vesicoureteral reflux, urinary tract obstruction, and renal calculi.

**Infants** with urinary tract infection may present with fever, vomiting, diarrhea, and jaundice. The jaundice is due to impaired bilirubin conjugation by *E. coli*. Older children present with classic signs and symptoms of cystitis (frequency, dysuria, and enuresis) or pyelonephritis (fever and flank tenderness). Asymptomatic bacteriuria is common in school-age girls.

The **diagnosis** is confirmed by culture of bacteria from the urine. Suprapubic puncture and catheterization are techniques used to obtain sterile urine specimens in infants and children. Specimens obtained from urine collection bags are frequently contaminated. Infants suspected of a urinary tract infection should also have a blood culture. Because pyuria can occur in the absence of urinary tract infection and urinary tract infection can occur without pyuria, the diagnosis should not be based solely on the presence or absence of leukocytes in the urine.

Because urinary tract infection is frequently the initial manifestation of these predisposing factors, children with urinary tract infection should undergo an evaluation of the genitourinary tract. Ultrasonography detects hydronephrosis, obstructive lesions, abscesses, and determines renal size, which is an indicator of chronic renal scarring. Voiding cystourethrography detects vesicoureteral reflux.

Differentiation of cystitis and pyelonephritis can be difficult, particularly in young children. Nuclear medicine scans and computerized tomography can be used to diagnose pyelonephritis.

**Infants** with urinary tract infection should be treated with **parenteral antibiotics**, the same treatment used in treating bacteremia.

**Older children** with urinary tract infection can be treated with **oral antibiotics**. A repeat urine culture should be obtained 1 week after treatment to document resolution.

Because of the frequency of recurrence in children, periodic urine cultures should be obtained, even in the absence of signs and symptoms. Children with recurrent urinary tract infections, vesicoureteral reflux, obstruction, or neurogenic bladder should receive antibiotic prophylaxis.

# RENAL DISEASE

Inadequate urine production during the fetal period results in oligohydramnios, which is associated with **Potter syndrome** and pulmonary hypoplasia. Potter syndrome consists of a combination of anomalies including epicanthal folds, low-set ears, flat nose, receding chin, and limb anomalies.

Although hematuria is a common manifestation of renal disease in children, most children with transient hematuria have no underlying renal pathology. Some children with hematuria have **idiopathic hypercalcuria**, defined as urinary calcium excretion of more than 4 mg/kg/day. Methods to distinguish glomerular from nonglomerular hematuria are listed in Table 15-1.

Nonpathologic proteinuria occurs in children with fever and with exercise (exercise-induced proteinuria) and in some older children with **orthostatic proteinuria.** Orthostatic proteinuria is a benign syndrome of unknown cause in which protein is found in urine collected when the child is upright and active but not when the child has been supine for a period of time.

## Alport Syndrome

Alport syndrome is the most common form of **hereditary nephritis**. It is much more severe in boys than in girls, suggesting an X-linked dominant mode of transmission in some cases. Children present with microscopic hematuria or episodes of gross hematuria. Sensorineural hearing loss and ocular defects, including cataracts, are associated with the syndrome. Boys with Alport syndrome may develop chronic renal failure in adolescence or early adulthood.

## Polycystic Kidney Disease

Autosomal recessive polycystic kidney disease, also called infantile polycystic disease, is a hereditary cystic disease of the **kidneys and liver**. Signs and symptoms of renal disease, which are not always

**TABLE 15-1.**

**Differentiation of Glomerular and Nonglomerular Hema-**

| Glomerular Hematuria | Urologic Hematuria |
|---|---|
| RBC casts | No RBC casts |
| Proteinuria | No proteinuria |
| Brown urine | Red urine |
| Never clots | Clots |
| Persistent | Sporadic or persistent |
| Throughout stream | Partial stream |
| RBC MCV <72 | RBC MCV >80 |

*MCV = mean corpuscular volume; RBC = red blood cells.*

detected in infancy, include bilateral renal masses, hematuria, hypertension, renal insufficiency, and ultimately chronic renal failure. The diagnosis is made by intravenous pyelogram and renal biopsy. The disease is also associated with congenital hepatic fibrosis, which can cause cirrhosis. Autosomal dominant polycystic kidney disease is rare in children.

## Acute Poststreptococcal Glomerulonephritis

Acute poststreptococcal glomerulonephritis (APSGN), which is characterized by the acute onset of edema, hypertension, gross hematuria, and renal insufficiency, is one of the nonsuppurative complications of group A beta-hemolytic streptococcal infection. Streptococcal pharyngitis precedes the onset of glomerulonephritis by 1 to 2 weeks; streptococcal skin infections have a latent period of 2 to 3 weeks. In contrast to rheumatic fever, early treatment of streptococcal infection does not prevent glomerulonephritis. The specific pathologic mechanism of acute streptococcal nephritis is not completely understood, but the condition probably represents an immunologic reaction to "nephritogenic" strains of group A beta-hemolytic streptococci, resulting in immune complex deposition within glomeruli.

Children with acute glomerulonephritis present with fever, lethargy, edema, hypertension, congestive heart failure, abdominal pain, and encephalopathy. Laboratory evaluation reveals hematuria, azotemia, elevated antistreptolysin O antibodies, and decreased levels of complement, particularly C3. Following skin infection, a rise in antibody titers to anti-DNase B is a more sensitive measure of preceding streptococcal infection.

Low serum complement levels are also found in membranoproliferative glomerulonephritis (MPGN) and systemic lupus erythematosus (SLE), but the hypocomplementemia in APSGN usually resolves by 8 weeks; persistence beyond this period should suggest another hypocomplementemic glomerulonephritis, particularly MPGN.

Acute poststreptococcal glomerulonephritis usually has a benign course. Most children recover within several weeks; however, microscopic hematuria can continue for as long as 2 years. Episodic hypertension during the acute phase can be severe and is a reason for hospitalization. Acute postinfectious glomerulonephritis may follow infections with organisms other than group A streptococci.

## IgA Nephropathy

IgA nephropathy, or **Berger disease**, is characterized pathologically by IgA deposition in the mesangium. Children, more often boys, present with microscopic hematuria or episodic gross hematuria. Complement levels are normal. One fifth of affected children develop chronic renal disease. The majority, however, have normal renal function with the exception of hematuria. The pathologic feature of IgA deposition is similar to the renal lesion in **Henoch-Schönlein purpura** in which the majority of children have only mild hematuria and proteinuria.

## Hemolytic-Uremic Syndrome

Hemolytic-uremic syndrome (**HUS**) is the most common cause of acute renal failure due to intrinsic kidney disease in children younger than 4 years old. It is characterized by anemia, thrombocytopenia, and acute renal failure. HUS is associated with a **preceding upper respiratory infection** or **bacterial or viral gastroenteritis**, especially due to *E. coli* 0157:H7.

Characterized pathologically by endothelial cell damage, red blood cells fragment as they pass through damaged vessels, causing a microangiopathic hemolytic anemia. The renal disease is characterized by hematuria, proteinuria, and acute renal failure with oliguria and azotemia. Intravascular coagulation may result in seizures or colitis. With supportive therapy most children recover normal renal function.

## Nephrosis

### Nephrotic Syndrome

The nephrotic syndrome is characterized by edema, proteinuria, hypoproteinemia, and hyperlipidemia. Typically, the child with nephrosis presents with the gradual onset of edema, which is often periorbital and dependent in distribution. Ascites, pleural effusions, and massive scrotal edema may also be seen. Children with nephrotic syndrome are at great risk of bacterial infections, particularly pneumococcal peritonitis.

The diagnosis is confirmed by documenting nephrotic range proteinuria, hypoalbuminemia, and hypercholesterolemia. Children with nephrosis have proteinuria of more than 1000 mg/m$^2$/day and hypoalbuminemia of less than 2.5 gm/dL.

### Minimal-Change Disease

Most children with nephrotic syndrome have minimal-change disease, a term used to describe the relative lack of pathologic findings on examination of renal biopsy material by light microscopy. Loss of epithelial foot processes can be seen by electron microscopy. The condition is more common in boys and in children between the ages of 2 to 6 years. Kidney biopsy is not indicated for children less than 8 years of age with typical features.

Children with minimal-change nephrosis are treated with corticosteroids to induce remission of the edema and proteinuria and to reduce the danger of infectious complications. With steroid therapy, the prognosis for children with minimal-change disease is excellent. The typical course is one of relapses until spontaneous remission occurs in late adolescence. One third of affected children never have a second relapse. Because of the danger of pneumococcal infections, especially pneumonococcal peritonitis, these children should receive the pneumococcal vaccine after a second relapse.

## Membranoproliferative Glomerulonephritis

Membranoproliferative glomerulonephritis is less common and is usually found in children older than 8 years of age. Patients may present with the nephrotic syndrome. For that reason, a renal biopsy is indicated for more precise diagnosis in older children and adolescents with this clinical syndrome.

## Renal Calculi

Children with **urolithiasis** present with hematuria, colicky flank pain, and urinary tract infection. Radiopaque calcium stones, which are most common in children in the United States, are due to hypercalcuria (greater than 4 mg Ca/kg/day) and can be diagnosed by abdominal radiograph.

Radiolucent uric acid stones are common in some parts of the world. Uric acid stones also occur in children treated for malignancies and those with **Lesch-Nyhan syndrome**, an inborn error of purine metabolism. Urinary tract infections caused by such urea splitting organisms as *Proteus* can produce an alkaline urine and the precipitation of struvite stones. Radiolucent cystine stones are found in cystinuria, an inborn error of metabolism. Radiolucent renal stones require ultrasonography or computerized tomography scan for diagnosis.

## Acute Renal Failure

In young children with diarrhea and dehydration, acute renal failure is often prerenal in origin and transient. The **fractional excretion of sodium** is a useful measure to differentiate prerenal from intrinsic renal failure. Other useful tests are listed in Table 15-2. The fractional excretion of sodium is the percentage of filtered sodium excreted in the urine and is calculated as:

$$\frac{\text{urine sodium}}{\text{serum sodium}} \times \frac{\text{serum creatinine}}{\text{urine creatinine}} \times 100$$

A fractional excretion of sodium of less than 1.0 suggests avid retention of sodium, decreased renal blood flow, and prerenal failure. A fractional excretion of sodium more than 2.0 suggests intrinsic renal failure.

**TABLE 15-2.**

**Acute Renal Failure: Differentiation of Prerenal Causes from Intrinsic Renal Disease**

|              | Prerenal | Intrinsic Renal Disease |
|--------------|----------|-------------------------|
| uOsm         | >500     | <300                    |
| uNa          | <20      | >40                     |
| FENa         | <1       | >2                      |
| Urine pH     | <6       | >6                      |
| uOsm/Posm    | >1.1     | <1.0                    |

*uOsm = urine osmolality; uNa = urinary sodium concentration; FENa = fractional excretion of sodium in the urine; Posm = plasma osmolality.*

*Postrenal failure is due to obstructive lesions or vesicoureteral reflux and can usually be diagnosed by ultrasonogram.*

The **glomerular filtration rate** (GFR), another measure of acute or chronic renal failure, can be estimated in children using the weight in kilograms, serum creatinine level, and the following formula:

$$\frac{\text{weight (kg)}}{\text{serum creatinine}} \times K = \text{GFR}$$

where K is 0.45 for infants less than 12 months of age and 0.55 for children up to 12 years of age. The GFR is expressed in mL/min/1.73 m$^2$.

# Renal Acidosis

## Renal Tubular Acidosis

Renal tubular acidosis (RTA), a defect in the acidification of urine, exists as three types: distal renal tubular acidosis (**type I**), proximal renal tubular acidosis (**type II**), and mineralocorticoid deficiency (**type IV**). The plasma bicarbonate level is low, and the children have a metabolic acidosis with a normal anion gap in all three types. The urine pH is low in types II and IV and high in type I RTA. Hyperkalemia is present in mineralocorticoid deficiency, while the serum potassium is low in types I and II.

## Proximal Renal Tubular Acidosis

Proximal RTA is more common in infants and is caused by a decreased proximal tubule threshold for bicarbonate with bicarbonate wasting. Normal infants have a lower renal tubular bicarbonate threshold than adults (18 mEq/L compared with 24 mEq/L in adults), but the threshold is decreased further in infants with proximal RTA (14 to 16 mEq/L). Infants with this defect usually present with failure to thrive.

Proximal RTA can be primary or associated with a number of other renal tubular disorders (**Fanconi syndrome**), including glucosuria, phosphaturia, and aminoaciduria. Galactosemia, hereditary fructose intolerance, tyrosinemia, Wilson disease, cystinosis (accumulation of cystine), and oculocerebrorenal (Lowe) syndrome (mental retardation, cataracts, glaucoma) represent secondary causes of proximal RTA and Fanconi syndrome. Proximal RTA is treated with bicarbonate supplementation.

# Chapter 16

# Immunologic and Rheumatologic Disorders

## PRIMARY IMMUNODEFICIENCIES

### Humoral Immunity Deficiencies

Deficiencies of **humoral immunity**, mediated by B cells, are characterized by pyogenic infections. Children with defects of cell-mediated immunity, regulated by T cells, often have **opportunistic infections**. However, because T cells play a critical role in regulating the immune response, T-cell defects can also result in deficiencies of humoral immunity.

#### X-Linked Agammaglobulinemia

X-linked agammaglobulinemia (**Bruton's disease**) is a genetic defect due to mutations in a cytoplasmic signal-transducing molecule that results in the lack of B cells and low or absent levels of IgG, IgA, and IgM. Passively acquired maternal IgG protects affected boys during the first year of life. Subsequently, these children present with frequent episodes of otitis media, sinusitis, pneumonia, and skin infections, usually due to *Streptococcus pneumoniae* and *Haemophilus influenzae*. Severe and persistent viral infections and arthritis may also occur. Recurrent episodes of pneumonia lead to chronic lung disease. Treatment consists of regular infusions of intravenous immune globulin.

#### IgA Deficiency

Children with IgA deficiency are often asymptomatic, but may have frequent respiratory tract infections and gastroenteritis. IgA deficiency is associated with autoimmune diseases and **IgG subclass deficiencies**. The clinical manifestations of children with IgG subclass deficiencies vary considerably, and many children are also asymptomatic. Children with deficiency of IgG2, the subclass important for humoral immunity against polysaccharide antigens, may be susceptible to bacterial infection with such encapsulated organisms as *S. pneumoniae* and *H. influenzae* type b.

*Common Variable Immunodeficiency*

Common variable immunodeficiency is used to describe a heterogenous group of disorders of antibody formation. B cells, although present, are immature and fail to produce antibodies, perhaps because of a defect in T-cell regulation. In the most common form, the disease presents during late childhood or adolescence with recurrent bacterial infections of the sinuses and lungs. Some patients develop opportunistic infections, recurrent herpes virus infections, lymphadenopathy, malabsorption, and malignancies.

## Severe Combined Immunodeficiency

Children with severe combined immunodeficiency (**SCID**) present early in infancy with failure to thrive, thrush, candidal diaper dermatitis, diarrhea, and such opportunistic infections as *Pneumocystis carinii* pneumonia. The most common form is X-linked, and results from genetic mutations of the interleukin receptors vital to the stimulation and differentiation of both T cells and B cells. Other forms are inherited as autosomal recessive disorders and are due to enzyme deficiencies, including adenosine deaminase. Affected children have marked lymphopenia, an absent thymus, dysfunctional B cells, and no cellular immunity. Treatment requires early recognition and bone marrow transplantation.

*Adenosine deaminase deficiency* has been successfully treated with gene therapy.

## DiGeorge Anomaly

DiGeorge anomaly is characterized by varying combinations of thymic abnormalities resulting in T-cell dysfunction, hypoparathyroidism, characteristic facies, congenital heart disease (coarctation of the aorta and truncus arteriosus), and genitourinary tract abnormalities. Newborns may present with hypocalcemic tetany. The immunodeficiency is usually mild and involves T-cell dysfunction and impaired immunoglobulin synthesis as a result of deficient T-helper function. Normal immune function usually develops later in life.

## Wiskott-Aldrich Syndrome

Wiskott-Aldrich syndrome is an **X-linked recessive disorder** characterized by repeated infections (both pyogenic and opportunistic), eczema, and thrombocytopenia. Severe thrombocytopenia occurs early in life and existing platelets are small. Serum IgM levels are diminished. Although levels of other immunoglobulin classes are normal or elevated, the antibody response to specific antigens is poor. T-cell numbers progressively decrease. Affected boys are prone to chronic otitis media, recurrent pneumonia, and malignancies. Some children have been successfully treated with bone marrow transplantation.

## Ataxia-Telangiectasia

Ataxia-telangiectasia is an autosomal recessive disorder characterized by progressive cerebellar ataxia, telangiectasia of the sclerae and skin, and a picture of mixed cellular and humoral deficiency. Children are prone to recurrent pneumonia, sinusitis, and lymphoma. The gene for ataxia-telangiectasia has been identified, and there is evidence that heterozygotes are at increased risk of malignancy.

## White Cell Immune Deficiencies

**Chronic granulomatous disease (CGD)** is a genetic condition, usually X-linked, and is characterized by impaired phagocytic function, specifically decreased production of superoxide anion, hydrogen peroxide, and hydroxyl radicals. The genetic defect in the X-linked form involves a component of the cytochrome b complex. Because of the defect in superoxide production, phagocytes from children with CGD cannot kill such catalase positive organisms as *Staphylococcus aureus*, *Serratia marcescens*, *Salmonella* species, *Pseudomonas* species, *Candida*, and *Aspergillus*. Catalase, the bacterial enzyme that breaks down hydrogen peroxide, is able to remove the hydrogen peroxide generated by bacterial metabolism, which could be used by host cells to destroy the bacteria. In contrast, catalase-negative organisms, such as streptococci and *H. influenzae*, are not typical pathogens for children with CGD.

Children present in the first 2 years of life with repeated bacterial infections: lymphadenitis, pneumonia, skin abscesses, and osteomyelitis. These children also have generalized lymphadenopathy and hepatosplenomegaly as well as granulomas and abscesses in lymph nodes, lungs, skin, bone, liver, and spleen. The diagnosis is confirmed by failure to reduce nitroblue tetrazolium (NBT test).

Children with CGD may benefit from long-term antibiotic prophylaxis with trimethoprim-sulfamethoxazole or gamma-interferon infusions.

Children with deficiencies of **early complement components** not only present with recurrent bacterial infections but also may have such autoimmune disorders as systemic lupus erythematosus (SLE). Children with deficiencies of **late complement components** (C6–C9) are prone to disseminated meningococcal and gonococcal infections.

# ACQUIRED IMMUNODEFICIENCIES

## Human Immunodeficiency Virus Infection

### Human Immunodeficiency Virus Type 1

Human immunodeficiency virus type 1 (**HIV-1**), the etiologic agent of the **acquired immunodeficiency syndrome (AIDS)**, is found in infants and children who are born to HIV-infected women or who have received HIV-contaminated blood or blood products. In some parts of the world, significant maternal-infant HIV transmission may occur through breast milk. In the United States, women and children form an increasing proportion of those infected with HIV. Risk factors for maternal HIV infection in the United States include intravenous drug use and sexual intercourse with men at risk of HIV infection.

Although all newborns born to HIV-infected women will be **HIV-antibody positive** because of the placental transfer of maternal antibody, in the United States only about 20% to 30% of these infants are infected with the virus; however, in some parts of the world the perinatal transmission rate may be as high as 40%.

Discrimination between newborns who are infected and those who are simply antibody-positive is not feasible at birth. Because the **passively acquired maternal antibody disappears at 15 to 18 months of age**, the presence of antibody to HIV beyond this age signifies infection. The techniques of HIV culture and polymerase chain reaction (PCR) can usually establish the presence of HIV infection within 3 to 6 months of life. **Detection of p24 antigen and anti-HIV IgA and IgM antibodies** in children less than 15 months of age have also been used with some success to establish the diagnosis.

The incubation period, from infection to disease, in perinatally infected children is much shorter than in adults. Some studies suggest two patterns of disease: one group presenting with severe symptoms early in infancy, and another group characterized by a later presentation of symptoms with a more chronic course.

*HIV infection can involve every organ system.* Infants with the disease commonly present with failure to thrive, persistent thrush, lymphadenopathy, hepatosplenomegaly, chronic diarrhea, anemia, and developmental delay. Infected children often have recurrent episodes of pneumonia, meningitis, sinusitis, and bacteremia. A defect in T-helper function to produce specific antibodies, even with elevated immunoglobulin levels, is probably the cause of the increased risk of bacterial infection.

**HIV-infected infants** are at **high risk** of the often fatal *P. carinii* pneumonia (**PCP**). Infants with PCP present with tachypnea, cough, and severe hypoxemia. Auscultatory findings may be minimal or absent. Chest radiographs typically show a diffuse alveolar infiltrate. PCP should be treated with trimethoprim-sulfamethoxazole (TMP-

SMX); children who cannot tolerate TMP-SMX can be treated with pentamidine. Some studies suggest a beneficial effect of early treatment with corticosteroids.

All newborns born to an HIV-infected woman should be placed on **trimethoprim-sulfamethoxazole prophylaxis** after the first month of life to protect them from *P. carinii* pneumonia. When the presence or absence of HIV infection is established, the prophylaxis can be discontinued for the uninfected group. Subsequent prophylactic therapy for PCP is based on the child's age and CD4 cell count.

**Lymphoid interstitial pneumonitis (LIP)** is a more indolent, chronic lung disease found in older HIV-infected children who present with wheezing and cough. On chest radiograph, a characteristic diffuse, nodular pattern is found. LIP frequently regresses with the development of marked lymphopenia in advanced HIV infection.

Other manifestations of pediatric HIV infection include skin infections, particularly varicella-zoster and candida; cardiomyopathy; and nephropathy, including the nephrotic syndrome.

**HIV encephalopathy**, which is not uncommon, presents with cognitive impairment, delayed development, and spasticity. Computerized tomography of the brain shows cortical atrophy and calcification of the basal ganglia. HIV-infected children rarely develop neoplasms such as lymphoma.

Children who survive to advanced AIDS with severe CD4 cell depletion are at risk for disseminated infection with *Mycobacterium avium*-complex as well as a wide variety of other opportunistic infections that may exist simultaneously.

The management of children infected with HIV includes vigorous therapy of infections, attention to nutrition, and support for the family and child. HIV-infected children, if possible, should attend school and otherwise be encouraged to lead as normal a life as possible. Treatment with monthly intravenous gamma globulin protects some children from serious bacterial infections. Zidovudine and other antiretroviral agents (DDI, DDC, ADD, 3TC) are also used for the treatment of HIV-infected children.

HIV-infected children should *not* receive live polio vaccine (OPV); instead, inactivated polio vaccine (IPV) should be administered. Other routine childhood vaccines should be given on schedule. HIV-infected children are also candidates for pneumococcal and influenza vaccines.

The primary prevention of pediatric HIV infection lies in the prevention of HIV infection in adolescent and adult women. Zidovudine therapy for HIV-infected women during pregnancy and delivery and for the infant until 6 weeks after birth substantially decreases the incidence of maternal-infant HIV transmission.

## Acquired Immunosuppression

Acquired immunosuppression can result from a variety of situations. Chemotherapy for the treatment of malignancy will cause children to become immunocompromised as a result of **neutropenia**. The underlying malignancy, especially **leukemia**, may contribute to the immunodeficiency. Children with organ transplantation and those receiving chronic, high-dose corticosteroids are also immunosuppressed. Those with organ transplantation are particularly prone to infection with cytomegalovirus (CMV), and those receiving corticosteroids are prone to disseminated varicella infection. Children with peripheral venous, arterial, and central venous catheters, urinary catheters, and those with cerebrospinal fluid shunts are at risk of bacterial and fungal infection.

Febrile children with absolute neutrophil counts less than $500/mm^3$ and especially those with counts less than $100/mm^3$ are at risk for serious and potentially fatal bacterial and fungal sepsis. In these situations, after cultures have been obtained, broad spectrum antibiotic therapy against both gram-positive and gram-negative organisms should be started empirically. Children who remain febrile and neutropenic despite antibiotics are at great risk of fungal sepsis, particularly with candida and aspergillus.

# RHEUMATOLOGIC DISORDERS

## Rheumatic Fever

Rheumatic fever is a systemic disease that represents a nonsuppurative complication of **group A beta-hemolytic streptococcal pharyngitis**. Early treatment of streptococcal pharyngitis, within 1 week of onset, prevents rheumatic fever and probably reduces the duration of symptoms. Unlike poststreptococcal glomerulonephritis, rheumatic fever does not follow streptococcal skin infection.

Rheumatic fever is more common in school-age children, the group most likely to acquire streptococcal pharyngitis. It has an attack rate of 3% in those with pharyngitis. The attack rate is much lower in streptococcal carriers and much higher in children with a previous episode of rheumatic fever. The latent period is 1 to 3 weeks following pharyngitis.

Rheumatic fever is diagnosed clinically using the Jones Criteria (Table 16-1). Although not all children with rheumatic fever meet the Jones criteria and not all children with the Jones criteria have rheumatic fever, these criteria make the diagnosis of rheumatic fever highly probable.

Children with rheumatic fever present with a **pancarditis**, which can cause first-degree heart block with a prolonged PR interval, mitral and aortic insufficiency, and congestive heart failure. These children also typically present with a migratory, extremely tender arthritis involving the elbows, knees, ankles, and wrists.

**Sydenham chorea** may occur several months following streptococcal pharyngitis, and it may be the only manifestation of

### TABLE 16-1.
### Duckett Jones Criteria for the Diagnosis of Rheumatic Fever

| Requirements for Diagnosis | Major Criteria | Minor Criteria |
| --- | --- | --- |
| Two major criteria, | Carditis | Previous rheumatic fever |
| *or* | Arthritis | Arthralgia |
| One major plus two minor criteria, | Chorea | Fever |
| *plus* | Erythema marginatum | Raised erythrocyte sedimentation rate |
| Evidence of previous streptococcal infection: (eg, elevated ASO titer) | Subcutaneous nodules | Elevated leukocyte count |
| | Prolonged PR interval | |
| | C reactive protein | |

ASO = antistreptolysin-0.
From Oski FA, et al., Principles and Practices of Pediatrics, 2nd ed., Philadelphia: J.B. Lippincott, 1994, p. 1629.

rheumatic fever. Early signs of chorea include clumsiness, deterioration of handwriting, and emotional lability.

All children with acute rheumatic fever should be treated with penicillin for the antecedent streptococcal infection. Once the diagnosis is established, the arthritis can be treated with salicylates. Corticosteroids are reserved for children with significant carditis and congestive heart failure. Congestive heart failure is managed with diuretics and digoxin, although low doses of digoxin should be used in children with acute rheumatic fever because of myocardial sensitivity.

Children with rheumatic fever should receive secondary prophylaxis, usually monthly intramuscular injections of benzathine penicillin, to prevent subsequent attacks.

## Juvenile Rheumatoid Arthritis

Juvenile rheumatoid arthritis (JRA) comprises a group of disorders of differing epidemiology, clinical manifestations, and prognosis (Table 16-2).

**Pauciarticular type I,** the most common form of JRA, usually presents before the age of 4 years in girls with an asymmetric pattern of arthritis involving the knees, ankles, and elbows. One third of these children will develop chronic iridocyclitis. Antinuclear antibodies (ANA) are almost always present.

**Pauciarticular type II** JRA, which affects older boys and is associated with HLA-B27, presents with arthritis in the large joints, particularly the hip and lower extremities. **Polyarticular JRA,** found primarily in girls, is a symmetric arthritis of multiple joints, typically the hands, elbows, knees, and ankles. The **rheumatoid factor-positive**

**TABLE 16-2.**

**Classification of Types of Onset of Juvenile Rheumatoid Arthritis**

| Sign/Symptom of Onset | Polyarthritis | Oligoarthritis (Pauciarticular Disease) | Systemic Disease |
|---|---|---|---|
| Frequency of cases | 40%–50% | 10%–20% | |
| Number of joints involved | ≥5 | ≤4 | Variable |
| Sex ratio (F:M) | 3:1 | 5:1 | 1:1 |
| Systemic involvement | Moderate involvement | Not present | Prominent |
| Occurrence of chronic uveitis | 5% | 20% | Rare |
| Frequency of seropositivity rheumatoid factors | 10% (increases with age) | Rare | Rare |
| Antinuclear antibodies | 40%–50% | 75%–85% | 10% |
| Course | Systemic disease is generally mild; articular involvement may be unremitting | Systemic disease is absent; major cause of morbidity is uveitis | Systemic disease is often self-limited; arthritis is chronic and destructive in 50% |
| Prognosis | Guarded to moderately good | | Moderate to poor |

From Oski FA, et al., Principles and Practices of Pediatrics, 2nd ed., Philadelphia: J.B. Lippincott, 1994, p. 246.

subtype resembles adult rheumatoid arthritis and occurs in older girls. A significant number of these children develop severe, debilitating arthritis. **Rheumatoid factor-negative** polyarticular JRA has a milder course, with less risk of the development of chronic arthritis. **Systemic onset JRA** is characterized by high fever, transient rash, hepatosplenomegaly, lymphadenopathy, pleuritis, and pericarditis. Although multiple joints are affected, the arthritis may not be obvious at the onset. Laboratory studies show leukocytosis and anemia.

Therapy requires medications to minimize joint inflammation, physical therapy to preserve joint function, careful ophthalmologic follow-up for children at risk of iridocyclitis, and long-term support of the child and family. **Aspirin** and **nonsteroidal anti-inflammatory agents** are commonly prescribed, but corticosteroids should rarely be used.

# Chapter 17

# Orthopedic Disorders

## CONGENITAL ANOMALIES

### Klippel-Feil Syndrome

Klippel-Feil syndrome is the congenital fusion of cervical vertebrae in which the neck is short and restricted in movement. Associated congenital anomalies are common.

### Atlantoaxial Instability

Atlantoaxial instability, which may be congenital or acquired, is a common feature of trisomy 21, because of odontoid dysplasia and ligamentous laxity. The serious complication of compression of the spinal cord may occur spontaneously or after minor trauma. The diagnosis is confirmed by careful radiographic examination of the neck.

### Sprengel Deformity

Sprengel deformity is the failure of the scapula to descend to its normal position. The shoulders appear asymmetric when viewed from the back; torticollis may be present.

### Metatarsus Adductus

Metatarsus adductus, the most common congenital foot deformity, is that in which the tarsometatarsal joints are subluxed medially and the anterior portion of the foot (metatarsals) is adducted. When the forefoot can be brought to the neutral position, the condition almost always resolves without treatment. When the position is fixed and persists, casting is required.

## Talipes Equinovarus

Talipes equinovarus, or clubfoot, another common congenital deformity of the foot, is bilateral in half of affected children. Uterine compression can produce mild talipes equinovarus; however, more severe forms are usually due to developmental defects. Treatment involves serial casts, starting in the first week of life. Severe talipes equinovarus requires surgical correction.

## Congenital Dislocation of the Hip

Congenital dislocation of the hip is a spectrum of **positional deformities** that includes subluxation, dislocatable hips, and dislocation. Oligohydramnios, breech presentation, neural tube defects, cerebral palsy, and a family history are all risk factors for congenital hip dislocation. One fifth of children have bilateral congenital dislocation of the hip.

**Subluxation** refers to a condition of malalignment of the femoral head and acetabulum in which the femoral head remains within the joint. A **dislocatable hip** is one in which the femoral head can be manipulated out of the acetabulum. Most newborns with subluxated or dislocatable hips will improve by 2 to 3 months of age with appropriate therapy. A **dislocated hip** is one in which the femoral head lies outside the acetabulum. During the neonatal period, the femoral head is often reducible, but if associated with such congenital anomalies as neural tube defects, a dislocated hip is often not reducible.

Infants with congenital dislocation of the hip have asymmetric gluteal folds, limitation on abduction of the hip, apparent shortening of the leg, and prominence and elevation of the greater trochanter of the femur. On flexion and abduction of the affected hip, a palpable "clunk" can be felt as the femoral head slips over the rim of the acetabulum (**Ortolani maneuver**). Ultrasonography can be used to confirm the diagnosis in difficult cases. Radiographs can be useful after 2 to 3 months of age, when normal ossification has progressed.

The treatment of children with congenital dislocation of the hip consists of the use of a splint or harness; more severe cases require casting and occasionally open surgical reduction.

## Slipped Capital Femoral Epiphysis

Slipped capital femoral epiphysis (SCFE) is a condition in which there is a displacement of the femoral head from the femoral neck prior to epiphyseal closure. A **fracture through the growth plate** allows for the displacement. The condition is most common in obese adolescent boys and is bilateral in a small proportion of cases. Children present with pain, limp, or refusal to walk. The pain may be referred to the knee or thigh. Avascular necrosis of the femoral head and chronic joint disease can develop. Children with slipped capital femoral epiphysis require urgent surgical fixation of the femoral head.

## Legg-Calve-Perthes Disease

Legg-Calve-Perthes disease, avascular necrosis of the femoral head, presents with joint stiffness, limp, and pain in the hip, thigh, knee, or groin of several weeks to months duration. Boys between the ages of 4 and 8 years are most commonly affected. On radiograph, a widened joint space is found early, with necrosis evident only later. The treatment includes casting the hip in abduction and surgical manipulation of the femoral head. Chronic degenerative arthritis can result.

## Osgood-Schlatter Disease

Osgood-Schlatter disease occurs in active children, particularly adolescent boys, and consists of the tearing of cartilage from the tibial tuberosity by the ligamentum patellae. The child presents with pain and swelling at the site of one or both tibial tubercles. The condition resolves with restricted physical activity.

## Toxic Synovitis

Toxic synovitis is a transient inflammatory arthritis of the hip, and is more common in children, especially boys, between the ages of 3 and 6 years. The child presents with a limp and pain of the hip, thigh, or knee. On examination, limitation of motion and pain are found on abduction and medial rotation of the hip. Because fever and an elevated sedimentation rate may be present, toxic synovitis may be confused with septic arthritis or osteomyelitis. Aspiration of the hip may be necessary to make the diagnosis. The condition resolves spontaneously.

## Scoliosis

Scoliosis, lateral and rotational curvature of the spine, may be due to such congenital anomalies of the spine as hemivertebrae or may be idiopathic.

### Idiopathic Scoliosis

Idiopathic scoliosis is familial. Severe forms are more frequent in adolescent girls. The signs and symptoms of scoliosis may be so subtle as to go undetected for some time.

The defect can be detected by having the child bend forward at the waist and observing an asymmetric curvature of the posterior thorax and discrepancy in the height of the shoulders. *Back pain is not a common symptom* of scoliosis. Radiographic examination of the spine determines the number, location, and severity of the curvature. Children with scoliosis that is likely to progress are often prescribed braces; severe, progressive scoliosis unresponsive to this therapy requires surgical correction.

## INFECTIONS OF THE BONES AND JOINTS

### Acute Osteomyelitis

Acute osteomyelitis usually begins with a **bacteremia** that establishes local infection at the **metaphyseal end of long bones**, an area in which blood pooling and reduced phagocytic activity predispose to infection. Osteomyelitis less commonly results from spread from a contiguous infection. In infants, blood vessels crossing the growth plate and connecting the metaphysis with the epiphysis allow for ready spread of the infection from the bone to the joint space, causing septic arthritis and damage to the growth plate. In older children, the growth plate prevents the spread of infection from the metaphysis to the epiphysis and surrounding joint. In such joints as the hip, shoulder, elbow, and ankle, in which the capsule inserts along the metaphysis, rupture of the infection through the periosteum can also result in septic arthritis.

*Staphylococcus aureus* is the most common bacterial pathogen in osteomyelitis. In neonates, group B streptococci and *Escherichia coli* can cause osteomyelitis; infants and young children are at risk for *Haemophilus influenzae* type b osteomyelitis. Although children with sickle cell disease are at risk of *Salmonella* osteomyelitis, *S. aureus* remains most common.

Infants with osteomyelitis present with fever, signs of sepsis, and limited motion of the affected limb (pseudoparalysis). Multifocal osteomyelitis, rare in older children, can occur in neonates. Older children present with fever, limp, voluntary guarding, local pain, tenderness, and swelling. Fever is not invariably present. Diffuse tenderness may be present if the infection has ruptured through the cortex and spread along the periosteum.

Most children with osteomyelitis have a **leukocytosis** with a left shift and an elevated erythrocyte sedimentation rate (ESR). Because the pathogenesis begins with bacteremia, blood cultures frequently reveal the causative pathogen. Arthrocentesis and needle aspiration of the bone can also be used to identify the causative agent. Radiographs of the bone do not show evidence of infection until 10 to 14 days after the onset, when the characteristic periosteal reaction and lytic lesions can be found. A three-phase bone scan can differentiate osteomyelitis from soft tissue infection. Treatment of acute osteomyelitis is with antibiotics directed against the most likely pathogens, particularly *S. aureus*.

## Septic Arthritis

Septic arthritis may accompany osteomyelitis (as previously discussed) but can also occur in isolation. Septic arthritis is usually monarticular and commonly involves the knee, hip, elbow, or ankle. *S. aureus* and *H. influenzae* type b are the most common pathogens seen in infants and young children. Gonococcal arthritis occurs in sexually active adolescents. As with osteomyelitis, **bacteremia precedes localized infection**. Neonates with septic arthritis present with fever and pseudoparalysis. Older children present with fever, limp, limited motion of the affected limb, and a tender, swollen warm joint. Children with septic arthritis of the hip frequently hold the thigh in flexion and external rotation; however, hip pain may be referred to the knee, obscuring the diagnosis. Adolescents with gonococcal arthritis have fever, rash, arthralgias, and a monarticular arthritis.

The **diagnosis** of septic arthritis is confirmed by arthrocentesis, which should be performed in every child suspected of septic arthritis. Because septic arthritis of the hip can cause a rapid increase in pressure within the joint, resulting in avascular necrosis of the femoral head, open surgical drainage is required.

# ORTHOPEDIC TRAUMA

## Fractures

Fractures, from falls, motor vehicle accidents, or child abuse, are common in children. Fractures through the growth plate usually involve separation of the epiphysis from the metaphysis with or without a small fracture of the metaphysis (Salter-Harris types 1 and 2). Because bones are more pliable in children, greenstick fractures are also common. Supracondylar fractures of the elbow result from falling on an outstretched arm. Injury to the neurovascular bundle (Volkmann contracture) can lead to paralysis and contracture.

## Subluxation of the Radial Head

Subluxation of the radial head ("nursemaid's elbow") occurs when the arm of a young child is suddenly pulled with the elbow extended. Supination of the forearm with the elbow in 90° of flexion often replaces the radial head.

# SKELETAL DYSPLASIAS

### Marfan's Syndrome

Marfan's syndrome is an autosomal dominant disorder with skeletal, ocular, and cardiovascular abnormalities. Approximately one third of cases represent new mutations. Children with Marfan's syndrome are typically tall and thin with joint laxity and arachnodactyly (long thin fingers). Children with this disorder have an arm span that is greater than their height; they also have a diminished upper segment to lower segment ratio. **Scoliosis is common**. The ocular abnormalities include blue sclera, lens dislocation, retinal detachment, and severe myopia. Progressive mitral valve prolapse and aortic root dilatation leading to aortic valve insufficiency can be found with associated congestive heart failure, arrhythmias, or bacterial endocarditis.

### Achondroplasia

Achondroplasia is an autosomal dominant disorder. Half of all cases are new mutations. Children with achondroplasia have markedly short stature; shortened proximal limbs; broad, short hands; lordosis; and a large head with frontal bossing and a flat nasal bridge. Cognitive development is usually normal. Hydrocephalus, recurrent otitis media, and hearing loss are complications of the condition.

### Osteogenesis Imperfecta

Osteogenesis imperfecta is a heterogenous group of genetic disorders characterized by osteoporosis and fractures. The condition results from a reduction in the synthesis of type I collagen and improves during puberty. The most common form, osteogenesis imperfecta type I, is an autosomal dominant disorder characterized by osteoporosis, fractures, blue sclerae, and conductive hearing loss. Recurrent fractures result in limb deformities.

### Caffey Disease

Caffey disease (infantile cortical hyperostosis) presents in the first few months of life with fever, swelling of the soft tissues of the face, and cortical thickening of bones. The disease can be confused with osteomyelitis and child abuse. The course is marked by a pattern of exacerbations and remissions with eventual resolution.

# Chapter 18

# Child Abuse and Neglect

Child **abuse** can take several forms, including physical, sexual, and emotional abuse or neglect, and it occurs in all socioeconomic groups. However, the incidence of physical abuse and neglect increases with poverty and is often associated with other intrafamilial problems such as domestic violence.

**Neglect** is probably the most common form of child abuse and occurs when the caretaker fails to provide adequate nutrition, nurturing, supervision, or medical care for a child. Hospitalization can be both diagnostic and therapeutic because a neglected infant will often rapidly grow and develop within the hospital.

In the United States, each year **physical abuse** results in the death of 1000 to 2000 children, most of whom are less than 5 years of age. Abused children present with histories that are not consistent with the physical findings; multiple bruises or fractures in different stages of healing; and lesions that are in the shape of an identifiable object, such as a hand, iron, or belt. Burns to the soles of both feet, which are unlikely to occur by a child stepping into hot water, suggest deliberate submersion.

"Bucket handle" **fractures** of the long bones, characterized by corner fractures and elevation of the periosteum, as well as posterior rib fractures, are highly suggestive of physical abuse. Subdural hematomas and cerebral contusions, particularly without external evidence of head trauma, are other signs of physical abuse. Because forceful blows to the chest or abdomen can cause retinal hemorrhages, careful ophthalmologic examination is required in all children suspected of physical abuse.

Examination of the child for evidence of **sexual abuse** requires a skilled examiner and a nonthreatening environment. Traumatic signs of sexual abuse, such as vaginal or perirectal lacerations, ecchymoses, and edema are not always present, particularly if the child is examined weeks or months after the abusive incident. Because of the normal wide variation in both the size and configuration of the hymen, measurement of a wide hymenal opening is not conclusive evidence of sexual abuse. However, normal hymens should be symmetric and have smooth rims without posterior tears or irregularities.

**Sexually transmitted infections** in children are also suggestive of abuse. Because of the possibility of cross-reaction with colonic bacteria, culture, rather than rapid antigen detection tests, should be used to diagnose chlamydial genital infection in children.

Most states in the United States have statutes that require health professionals to report all cases of suspected child abuse to either child welfare or legal authorities. The treatment of abused children and their families usually involves a multidisciplinary team to deal with the deep rooted social and familial problems usually present. The long-term sequelae of child abuse are emotional and social maladjustment.

# Chapter 19

# Ophthalmologic Disorders

## CONGENITAL ANOMALIES

### Strabismus

Strabismus, the malalignment of the visual axes, can be latent (phoria), occurring only under conditions of stress or fatigue, or manifest (tropia). Alternating strabismus occurs when either eye is used for fixation; in this situation amblyopia is unlikely. However, in the instance of monocular strabismus in which one eye is used exclusively for fixation, amblyopia is likely and requires urgent attention.

The treatment of strabismus involves the correction of any underlying ocular abnormality, including refractive errors; occlusion therapy for amblyopia; and surgical correction of ocular malalignment.

### Amblyopia

Amblyopia refers to decreased visual acuity that is not due to a correctable error of refraction. The "rule of fours" serves as a guide to normal visual acuity in children: At 4 days, neonates have an aversion to light; at 4 weeks, infants can recognize their mother's face; at 4 months, infants can fixate and follow; and at 4 years, children develop normal adult visual acuity. Because the development of normal visual acuity depends on the formation of a clear retinal image, interference with this process can result in amblyopia of the affected eye.

The risk of amblyopia is greatest in the first 3 years of life, especially in the first months of life, but can occur up to 7 years of age. Unilateral **cataracts**, **anisometropia** (marked difference in refractive power between the two eyes) and **strabismus** are common causes of amblyopia. In these instances the retinal image from the *bad* eye is suppressed, with resulting amblyopia. The treatment of amblyopia involves correcting the underlying problem and forcing the child to use the *bad* eye by occluding the *good* eye.

## Cataracts

Cataracts in infants and children can be caused by congenital infections (rubella, syphilis, cytomegalovirus [CMV], toxoplasmosis), metabolic disorders (galactosemia, mucopolysaccharidoses), chromosomal abnormalities (trisomies 21, 18, and 13, Turner syndrome), drugs (corticosteroids), and trauma. Cataracts may also be inherited in isolation without other anomalies. The treatment of cataracts in children involves surgical removal of the cataract, correction of the refractive error, and treatment of residual amblyopia.

## Glaucoma

Glaucoma is usually caused by residual tissue obstructing the filtration angle in the anterior chamber at the site of the canal of Schlemm. It results in the **elevation of intraocular pressure**. Glaucoma is also found in children with retinopathy of prematurity and neurocutaneous syndromes. Infants and children with glaucoma present with enlargement of the eye (buphthalmos), tearing, photophobia, and corneal clouding. Untreated glaucoma can result in blindness from damage to the optic nerve. The treatment is surgical opening of the canal, allowing drainage of the aqueous humor.

## Dacryostenosis

Dacryostenosis is partial or complete obstruction of the drainage system of the eye caused by congenital narrowing or failure of canalization of the lacrimal duct. It presents as excessive tearing of the affected eye. In most children, the condition resolves in the first year of life, with routine nasolacrimal massage several times a day. Infection of the nasolacrimal sac, **dacryocystitis**, requires antibiotic therapy. Excessive tearing may also result from glaucoma, corneal abrasion or ocular foreign body.

# INFECTIONS OF THE EYE

## Acute Purulent Conjunctivitis

Acute purulent conjunctivitis in children beyond the neonatal period is usually due to staphylococci, pneumococci, streptococci and *Haemophilus influenzae*. When *H. influenzae* is the etiologic agent, otitis media may also be present (the otitis-conjunctivitis syndrome). Conjunctivitis due to viral infections (adenovirus, enterovirus, measles) is usually not purulent, and is characterized by small follicles of lymphocytes on the palpebral conjunctivae.

## Epidemic Keratoconjunctivitis

Epidemic keratoconjunctivitis, which is caused by a specific adenovirus (type 8), can cause corneal damage. Keratoconjunctivitis can also occur with primary or recurrent herpes simplex infection, which can cause corneal scarring and blindness.

## Trachoma

Trachoma, a leading cause of blindness in some countries, is caused by infection with *Chlamydia trachomatis*.

## Allergic Conjunctivitis

Allergic conjunctivitis must be distinguished from infectious conjunctivitis. Pruritus, tearing, and seasonality are characteristic features of allergic conjunctivitis.

## Periorbital Cellulitis

Periorbital cellulitis is a **bacterial infection of the preseptal tissue**, resulting from trauma or hematogenous spread. Trauma leads to local infection with *Staphylococcus aureus* or group A streptococci. Hematogenous periorbital cellulitis most commonly occurs in young children as a consequence of *H. influenzae* type b bacteremia, but pneumococci can cause a similar clinical picture.

The signs and symptoms of periorbital cellulitis include the acute onset of unilateral eyelid edema, erythema, and tenderness. **Fever** and **leukocytosis** are often present. The *extraocular movements of the eye are normal*, a finding that distinguishes periorbital from orbital cellulitis. Periorbital cellulitis due to *H. influenzae* type b often has a characteristic purple hue. Children with periorbital cellulitis should be treated with parenteral antibiotics.

The differential diagnosis of periorbital cellulitis includes insect bites, conjunctivitis with lid chemosis, orbital cellulitis, and sinusitis. Sinusitis may result in inflammatory edema, which mimics periorbital cellulitis without causing a true infection of the preseptal space.

## Orbital Cellulitis

Orbital cellulitis, or **infection posterior to the orbital septum**, occurs commonly as a result of contiguous spread of infection from adjacent sinuses. The ethmoid sinuses are commonly involved because only a thin layer of bone (the lamina papyracea) separates the sinus from the orbit of the eye. The organisms that cause sinusitis, *Streptococcus pneumoniae*, nontypable *H. influenzae*, *S. aureus*, and streptococci are common causes of orbital cellulitis.

The onset of orbital cellulitis is often insidious. Children with orbital cellulitis present with proptosis, pain on movement of the eye, decreased ocular mobility, and loss of visual acuity due to increased intraorbital pressure, which damages the optic nerve.

Computerized tomography of the orbit and sinuses confirms the diagnosis. After appropriate blood cultures, parenteral antibiotic therapy is indicated. Surgical drainage of the sinuses or orbital abscess may be necessary.

# Chapter 20

# Skin Disorders

## CONGENITAL ANOMALIES

Anal or **presacral dimples** are small pits that are usually of no consequence when covered with skin. **Preauricular sinuses and pits** are often familial and may become infected, requiring excision. **Supernumerary nipples** in various stages of development occur along the nipple line, descending to the inguinal region, and may be associated with genitourinary tract anomalies. **Branchial cleft cysts**, a result of failure in closure of the first and second branchial clefts, occur on the lateral neck, and may become infected or form sinus tracts. **Thyroglossal duct cysts** are midline in location, may extend to the base of the tongue, and often contain thyroid tissue. Because this ectopic thyroid may represent the only thyroid in the child, surgical excision must involve preservation of the thyroid tissue. **Cystic hygromas**, lymphangiomas frequently located on the head and neck and sometimes extending into the thorax, require surgical excision.

## DERMATITIS

### Chronic Dermatitis

*Atopic Dermatitis*

Atopic dermatitis affects approximately 5% of children and usually begins in infancy as an erythematous, pruritic scaly rash on the cheeks. The rash spreads to involve the face, hands, abdomen, and extensor surfaces of the extremities. In older children, the flexural surfaces are commonly involved. The intense pruritus causes the child to scratch, resulting in crusting and weeping. Lesions may become secondarily infected, particularly with staphylococci, streptococci, and herpes simplex virus (eczema herpeticum). Chronic atopic dermatitis causes lichenification of the skin; some children develop linear skin folds below the eyelids (Dennie lines or Morgan folds).

Atopic dermatitis is associated with elevated serum IgE levels, eosinophilia, hypersensitivity reactions to foods, asthma and allergic rhinitis.

Treatment involves avoiding soaps and frequent bathing, both of which dry the skin; the use of oils and creams to keep the skin moist after bathing; wet dressings with Burrow solution; and topical corticosteroids. A primary goal of treatment is to prevent scratching, which perpetuates the dermatitis.

### Seborrheic Dermatitis

Seborrheic dermatitis is a dermatitis of unknown etiology that commonly occurs in infants and adolescents. Infants may develop scaling and crusting of the scalp, **cradle cap**, or a greasy, scaly, erythematous rash on the ears, nasolabial folds, eyebrows, or diaper area. Occasionally, the entire body is involved. In contrast to atopic dermatitis, pruritus is usually minimal or absent. Severe seborrhea may occur in infants with Leiner disease (chronic diarrhea and failure to thrive), Langerhans' cell histiocytosis, and human immunodeficiency virus (HIV) infection.

Adolescents with seborrheic dermatitis have involvement of the scalp and intertriginous areas. Treatment is with an antiseborrheic shampoo and topical corticosteroids.

### Contact Dermatitis

Contact dermatitis is common in children, and may be due to irritants or an allergic reaction. Common irritants are saliva (perioral dermatitis) and soaps. **Diaper dermatitis** is an irritant contact dermatitis due to prolonged contact with urine and feces, and must be distinguished from candidal diaper dermatitis.

**Postinflammatory pigmentary changes** are common in children, particularly those with dark skin. Both hypopigmentation and hyperpigmentation can occur and resolve without treatment within several weeks to months.

## Erythema Multiforme

Erythema multiforme is a hypersensitivity reaction to infections or drugs. Herpes simplex is a common precipitating infection. The severity varies, ranging from mild skin and mucous membrane lesions to severe multisystem disease. The rash, often involving the palms and soles, consists of petechiae, macules, wheals, vesicles, and bullae. The characteristic iris or target lesions may progress to form a series of concentric rings.

In **Stevens-Johnson disease**, the severe form of erythema multiforme, children present with fever, malaise, myalgias, and crusting, ulcerative bullae on the skin and mucous membranes, particularly the mouth, conjunctivae, and genitalia. Ocular involvement can lead to corneal ulceration and blindness.

## Pityriasis Alba

Pityriasis alba is a rash on the face, neck, upper chest, and arms of unknown etiology. It is characterized by hypopigmented, round macules with fine scales and indistinct margins. The hypopigmentation resolves in several weeks or months.

## Pityriasis Rosea

Pityriasis rosea, a rash common in children, also is of unknown etiology. The typical rash begins with a single, 1- to 10-cm oval herald patch, followed by the eruption of multiple, oval, small (less than 1 cm), fine scaly lesions on the trunk and upper arms. The lesions are arranged on the trunk so that the long axis is aligned with the cleavage lines, creating a "Christmas tree" pattern. The rash resolves in several weeks without treatment.

## Acne Vulgaris

Acne vulgaris, a common rash of adolescents, begins with the development of comedones, sebaceous follicles impacted with keratin. When the impacted follicle ruptures into the dermis, inflammatory papules and nodules form. Bacteria, particularly *Propionibacterium acnes*, exacerbate the inflammatory response. Acne frequently involves the face, but lesions may be found on the back and chest. Scarring may result from severe, chronic acne. Treatment of mild acne is with topical keratolytic agents such as benzoyl peroxide. Topical retinoic acid also decreases keratin plugging of sebaceous follicles. Topical antibiotics are sometimes used to suppress the growth of *P. acnes*. More severe forms of acne, particularly nodulocystic acne, require the addition of systemic antibiotics, usually tetracycline or erythromycin.

# VASCULAR LESIONS

## Hemangiomas

### Capillary Hemangiomas

Capillary hemangiomas, also called strawberry nevi, are small, superficial, bright red lesions, which are due to the proliferation of vascular endothelium. Most progress rapidly and then involute after a period of stasis. Almost all involute by the age of 10 years.

### *Cavernous Hemangiomas*

Cavernous hemangiomas that extend deeper into the subcutaneous tissues also grow rapidly and then involute. However, depending upon their location, they may compress the airway or impair feeding or vision, requiring treatment with corticosteroids or laser therapy.

The Kasabach-Merritt syndrome occurs in children with large cavernous hemangiomas that sequester platelets, causing thrombocytopenia, hemorrhage, and anemia. The two other syndromes that are associated with vascular lesions are Klippel-Trenaunay-Weber syndrome (port-wine nevus, soft tissue hypertrophy, and venous varicosities, usually involving the leg) and Osler-Weber-Rendu disease (hemorrhagic telangiectasias, usually of the nose and mouth).

# BACTERIAL SKIN INFECTIONS

## Impetigo

Impetigo is a superficial infection of the skin consisting of vesicles, pustules, and bullae, which easily rupture, leaving crusts. Group A beta-hemolytic streptococci and *Staphylococcus aureus* are the etiologic agents. **Bullous impetigo**, caused by specific strains of *S. aureus*, is common in the diaper area in neonates. Cleansing, compresses, and topical antibiotics are usually effective in treating impetigo.

## Cellulitis

Cellulitis, a deeper infection involving the skin and subcutaneous tissues, usually follows local trauma and is generally caused by staphylococci or streptococci. Streptococcal skin infections include **erysipelas**, **blistering distal dactylitis** (infection of the fingertips), and **perianal streptococcal cellulitis**. *Haemophilus influenzae* type b bacteremia can also cause cellulitis, particularly in the periorbital and buccal regions (**periorbital cellulitis** and **buccal cellulitis**). Lymphangitis and regional lymphadenopathy frequently are associated with more severe cellulitis.

## Staphylococcal Scalded Skin Syndrome

Staphylococcal scalded skin syndrome occurs in young children following infection with phage group 2 *S. aureus*. Phage group 2 produces an extracellular, exfoliative toxin that causes a diffuse macular erythema followed by widespread bullae and crusting. Facial edema, conjunctivitis, and pharyngitis may be present. Stroking the skin results in epithelial separation (Nikolsky sign). Staphylococci cannot be cultured from the bullae but can be found at other sites. Treatment is with systemic antibiotic therapy. The denuded areas of skin heal rapidly.

## Toxic Epidermal Necrolysis

Toxic epidermal necrolysis resembles staphylococcal scalded skin syndrome but follows drug ingestion and causes exfoliation of the entire epidermis.

# VIRAL SKIN INFECTIONS

## Warts

Warts are caused by papillomavirus infection of the skin or mucous membranes. The papillomavirus is probably transmitted by person-to-person contact; autoinoculation then spreads the infection on the individual. Warts can occur anywhere but typically are found on the fingers, hands, face, knees, and elbows. In a prepubertal child, warts on the genitalia or perianal region (**condylomata acuminata**) suggest the **possibility of sexual abuse**. Condylomata acuminata is usually treated with topical application of podophyllin.

## Molluscum Contagiosum

Molluscum contagiosum, also of viral etiology (a poxvirus), consists of small, skin-colored papules with central umbilication and are commonly found on the face, neck, and axillae. Disseminated molluscum contagiosum can occur in immunocompromised children, particularly those with HIV infection or acute lymphocytic leukemia. Treatment is with curettage or application of liquid nitrogen.

## Herpes Simplex Virus

Herpes simplex virus infections in children are found in a variety of forms. Most herpes simplex virus infections are asymptomatic, the virus becomes latent, and infected individuals continue to be contagious. Herpes simplex infections in children usually involve the skin and mucous membranes. The skin lesions are vesicles morphologically indistinguishable from varicella.

### Acute Herpetic Gingivostomatitis

Acute herpetic gingivostomatitis occurs most commonly in children 1 to 3 years of age who present with the abrupt onset of high fever, oral pain, refusal to feed, and drooling. Vesicles quickly rupture, creating ulcers on the tongue, gums, and buccal mucosa. Lymphadenopathy of the submaxillary glands is common. Tzanck preparation of herpes-simplex-infected skin reveals multinuclear giant cells and intranuclear inclusions. The treatment of children with herpetic gingivostomatitis is largely supportive. There is little or no evidence that acyclovir shortens the duration of symptoms or reduces the rate of recurrence.

### Varicella

Varicella, or **chickenpox**, is a common and **highly contagious herpesvirus infection**. Children with chickenpox present with fever, malaise, and the appearance of a rash consisting of crops of small vesicles on an erythematous base, which begins on the trunk and spreads to the face and extremities. The vesicles continue to appear for 3 to 4 days; characteristically the lesions are in various degrees of development, ranging from papules, to vesicles, to crusted lesions. The incubation period ranges from 11 to 21 days, and children with the disease are infectious from 1 day before the rash appears until all lesions are crusted.

The complications of varicella include secondary bacterial infection, pneumonia, and postinfectious encephalitis with cerebellar ataxia. Immunocompromised children, particularly those receiving corticosteroids, with leukemia, or with HIV infection, are at risk of fatal disseminated varicella. Varicella can be prevented with active **immunization** or passive administration of **varicella immunoglobulin** (VZIG). Acyclovir can be used as treatment in immunocompromised children or those who develop such serious complications as pneumonia. Hospitalized children with varicella should be isolated from other children.

Children with a history of varicella can develop **herpes zoster**, but immunocompromised children and those exposed to varicella at the time of delivery are at particularly high risk.

## FUNGAL SKIN INFECTIONS

**Candidal infections** in infants frequently involve the oral cavity (thrush) and diaper area. **Thrush** is manifested as white plaques on the buccal mucosa and tongue. Scraping the white membrane leaves an erythematous base. **Candidal diaper dermatitis** consists of a "beefy" red plaque with well demarcated borders and satellite pustules. The intertriginous folds in the groin are usually involved. Potassium hydroxide (KOH) preparation confirms the diagnosis. Treatment is with antifungal agents.

**Tinea capitis** is a dermatophyte infection of the scalp, characterized by one or multiple pruritic, erythematous, scaly, circular plaques with alopecia. A **kerion** is a boggy, inflammatory mass that sometimes accompanies the primary lesion. Tinea capitis should be treated with griseofulvin taken orally for 2 to 3 months.

**Tinea corporis** is a dermatophyte infection of the skin that typically forms an annular lesion with raised margins and central clearing. Tinea corporis is treated with a topical antifungal cream for several weeks.

**Tinea pedis and tinea cruris** are fungal infections of the feet and inguinal region, and are more common in adolescents.

**Tinea versicolor**, a superficial fungal infection caused by *Malassezia furfur*, is also more common in adolescents. The scaly, macular lesions can be either hyperpigmented or hypopigmented and occur on the neck, chest, and upper arms. The diagnosis can be confirmed by Wood lamp examination (gold fluorescence) and KOH preparation of skin scrapings. Because the causative agent is part of the normal skin flora, recurrences are common even after treatment.

# PARASITIC SKIN INFECTIONS

## Scabies

Scabies is a pruritic, papular rash caused by infection with the gravid female mite *Sarcoptes scabiei*. Burrows may also be seen. In older children, the lesions are commonly found on the fingers, wrists, axillae, buttocks, and groin. The palms, soles, and head can be involved in infants. The diagnosis is confirmed by microscopic examination of skin scrapings after the application of mineral oil to a burrow or fresh papule. Treatment is the application of a scabicide to the entire body from the neck down. Potentially neurotoxic 1% gamma benzene hexachloride should not be used in young infants. Family members should also be treated, and clothing, bed linen, and towels cleaned.

## Lice

Infestation with lice can involve the scalp (pediculosis capitis), groin (pediculosis pubis), or body (pediculosis corporis). **Pediculosis capitis** is most common in children. The lice are not frequently visible, but nits may be seen on the hair shafts. Treatment is with a pediculicide such as permethrin.

# Chapter 21

# Preventive Pediatrics

The physician who cares for children must not only provide curative medical care but must also be involved in the prevention of disease and disability. Because children are growing and developing, the physician's focus on prevention will vary with the child's age. Although all encounters with children present opportunities for preventive care, most preventive pediatrics takes place during the well-child visit. Well-child care visits are recommended in the prenatal period, newborn period, at 2 weeks, and at 2, 4, 6, 9, 12, 15, 18, and 24 months. Well-child visits take place yearly between 3 and 6 years, and every 2 years thereafter.

Preventive pediatrics includes **psychosocial assessment** of the child within the context of the family; assessment of diet and nutrition; monitoring growth and development; screening with physical examination and laboratory tests (anemia, lead poisoning, vision and hearing); immunization; and anticipatory guidance. Anticipatory guidance is directed at normal developmental processes (changes in growth and appetite, weaning, toilet training), age-related behavioral problems (pica, night terrors), and accident prevention.

## DENTAL CARE

**Dental caries** and **periodontal disease** can be prevented through fluoride supplementation, good oral hygiene, and good dietary habits. Fluoridation of the water supply represents the most effective means of primary prevention, but children who live in areas without fluoridation of the water should receive supplemental fluoride daily.

Parents of children under 10 years of age should assist with brushing and flossing of the teeth. Avoidance of carbohydrate snacks diminishes the formation of organic acids by bacterial fermentation (particularly by *Streptococcus mutans*) and erosion of the tooth enamel. A severe form of dental caries, typically of the incisors, occurs when infants sleep with a bottle containing milk or other carbohydrate-containing fluids (baby bottle caries).

# POISONING

Poisonings are common in two age groups: toddlers and adolescents. Children less than the age of 5 years, especially toddlers, are particularly susceptible to accidental ingestion, whereas adolescents ingest toxic substances, usually medications, to attempt or commit suicide. When completing the history, information about what, how much, and the timing of the ingestion is critical, but, especially in adolescent ingestions, the information may be very inaccurate.

If ipecac is available, emesis can be induced at home in young children if there are no contraindications and the ingestion was recent. The contraindications to emesis are the presence of a depressed gag reflex or coma, ingestion of an acid or alkali, and ingestion of most hydrocarbons. Emergency management of poisoning includes cardiopulmonary resuscitation and supportive care, general measures such as the administration of activated charcoal and cathartics, and treatment regimens specific to the type of poisoning. Common serious poisonings include acetaminophen, salicylates, iron, hydrocarbons, and organophosphates. *N*-acetyl-L-cysteine is a specific antidote for acetaminophen poisoning. Children with organophosphate poisoning should be treated with atropine.

## Lead Poisoning

Lead poisoning continues to be a serious hazard for many children in the United States. Dust and plaster in older housing that has been painted with lead-based paints are the major sources of lead. Children ingest lead by putting contaminated hands into their mouths. **Pica**, the repetitive ingestion of paint chips and plaster, is a cause of more severe lead poisoning. Young children absorb lead much more readily than adults. Diets high in fat and low in minerals (iron, calcium) also increase lead absorption. Because lead is deposited in bone and soft tissues, the slow release of lead from bone can maintain elevated blood lead levels long after ingestion.

Because the symptoms of lead poisoning can be very subtle and early detection is crucial, routine screening, using blood lead levels, is recommended for all children residing in areas in which there is the potential for exposure to excessive amounts of lead. Children with moderate to severe lead poisoning typically present with anemia, encephalopathy, and colic. Acute lead encephalopathy can result in cerebral edema, manifested as vomiting, seizures, and coma. Chronic lower levels of lead cause cognitive and behavioral deficits. In some children, radiopaque paint chips may be seen in the intestine on abdominal radiograph. "Lead lines" may be seen as increased areas of calcification at the metaphyses of long bones.

The treatment of chronic lead poisoning includes removal of the child and siblings from the environment containing lead. In children with significantly elevated lead levels, chelation therapy with dimercaptosuccinic acid (DMSA) is recommended. An alternative chelating agent is CaEDTA, which requires intravenous administration.

## Carbon Monoxide Poisoning

Carbon monoxide poisoning occurs in children exposed to smoke and fire. Carbon monoxide displaces oxygen from hemoglobin, greatly reducing the oxygen content of blood. Standard measures of oxygenation, such as arterial blood gas analysis of $PO_2$ and pulse oximetry determination of oxygen saturation, give misleading results. The $PO_2$, a measure of dissolved oxygen, is normal in children with carbon monoxide poisoning. The pulse oximeter cannot distinguish oxyhemoglobin from carboxyhemoglobin. Carbon monoxide poisoning must be diagnosed by **direct measurement of carboxyhemoglobin**.

The symptoms of carbon monoxide poisoning include dyspnea, nausea, and central nervous system dysfunction. Therapy for any child suspected of having carbon monoxide poisoning is administration of 100% oxygen. Hyperbaric oxygen therapy is useful for children with severe carbon monoxide poisoning.

## Prevention of Poisoning

Accidental poisoning can be prevented by instructing caretakers to place all toxic substances, including household cleaners and medications, out of reach and preferably in a locked cabinet. The development of **child-proof containers** has greatly reduced the accidental ingestion of medications.

# AUTOMOBILE ACCIDENTS

**Automobile accidents**, both pedestrian and vehicular, continue to be the most common cause of death in children in the United States. Physicians should do everything possible to make certain that parents obtain car seats for infants and young children and that they establish the habit of using seat belts for all members of the family. State regulations mandating the use of **bicycle helmets** for children should be supported, and their use promoted during well-child visits.

## DROWNING

Drowning is a common accidental cause of childhood death and injury and can be prevented through the promotion of water and household safety with close supervision of children. Drowning, most common in children between 1 and 4 years of age, frequently occurs in bathtubs and swimming pools.

## BURNS

**Burns**, which are common accidental injuries in children, are a frequent cause of morbidity and death. To prevent burn injuries, parents should be educated on the storage of matches and flammable liquids, the value of flame-retardant fabrics, and the regulation of proper temperature for home water heaters.

The management of moderate or severe burns in children requires hospitalization and the expertise of specialists. Children with burns of the face, hands, feet, or genitalia should also be hospitalized. The management of burns requires meticulous nursing care, precise fluid and electrolyte therapy, proper nutrition, aggressive treatment of infection, and intensive monitoring for complications. **Sepsis** is the leading cause of death in children with burns.

## CHILDHOOD IMMUNIZATIONS

The incidence of preventable childhood diseases, such as diphtheria, pertussis, tetanus, measles, mumps, and rubella, has declined dramatically since the introduction of effective vaccines. Although **poliomyelitis** has been eradicated in the western hemisphere, it continues to be a debilitating childhood infection in parts of Africa and Asia, and can still occur as a consequence of the live viral vaccine. Recent recommendations on the use of the inactivated polio vaccine for the first two doses are intended to prevent this complication. The current recommended schedule of immunizations during childhood is provided in Table 21-1. Revisions are made frequently as new information and new vaccines become available. The characteristics of some vaccines are listed in Table 21-2.

Outbreaks of **vaccine-preventable diseases** still occur. Recent epidemics in the United States include measles, mumps, pertussis, and congenital rubella. Although greater than 95% coverage has been achieved in school-age children, many areas within the United

## TABLE 21-1.
## Recommended Childhood Immunization Schedule, United States, Jan.–Dec. 1997

### Recommended Childhood Immunization Schedule
### United States, January – December 1997

Vaccines[1] are listed under the routinely recommended ages. **Bars** indicate range of acceptable ages for vaccination. **Shaded bars** indicate *catch-up vaccination:* at 11-12 years of age, hepatitis B vaccine should be administered to children not previously vaccinated, and Varicella vaccine should be administered to children not previously vaccinated who lack a reliable history of chickenpox.

| Age ▶<br>Vaccine ▼ | Birth | 1 mo | 2 mos | 4 mos | 6 mos | 12 mos | 15 mos | 18 mos | 4–6 yrs | 11–12 yrs | 14–16 yrs |
|---|---|---|---|---|---|---|---|---|---|---|---|
| Hepatitis B[2,3] | Hep B-1 | Hep B-2 | | | Hep B-3 | | | | | Hep B[3] | |
| Diphtheria, Tetanus, Pertussis[4] | | | DTaP or DTP | DTaP or DTP | DTaP or DTP | | DTaP or DTP[4] | | DTaP or DTP | Td | |
| H. influenzae type b[5] | | | Hib | Hib | Hib[5] | Hib[5] | | | | | |
| Polio[6] | | | Polio[6] | Polio | | Polio[6] | | | Polio | | |
| Measles, Mumps, Rubella[7] | | | | | | MMR | | | MMR[7] or MMR[7] | | |
| Varicella[8] | | | | | | Var | | | | Var[8] | |

Approved by the Advisory Committee on Immunization Practices (ACIP), the American Academy of Pediatrics (AAP), and the American Academy of Family Physicians (AAFP).

[1] This schedule indicates the recommended age for routine administration of currently licensed childhood vaccines. Some combination vaccines are available and may be used whenever administration of all components of the vaccine is indicated. Providers should consult the manufacturers' package inserts for detailed recommendations.

[2] Infants born to HBsAg-negative mothers should receive 2.5 µg of Merck vaccine (Recombivax HB) or 10 µg of SmithKline Beecham (SB) vaccine (Engerix-B). The 2nd dose should be administered ≥ 1 mo after the 1st dose.
Infants born to HBsAg-positive mothers should receive 0.5 mL hepatitis B immune globulin (HBIG) within 12 hrs of birth, and either 5 µg of Merck vaccine (Recombivax HB) or 10 µg of SB vaccine (Engerix-B) at a separate site. The 2nd dose is recommended at 1-2 mos of age and the 3rd dose at 6 mos of age.
Infants born to mothers whose HBsAg status is unknown should receive either 5 µg of Merck vaccine (Recombivax HB) or 10 µg of SB vaccine (Engerix-B) within 12 hrs of birth. The 2nd dose of vaccine is recommended at 1 mo of age and the 3rd dose at 6 mos of age. Blood should be drawn at the time of delivery to determine the mother's HBsAg status; if it is positive, the infant should receive HBIG as soon as possible (no later than 1 wk of age). The dosage and timing of subsequent vaccine doses should be based upon the mother's HBsAg status.

[3] Children and adolescents who have not been vaccinated against hepatitis B in infancy may begin the series during any childhood visit. Those who have not previously received 3 doses of hepatitis B vaccine should initiate or complete the series during 11-12 year-old visit. The 2nd dose should be administered at least 1 mo after the 1st dose, and the 3rd dose should be administered at least 4 mos after the 1st dose and at least 2 mos after the 2nd dose.

[4] DTaP (diphtheria and tetanus toxoids and acellular pertussis vaccine) is the preferred vaccine for all doses in the vaccination series, including completion of the series in children who have received ≥1 dose of whole-cell DTP vaccine. Whole-cell DTP is an acceptable alternative to DTaP. The 4th dose of DTaP may be administered as early as 12 months of age, provided 6 months have elapsed since the 3rd dose, and if the child is considered unlikely to return at 15-18 mos of age. Td (tetanus and diphtheria toxoids, absorbed, for adult use) is recommended at 11-12 years of age if at least 5 years have elapsed since the last dose of DTP, DTaP, or DT. Subsequent routine Td boosters are recommended every 10 years.

[5] Three *H. influenzae* type b (Hib) conjugate vaccines are licensed for infant use. If PRP-OMP (PedvaxHIB [Merck]) is administered at 2 and 4 mos of age, a dose at 6 mos is not required. After completing the primary series, any Hib conjugate vaccine may be used as a booster.

[6] Two poliovirus vaccines are currently licensed in the US: inactivated poliovirus vaccine (IPV) and oral poliovirus vaccine (OPV). The following schedules are all acceptable by the ACIP, the AAP, and the AAFP, and parents and providers may choose among them:
1. IPV at 2 and 4 mos; OPV at 12-18 mos and 4-6 yr
2. IPV at 2, 4, 12-18 mos and 4-6 yr
3. OPV at 2, 4, 6-18 mos and 4-6 yr

The ACIP routinely recommends schedule 1. IPV is the only poliovirus vaccine recommended for immunocompromised persons and their household contacts.

[7] The 2nd dose of MMR is routinely recommended at 4-6 yrs of age or at 11-12 yrs of age, but may be administered during any visit, provided at least 1 month has elapsed since receipt of the 1st dose and that both doses are administered at or after 12 months of age.

[8] Susceptible children may receive Varicella vaccine (Var) at any visit after the first birthday, and those who lack a reliable history of chickenpox should be immunized during the 11-12 year-old visit. Children ≥ 13 years of age should receive 2 doses, at least 1 mo apart.

### TABLE 21-2. Characteristics of Childhood Vaccines

| Vaccine | Type | Route | Adverse Reaction | Comments |
|---|---|---|---|---|
| DTP | Toxoids (DT) and inactivated bacteria (P) | IM | Local redness, fever, anaphylaxis, crying, shock | Pertussis vaccine has not been proven to be a cause of brain damage |
| DTaP | Toxoids and bacterial products (aP) | IM | Above reactions, but more diminished than with DTP | Licensed for use at all ages |
| MMR | Live attenuated viruses | SC | Fever | Two doses recommended |
| Oral polio vaccine (OPV/Sabin) | Live attenuated virus | Oral | Paralysis | Induces intestinal immunity and can immunize contacts |
| Inactivated polio vaccine (IPV/Salk) | Inactivated virus | SC | No serious reactions | For use in immunocompromised children; also recommended as sole vaccine or for sequential use |
| Hib conjugates | Saccharide-protein conjugate | IM | Local inflammation | Different manufacturers use different protein conjugates |
| Hepatitis B | Yeast-derived recombinant | IM | Local pain and fever | Unimmunized adolescents should also receive the vaccine |
| Varicella | Live attenuated virus | SC | Local inflammation | 70% protection against varicella; greater than 95% protection against severe disease |
| Influenza | Inactivated virus or viral components | IM | Infrequent fever | Only "split"-virus vaccines should be used in children less than 13 years |
| Pneumococcal | Polysaccharide | IM/SC | Local inflammation | Antigens of 23 pneumococcal serotypes |
| Meningococci | Polysaccharide | SC | Local inflammation | Against serogroups A, C, Y, and W-135 |

*DTaP = diphtheria and tetanus toxoids and acellular pertussis; DTP = diphtheria tetanus pertussis; Hib = Haemophilus influenzae type b; IM = intramuscularly; MMR = measles, mumps, rubella; SC = subcutaneously.*

States have failed to reach the national goal of 90% coverage for children under 2 years of age. Reasons for the low coverage rate, and thus consequent epidemics, include missed opportunities for immunization, poor access to health care services, and lack of public awareness. Missed opportunities are the fault of health care providers, and are often due to a misunderstanding of the contraindications for immunization and a reluctance to give multiple vaccines at the same well-child visit. Contraindications to immunization are listed in Table 21-3. Mild illnesses, including otitis media and upper respiratory tract infections, local soreness, and prematurity, are *not* contraindications to immunization.

**TABLE 21-3.**

**Contraindications to Childhood Immunizations**

Previous anaphylactic reaction to the specific vaccine

Severe anaphylactic reaction to a vaccine constituent

Concurrent moderate or severe illness

In general, live virus vaccines should not be given to immunocompromised children or pregnant women. Exceptions include the use of live measles-mumps-rubella vaccine in HIV-infected children.

*Adapted from Peter G. Childhood immunizations.* N Engl J Med *1992; 327:1795.*

Recent progress in childhood immunization includes the development of protein-polysaccharide conjugate *Haemophilus influenzae* type b vaccines and the development of new acellular pertussis vaccines. The development of **protein-polysaccharide conjugate vaccines** allows for the stimulation of humoral immunity in children less than 2 years of age. Children of this age do not develop a strong humoral response to polysaccharide antigens, but are at greatest risk of infection from *H. influenzae* type b (in part because of their poor humoral response). Examples of the protein conjugates are diphtheria and tetanus toxoids. Concern about adverse effects of whole-cell pertussis vaccines has stimulated development of new acellular vaccines. When combined with diphtheria and tetanus toxoids, the acellular vaccines are termed DTaP. Acellular pertusis vaccine is recommended for use at all ages.

The American Academy of Pediatrics recommends that all children in the United States be immunized against both **hepatitis B and varicella**. Hepatitis B vaccine should be administered as three doses in infancy. Varicella vaccine should be administered as a single dose between 12 and 18 months of age. Older children should also receive these vaccines.

Other vaccines used in children in the United States include pneumococcal vaccine (children with sickle cell disease, the nephrotic syndrome, HIV infection), and influenza vaccine (children with cystic fibrosis, severe congenital heart disease, HIV infection).

# PEDIATRICS QUESTIONS

**DIRECTIONS:** Each of the numbered items or incomplete statements in this section is followed by answers or by completions of the statement. Select the ONE lettered answer or completion that is BEST in each case.

1. An 8-month-old boy presents with failure to thrive, thrush, lymphadenopathy, and *Pneumocystis carinii* pneumonia. He most likely has

    (A) acute lymphoblastic leukemia
    (B) chronic granulomatous disease
    (C) human immunodeficiency virus (HIV) infection
    (D) IgA deficiency
    (E) X-linked hypogammaglobulinemia

2. Which of the following features most accurately describes Turner syndrome?

    (A) Can be established using buccal smear
    (B) Is associated with advanced maternal age
    (C) Often presents with short stature and primary amenorrhea
    (D) Rarely results in spontaneous abortion
    (E) Usually is due to deletion of the short arm of the X chromosome

3. A 6-year-old boy presents with fever and malaise, followed by headache and back pain. On examination, an asymmetric flaccid paralysis of the muscles of the lower extremities is found. This child most likely has

    (A) Charcot-Marie-Tooth disease
    (B) Duchenne muscular dystrophy
    (C) Guillain-Barré syndrome
    (D) Kugelberg-Welander disease
    (E) Poliomyelitis

4. The most common cause of bacterial pneumonia in children is

   (A) group A streptococci
   (B) *Haemophilus influenzae*
   (C) *Mycobacterium tuberculosis*
   (D) *Staphylococcus aureus*
   (E) *Streptococcus pneumoniae*

5. In the United States, the most common cause of death in children is

   (A) acquired immunodeficiency syndrome (AIDS)
   (B) automobile accidents
   (C) malignancy
   (D) poisoning
   (E) sudden infant death syndrome

6. Which of the following phrases about tuberculosis in children is correct?

   (A) It can be difficult to diagnose because of prior immunization with bacille Calmette-Guérin (BCG) vaccine
   (B) It is almost always symptomatic
   (C) It is highly contagious
   (D) It should prompt identification and treatment of the source case
   (E) It usually results from reactivation of latent disease

7. In children, midline cysts of the neck that move with swallowing are most likely

   (A) branchial cleft cysts
   (B) cavernous hemangiomas
   (C) cystic hygromas
   (D) Langerhans' cell histiocytosis
   (E) thyroglossal duct cysts

8. Which of the following features is associated with external otitis media?

   (A) Can progress to mastoiditis
   (B) Is most commonly due to infection with *Staphylococcus aureus*
   (C) Presents with ear pain exacerbated by pressure on the tragus
   (D) Requires systemic antibiotic therapy
   (E) Requires visualization of the tympanic membrane

9. Which of the following features is true of all infants born to HIV-infected women?

   (A) They will develop AIDS
   (B) They will be infected with HIV
   (C) They will be protected by maternal antibodies
   (D) They will have antibodies to HIV
   (E) They have low CD4 cell counts

10. Which of the following is characteristic of slipped capital femoral epiphysis?

    (A) Always resolves without long-term sequelae
    (B) Is associated with a fracture through the growth plate
    (C) Is best treated by casting the hips in abduction
    (D) Is most common in school-age girls
    (E) Is never bilateral

11. The most serious complication of rubella infection is

    (A) chronic arthritis
    (B) congenital rubella syndrome
    (C) iridocyclitis
    (D) meningoencephalitis
    (E) myocarditis

12. Congenital hypothyroidism most often results from

    (A) congenital pituitary insufficiency
    (B) defective synthesis of thyroxine
    (C) maternal radioiodine intake
    (D) thyroid aplasia or ectopic thyroid
    (E) thyrotropin unresponsiveness

13. Fever and petechiae in a child warrant careful evaluation because of the possibility of

    (A) autoimmune thrombocytopenia
    (B) enteroviral infection
    (C) Henoch-Schönlein purpura
    (D) meningococcemia
    (E) Kawasaki disease

14. The metaphyseal ends of long bones are common sites of osteomyelitis. This condition occurs because

    (A) relative anoxia promotes bacterial growth
    (B) there is blood pooling and reduced phagocytic activity
    (C) they are closer to the skin surface
    (D) they are common sites of trauma
    (E) they have minimal lymphoid tissue

15. Which of the following statements about children with cerebral palsy is correct?

    (A) They are all mentally retarded
    (B) They have low Apgar scores
    (C) They have nonprogressive disorders of motor function
    (D) They infrequently have seizures
    (E) Their mothers usually have had poor obstetric care

16. A 4-day-old infant of a diabetic mother develops irritability, lethargy, and seizures. The most likely cause of these symptoms is

    (A) hypocalcemia
    (B) hypoglycemia
    (C) intraventricular hemorrhage
    (D) meningitis
    (E) subdural hematoma

17. The most common type of leukemia found in children is

   (A) acute lymphocytic leukemia
   (B) acute myelogenous leukemia
   (C) acute nonlymphocytic leukemia
   (D) chronic lymphocytic leukemia
   (E) chronic myelogenous leukemia

18. Orbital cellulitis most commonly results from local extension of infection from the

   (A) cavernous sinus
   (B) conjunctivae
   (C) ethmoid sinus
   (D) maxillary sinus
   (E) preseptal space

19. Which of the following causes cerebral malaria?

   (A) An autoimmune reaction triggered by malarial parasites
   (B) Communicating hydrocephalus
   (C) Hemolysis within cerebral vessels
   (D) Infection of neurons by malarial parasites
   (E) Obstruction of cerebral capillaries by infected erythrocytes

20. A 10-year-old boy has proteinuria in the afternoon but not on the first voided morning urine. He most likely has

   (A) Alport syndrome
   (B) early chronic renal failure
   (C) IgA nephropathy
   (D) membranoproliferative glomerulonephritis
   (E) orthostatic proteinuria

## PEDIATRICS

**21.** Which of the following statements best describes glucose-6-phosphate dehydrogenase deficiency?

(A) It is a cause of megaloblastic anemia in children
(B) It is a cause of immediate hemolysis after ingestion of drugs with oxidant properties
(C) It is associated with severe hemolytic crises in children with sickle cell anemia
(D) It is diagnosed with the osmotic fragility test
(E) It is inherited as an autosomal recessive trait

**22.** Boys with chronic granulomatous disease (CGD) are prone to infection with

(A) group A streptococci
(B) *Haemophilus influenzae*
(C) pneumococci
(D) *Pneumocystis carinii*
(E) *Staphylococcus aureus*

**23.** Maternal varicella results in severe neonatal varicella when maternal infection takes place during

(A) the first trimester
(B) the second trimester
(C) early in the third trimester
(D) the 1-week period prior to and after delivery
(E) delivery

**24.** Nontyphoidal salmonella gastroenteritis should be treated with antibiotics when it occurs in

(A) infants less than 3 months of age
(B) children who are chronic carriers
(C) children with high fever
(D) children with severe dehydration
(E) all children

**25.** An iris or target lesion is characteristic of

(A) erythema infectiosum
(B) erythema multiforme
(C) pityriasis alba
(D) pityriasis rosea
(E) tinea versicolor

**26.** The three most common malignancies in children are

  (A) leukemia, lymphoma, and bone tumors
  (B) leukemia, lymphoma, and central nervous system tumors
  (C) leukemia, Wilms' tumor, and neuroblastoma
  (D) leukemia, Wilms' tumor, and rhabdomyosarcoma
  (E) Wilms' tumor, neuroblastoma, and rhabdomyosarcoma

**27.** Which of the following phrases accurately describes rheumatic fever?

  (A) It can be confirmed by demonstrating antistreptolysin O antibodies
  (B) It cannot be prevented with early antibiotic therapy
  (C) It follows both streptococcal pharyngitis and skin infection
  (D) It is a complication of group A streptococcal pharyngitis
  (E) It occurs simultaneously with streptococcal pharyngitis

**28.** Which statement best describes Meckel's diverticulum?

  (A) It can present as rectal bleeding or intestinal volvulus
  (B) It frequently connects the small intestine with the ligament of Treitz
  (C) It is a predisposing factor for carcinoma of the intestine
  (D) It is a fibrous remnant of Wharton's jelly
  (E) It should be treated with $H_2$-receptor antagonists and antacids

**29.** Folic acid supplementation is recommended for women of reproductive age to prevent

  (A) anemia of prematurity
  (B) Klumpke's paralysis
  (C) neural tube defects
  (D) retinopathy of prematurity
  (E) small left colon syndrome

30. A 6-week-old infant presents with a 1-day history of fever, cough, and rapid breathing. On examination, the infant has a fever of 102°F and a respiratory rate of 60/minute. There are intercostal and subcostal retractions, fair air entry into the lungs, prolongation of the expiratory phase of respiration, and generalized wheezing. The reason for the severity of this infant's respiratory distress is

    (A) edema and inflammation of respiratory infections compromise the airways because of their size
    (B) the epiglottis is more anterior in young infants
    (C) the respiratory rate of young infants is higher than that of older children and adults
    (D) young infants are obligate nasal breathers
    (E) young infants breathe primarily using the diaphragm

31. A ventricular septal defect may not be apparent until several weeks after birth. This is because

    (A) most ventricular septal defects remain asymptomatic unless associated with other cardiac lesions
    (B) symptoms do not occur until the child's cardiac output increases beyond a critical threshold
    (C) symptoms do not occur until the ductus arteriosus has fully closed
    (D) the relatively high pulmonary vascular resistance diminishes the left-to-right shunt
    (E) the ventricular septal defect usually enlarges as the child grows

32. Which of the following phrases about condylomata acuminata in children is accurate?

    (A) Can progress to malignancy
    (B) Due to a pox virus
    (C) Require surgical excision
    (D) Skin-colored papules with central umbilication
    (E) Suggest the possibility of sexual abuse

33. A newborn infant is evaluated at 1 minute with the following signs:
    heart rate present but less than 100 beats/min
    slow respiratory rate
    some flexion of extremities
    grimaces when suctioned
    blue extremities
    This infant has an Apgar score of

    (A) 4
    (B) 5
    (C) 6
    (D) 7
    (E) 8

34. Which of the following neonatal skin rashes requires therapy?

    (A) Acrocyanosis
    (B) Bullous impetigo
    (C) Erythema toxicum
    (D) Milia
    (E) Miliaria

35. A correct statement about the immunologic system of the newborn is

    (A) all newborns with neonatal sepsis will have an elevated white blood cell count
    (B) IgG antibody crosses the placenta beginning at 20 weeks gestation
    (C) IgM and IgA antibodies are passively transferred from the mother to the infant
    (D) maternal antibodies disappear by 3 months of age
    (E) the infant's humoral system begins to function at 12 to 18 months of age

36. Which feature best distinguishes bacterial gastroenteritis from viral gastroenteritis?

    (A) Abdominal pain
    (B) High fever
    (C) Presence of blood, mucous, and leukocytes in the stool
    (D) Severe dehydration

37. Suctioning of the airway at birth through an endotracheal tube can prevent

    (A) bronchopulmonary dysplasia
    (B) hyaline membrane disease
    (C) meconium aspiration syndrome
    (D) pneumonia
    (E) respiratory distress syndrome

38. Which of the following is an unusual feature of neuroblastoma?

    (A) A high rate of spontaneous regression occurs in early infancy
    (B) It can metastasize to any organ in the body
    (C) It can occur at any age
    (D) It usually occurs both above and below the diaphragm
    (E) It is treated with a single chemotherapeutic agent

39. The estimated water requirement of a 12-kg child with normal body temperature and normal renal function is

    (A) 800 mL
    (B) 1000 mL
    (C) 1100 mL
    (D) 1200 mL
    (E) 1500 mL

40. Which of the following statements best describes retinopathy of prematurity?

    (A) It is associated with prolonged hypoxia
    (B) It is a common cause of amblyopia
    (C) It is common in infants of diabetic mothers
    (D) It is common in sick, premature infants
    (E) It is a precursor to retinoblastoma

41. The most common cause of the nephrotic syndrome in children is

    (A) acute poststreptococcal glomerulonephritis
    (B) Alport syndrome
    (C) IgA nephropathy
    (D) membranoproliferative glomerulonephritis
    (E) minimal change disease

**42.** Complications of thalassemia and its treatment include

(A) cerebral infarction
(B) iron deposition in the heart and liver
(C) pneumococcal sepsis
(D) priapism
(E) splenic sequestration

**43.** Infants with homocystinuria have features resembling those associated with

(A) Fanconi syndrome
(B) Marfan syndrome
(C) trisomy 18
(D) Turner syndrome
(E) Williams syndrome

**44.** Intraventricular hemorrhage in the newborn

(A) is due to vitamin K deficiency
(B) most commonly occurs in the subependymal germinal matrix
(C) most commonly occurs in full-term infants with large heads
(D) requires computerized tomography for diagnosis
(E) should be suspected in all infants with cephalhematomas

**45.** Precocious pseudopuberty differs from true precocious puberty in that precocious pseudopuberty

(A) begins with breast development in girls
(B) is always heterosexual
(C) is always isosexual
(D) is independent of gonadotropin function
(E) may be caused by gonadal tumors

**46.** The syndrome of neonatal systemic lupus erythematosus is characterized by

(A) alopecia
(B) arthritis
(C) glomerulonephritis
(D) heart block
(E) peripheral neuropathy

47. Which of the following most often causes anemia in children?

   (A) Glucose-6-phosphate dehydrogenase deficiency
   (B) Iron deficiency
   (C) Sickle cell anemia
   (D) Thalassemia
   (E) Vitamin B12 deficiency

48. A newborn develops symptoms of irritability, tremors, and poor feeding during the first few days of life. The most likely maternal cause of these symptoms is habitual use of

   (A) alcohol
   (B) cigarettes
   (C) hallucinogens
   (D) marijuana
   (E) methadone

49. Neonatal bacterial sepsis is most commonly caused by which one of the following organisms?

   (A) *Haemophilus influenzae*
   (B) Group A beta-hemolytic streptococci
   (C) Group B beta-hemolytic streptococci
   (D) *Klebsiella pneumoniae*
   (E) *Streptococcus pneumoniae*

50. Red blood cells in children with sickle cell anemia contain which form of hemoglobin?

   (A) Hemoglobin S and hemoglobin C
   (B) Hemoglobin S and hemoglobin A
   (C) Hemoglobin S and hemoglobin F
   (D) Hemoglobin S, hemoglobin F, and hemoglobin A
   (E) Only hemoglobin S

51. Teratogenic drugs are most likely to result in congenital malformations when taken during the period of

    (A) conception
    (B) delivery
    (C) late pregnancy
    (D) organogenesis
    (E) second trimester

52. A correct statement about the normal full-term newborn is

    (A) extremities and hips are usually held in flexion
    (B) palpable kidneys are abnormal
    (C) palpable liver is abnormal
    (D) palpable spleen is abnormal
    (E) patent anterior fontanelle is abnormal

53. Which statement best describes acute splenic sequestration?

    (A) It can result in rapid intravascular blood loss and shock
    (B) It is a consequence of autoinfarction of the spleen
    (C) It is a consequence of Salmonella infection in children with sickle cell anemia
    (D) It occurs in older children with sickle cell anemia
    (E) It usually occurs in infants less than 6 months of age with sickle cell anemia

54. Which of the following statements best describes testicular feminization syndrome?

    (A) It causes gynecomastia in adolescent boys
    (B) It is an autosomal recessive disorder
    (C) It is due to insufficient androgen production
    (D) It may present as an inguinal hernia in a girl
    (E) It predisposes to carcinoma of the uterus

55. A 4-year-old boy presents with a retropharyngeal abscess. His physician tells the boy's parents that this condition occurs primarily in young children because of

   (A) dental caries
   (B) frequent episodes of pharyngitis
   (C) frequent minor injury to the pharynx
   (D) lymph nodes between the posterior pharyngeal wall and the prevertebral space
   (E) relatively immunocompromised system

56. The lecithin:sphingomyelin ratio in the amniotic fluid can be used to assess

   (A) fetal growth
   (B) fetal karyotype
   (C) fetal lung maturity
   (D) multiple gestational pregnancies
   (E) presence of neural tube defects

57. Which of the following statements about Wilms' tumor is correct?

   (A) It causes hypertension by releasing catecholamines
   (B) It commonly presents with proteinuria
   (C) It is more common in older children and adolescents
   (D) It is usually bilateral
   (E) It sometimes is associated with hemihypertrophy and aniridia

58. Which of the following statements best describes craniosynostosis?

   (A) It causes delayed closure of the fontanelles
   (B) It is associated with intraventricular hemorrhage
   (C) It is a common cause of cephalopelvic disproportion
   (D) It is a common cause of molding of the newborn's head
   (E) It is a condition of premature closure of the cranial sutures

59. Children with retinoblastoma usually present with which of the following clinical features?

    (A) Amblyopia
    (B) Blindness
    (C) Leukokoria
    (D) Ptosis
    (E) Seizures

60. True statements about infantile spasms include which of the following?

    (A) They are not associated with other neurologic conditions
    (B) They are not true seizures but are due to a defect of the neuromuscular junction
    (C) They consist of brief, repetitive flexion and extensor spasms
    (D) They are usually associated with a normal neurologic outcome
    (E) They have nonspecific electroencephalogram (EEG) findings

61. Kernicterus can best be described as

    (A) a major cause of blindness in newborns
    (B) an unpreventable consequence of hemolysis
    (C) the deposition of conjugated bilirubin in the brain
    (D) the deposition of unconjugated bilirubin in the skin and sclerae
    (E) the deposition of unconjugated bilirubin in the basal ganglia and cerebellum

**PEDIATRICS**

62. Which statement regarding the treatment of children with febrile seizures is correct?

    (A) Children with febrile seizures should receive phenobarbital to prevent recurrence
    (B) Most children with febrile seizures require anticonvulsant therapy
    (C) Prolonged use of phenobarbital for the treatment of febrile seizures is associated with cognitive and behavioral abnormalities
    (D) The use of antipyretics during febrile illnesses is ineffective in preventing recurrence
    (E) The use of rectal or oral diazepam is the ideal preventive therapy because the drug has no adverse effects

63. Premature infants are at greater risk of iron deficiency anemia than full-term infants because

    (A) iron intake is less in premature infants
    (B) gastrointestinal absorption of iron is reduced
    (C) premature infants have a higher rate of blood loss
    (D) premature infants have a higher rate of postnatal growth
    (E) premature infants have proportionally less iron per body weight than full-term infants

64. Bacterial meningitis in children is most commonly caused by

    (A) group A streptococcus, *Haemophilus influenzae* type b, and *Neisseria meningitidis*
    (B) group A streptococcus, *H. influenzae* type b, and *Staphylococcus aureus*
    (C) *Streptococcus pneumoniae*, *Escherichia coli*, and *N. meningitidis*
    (D) *S. pneumoniae*, *H. influenzae* type b, and *Neisseria meningitidis*
    (E) *S. pneumoniae*, *H. influenzae* type b, and *S. aureus*

**65.** A maternal marker for the increased risk of transmission of hepatitis B virus to the infant is

(A) antibodies to the Australia antigen
(B) antibodies to hepatitis B surface antigen
(C) hepatitis B core antigen
(D) hepatitis B e antigen
(E) hepatitis B surface antigen

**66.** A 6-week-old infant presents with a history of poor feeding and generalized weakness. On examination, the infant weighs below the fifth percentile for weight, has no head control, and has generalized hypotonia. No deep tendon reflexes are elicited and fasciculations of the tongue are seen. The most likely diagnosis of this infant is

(A) Becker muscular dystrophy
(B) Duchenne muscular dystrophy
(C) myotonic dystrophy
(D) Sydenham chorea
(E) Werdnig-Hoffmann disease

**67.** The urgency in evaluating a child with fever and seizures is because of the possibility of

(A) brain tumors
(B) epilepsy
(C) febrile seizures
(D) intracranial hemorrhage
(E) meningitis

**68.** The clinical sign that frequently distinguishes upper airway obstruction from lower airway disease is

(A) cough
(B) dyspnea
(C) stridor
(D) supraclavicular retractions
(E) tachypnea

69. Which of the following best characterizes infantile botulism?

    (A) It affects primarily the distal muscles of the arms and legs
    (B) It is associated with contaminated pork
    (C) It is caused by *Clostridium botulinum* bacteremia
    (D) It is caused by ingestion of a preformed toxin
    (E) It occurs in infants with infected wounds

70. A 6-month-old infant who presents with crises consisting of persistent vomiting, irritability, sweating, flushing, and hypertension will be diagnosed with which one of the following conditions?

    (A) Critical coarctation of the aorta
    (B) Familial dysautonomia
    (C) Myasthenia gravis
    (D) Reye's syndrome
    (E) Tetralogy of Fallot

71. Which statement best describes sarcoma botryoides?

    (A) It is due to infection with *Echinococcus granulosus*
    (B) It is due to rhabdomyosarcoma extending into a body cavity such as the vagina or bladder
    (C) It is due to vaginal infection with papillomavirus
    (D) It is a highly malignant form of osteogenic sarcoma
    (E) It is a rare complication of non-Hodgkin's lymphoma

72. An adolescent presents with pneumonia, malaise, sore throat, and a positive test for cold hemagglutinins. She most likely is infected with

    (A) group A streptococci
    (B) *Haemophilus influenzae*
    (C) *Mycoplasma pneumoniae*
    (D) *Staphylococcus aureus*
    (E) *Streptococcus pneumoniae*

**73.** Which statement accurately describes children with acute appendicitis?

(A) They are hungry and willing to eat
(B) They have localized pain to the left lower quadrant
(C) They may have diarrhea or pyuria
(D) They are usually less than 2 years of age
(E) They usually have normal temperatures

**74.** Which statement regarding the treatment of asthma in children is correct?

(A) Cromolyn sodium is contraindicated in children less than 13 years of age
(B) Corticosteroids should be reserved for children with severe, refractory asthma
(C) Inhaled beta$_2$-agonists should be reserved for children with severe asthma
(D) Inhaled corticosteroids reduce the likelihood of complications from chronic steroid use
(E) Theophylline is the drug of choice

**75.** Poststreptococcal glomerulonephritis must be distinguished from which of the following causes of glomerulonephritis and a low serum complement level?

(A) Hemolytic-uremic syndrome
(B) Henoch-Schönlein purpura
(C) IgA nephropathy
(D) Membranoproliferative glomerulonephritis
(E) Minimal change disease

**76.** Which of the following is the most common congenital heart lesion?

(A) Atrial septal defect
(B) Coarctation of the aorta
(C) Tetralogy of Fallot
(D) Transposition of the great vessels
(E) Ventricular septal defect

77. Which of the following is characteristic of pertussis?

    (A) Easily diagnosed
    (B) Elevated neutrophil count
    (C) Fecal-oral transmission
    (D) Parainfluenza viral infection
    (E) Repetitive coughs followed by an inspiratory whoop

78. Chemoprophylaxis should be considered for some families of children with meningitis caused by

    (A) group B streptococcus
    (B) group A streptococcus
    (C) *Haemophilus influenzae* type b
    (D) pneumococcus
    (E) *Staphylococcus aureus*

79. Prostaglandin E should be used in infants with congenital heart disease to maintain a patent ductus arteriosus. Prostaglandin E is given when

    (A) the development of Eisenmenger syndrome is likely
    (B) there is anomalous origin of the left coronary artery
    (C) there is a hypoplastic left ventricle
    (D) there is a large ventricular septal defect
    (E) there is severe restriction to pulmonary blood flow

80. Which of the following phrases most accurately describes testicular torsion?

    (A) It is characterized by a "blue dot" sign visible on the scrotum
    (B) It is a surgical emergency
    (C) It is due to failure of the proximal part of the processus vaginalis to close in late fetal life
    (D) It is due to trauma producing rotational forces on the testes
    (E) It occurs in boys with inguinal hernias

81. Eisenmenger syndrome is best described as

    (A) a left-to-right shunt through a ventricular septal defect resulting from severe aortic stenosis
    (B) a right-to-left shunt through a ventricular septal defect resulting from pulmonary hypertension
    (C) the association of supravalvular aortic stenosis and hypercalcemia
    (D) the association of transposition of the great vessels and elfin facies
    (E) the coexistence of a ventricular septal defect and atrial septal defect

82. Which of the following statements best describes Guillain-Barré syndrome?

    (A) Paresthesia begins with the muscles of the head and neck
    (B) It is characterized by exaggerated deep tendon reflexes
    (C) It is characterized by normal cerebrospinal fluid
    (D) It is a demyelinating polyneuropathy
    (E) It is usually more severe in children than adults

83. A 3-month-old infant presents with afebrile pneumonitis and eosinophilia. She most likely is infected with

    (A) *Chlamydia trachomatis*
    (B) group B streptococcus
    (C) respiratory syncytial virus
    (D) *Listeria monocytogenes*
    (E) ascariasis

84. A widely split second heart sound that is fixed in both inspiration and expiration is characteristic of which lesion?

    (A) Aortic stenosis
    (B) Atrial septal defect
    (C) Ebstein anomaly
    (D) Pulmonary valve stenosis
    (E) Ventricular septal defect

85. Correct statements about pyloric stenosis include which of the following?

    (A) It is due to membranous remnants obstructing the stomach antrum
    (B) It presents with projectile, bilious vomiting
    (C) It results in anorexia and poor feeding
    (D) It results in a metabolic alkalosis and hypokalemia
    (E) It usually presents in the first 3 days after birth

86. Which of the following statements most accurately describes occult bacteremia?

    (A) It can be confirmed on the basis of clinical findings
    (B) It is most common in children over 2 years of age
    (C) It is most commonly due to *Streptococcus pneumoniae*
    (D) It never progresses to localized infection
    (E) It should always be treated with parenteral antibiotics

87. A positive Ortolani maneuver indicates the presence of

    (A) dislocation of the hip
    (B) dislocatable hip
    (C) Legg-Calve-Perthes disease
    (D) slipped capital femoral epiphysis
    (E) subluxation of the hip

88. Which of the following is most characteristic of undescended testes?

    (A) Always unilateral
    (B) Associated with normal fertility
    (C) Caused by failure of testicular descent in the first trimester
    (D) Rarely associated with indirect inguinal hernias
    (E) Risk of testicular malignancy

89. Which phrase best defines a kerion?

    (A) Boggy mass associated with tinea capitis
    (B) Excessive growth of scar tissue
    (C) Parasitic infection
    (D) Soft tissue tumor
    (E) Stage of dental plaque

90. Bilious vomiting can be caused by

   (A) hepatitis
   (B) increased intracranial pressure
   (C) intestinal malrotation
   (D) pyloric stenosis
   (E) rotavirus gastroenteritis

91. Which of the following best describes protein-polysaccharide conjugate vaccines for *Haemophilus influenzae* type b?

   (A) They allow for combination vaccines
   (B) They allow for the stimulation of humoral immunity in children less than 2 years of age
   (C) They are designed to stimulate cell-mediated immunity
   (D) They are live-attenuated vaccines
   (E) They reduce the incidence of adverse effects

92. The most common bacterial cause of osteomyelitis in children is

   (A) group A beta hemolytic streptococci
   (B) *Haemophilus influenzae* type b
   (C) pneumococci
   (D) Salmonella
   (E) *Staphylococcus aureus*

93. Which of the following is associated with the occurrence of trisomy 21 in younger women?

   (A) Higher rate of exposure to infectious diseases
   (B) Higher rate of exposure to radiation
   (C) Maternal nondisjunction during meiosis
   (D) Maternal nondisjunction during mitosis
   (E) Translocation or paternal nondisjunction

94. Urinary tract obstruction in boys is most commonly caused by

   (A) posterior urethral valves
   (B) renal stones
   (C) ureteropelvic junction obstruction
   (D) ureterovesicular junction obstruction
   (E) urethral obstruction

**95.** Which of the following phrases about infants infected with hepatitis B virus is correct?

(A) Almost always develop jaundice
(B) Are at high risk of developing subsequent cirrhosis or hepatocellular carcinoma
(C) Are highly infectious to other children in day-care centers
(D) Are usually infected by mothers who are hepatitis e antigen negative
(E) Usually develop liver failure by the end of the first decade of life

**96.** Diarrhea in infants and young children is most commonly caused by

(A) enteric adenovirus
(B) Norwalk virus
(C) rotavirus
(D) salmonella
(E) shigella

**97.** Septic arthritis of the hip is particularly dangerous because

(A) arthrocentesis can damage the femoral nerve
(B) infection can spread to the peritoneal cavity
(C) increased pressure can cause avascular necrosis of the femoral head
(D) osteomyelitis is frequently present
(E) slipped capital femoral epiphysis is a long-term complication

**98.** Recommendations for treating children less than 8 years of age with the nephrotic syndrome include which of the following?

(A) Corticosteroid therapy to prevent chronic renal failure
(B) Corticosteroid therapy to reduce the proteinuria and infectious complications
(C) Place on a high protein diet
(D) Prepare for chronic dialysis therapy
(E) Perform kidney biopsy to confirm diagnosis

**99.** Lactase deficiency is best described by which statement?

(A) It can be confirmed by identifying a reducing sugar in the stool
(B) It is a common congenital defect in infants
(C) It frequently requires the use of a lactose-free formula
(D) It is more common in infants than in adults
(E) It occurs in children with pancreatic insufficiency

**100.** Which of the following statements about children with severe combined immunodeficiency (SCID) is most accurate?

(A) It occurs more often in girls than in boys
(B) They are at high risk of pneumococcal infection
(C) They have defects in both humoral immunity and complement
(D) They present with failure to thrive, diarrhea, and opportunistic infections
(E) They should be treated with gamma globulin infusions

**101.** Children treated for leukemia are at increased risk of serious bacterial infection. The primary cause is

(A) complement deficiency
(B) hypogammaglobulinemia
(C) neutropenia
(D) T-cell dysfunction
(E) venous catheters

**102.** Which of the following is associated with systemic onset juvenile rheumatoid arthritis?

(A) Corticosteroids are the treatment of choice
(B) HLA-B27 is a common association
(C) Iridocyclitis is common
(D) Rheumatoid factor is frequently present
(E) Systemic symptoms may precede its onset

# PEDIATRICS

**103.** Which of the following disorders is commonly associated with trisomy 21?

(A) Atlantoaxial instability
(B) Congenital dislocation of the hip
(C) Klippel-Feil syndrome
(D) Osgood-Schlatter disease
(E) Sprengel deformity

**104.** Amblyopia is most likely to occur in children with

(A) monocular strabismus
(B) alternating strabismus
(C) bilateral cataracts
(D) retinopathy of prematurity

**105.** A 6-week-old infant presents for a routine health maintenance visit. The mother complains of a rash on the infant's scalp. Examination reveals scaling crusty lesions of the scalp and greasy scaling erythematous lesions behind the ears and eyebrows. The most likely diagnosis of this infant's condition is

(A) candidal dermatitis
(B) eczema herpeticum
(C) impetigo
(D) seborrheic dermatitis
(E) tinea capitis

**106.** Which of the following phrases is true about sexual abuse of prepubertal girls?

(A) Can be excluded if the genital examination is normal
(B) Is confirmed by measuring the size of the hymenal opening
(C) Is confirmed by a positive antigen detection test for chlamydia
(D) Is suggested by posterior tears and irregularities of the hymen
(E) Is without long-term sequelae

## Pediatrics Questions

**107.** Which of the following features is most closely associated with carbon monoxide poisoning?

(A) It can be diagnosed by measurement of carboxyhemoglobin
(B) It can be diagnosed by measurement of $PO_2$
(C) It can be diagnosed by pulse oximetry
(D) It greatly reduces the dissolved oxygen in the blood
(E) It is treated with 50% oxygen delivered by a positive pressure mask

**108.** Which of the following accurately describes Fragile X syndrome?

(A) It causes testicular feminization
(B) It causes undescended testicles
(C) It is associated with hypogonadism
(D) It is a common cause of mental retardation
(E) It predisposes to testicular malignancy

**109.** A young child presents with a fever of 40°C that resolves with the onset of a generalized erythematous rash. She most likely has

(A) erythema infectiosum
(B) measles
(C) meningococcemia
(D) occult bacteremia
(E) roseola

**110.** Which of the following statements about boys with X-linked agammaglobulinemia is most accurate?

(A) They are at risk of infection from such opportunistic organisms as *Pneumocystis carinii*
(B) They are most prone to infection in the first year of life
(C) They are prone to infection with *Streptococcus pneumoniae* and *Haemophilus influenzae* type b
(D) They are protected by the transfer of maternal B cells
(E) They should be treated with plasma exchange therapy

111. Which of the following is the most prevalent nematode infection in the United States?

   (A) *Ancylostoma duodenale*
   (B) *Ascaris lumbricoides*
   (C) *Enterobius vermicularis*
   (D) *Necator americanus*
   (E) *Strongyloides stercoralis*

112. The most common bacterial causes of acute otitis media are

   (A) group A beta hemolytic streptococci, *Haemophilus influenzae* type b, and *Staphylococcus aureus*
   (B) *H. influenzae* type b, *Streptococcus pneumoniae*, and *S. aureus*
   (C) *S. pneumoniae*, group A beta hemolytic streptococci, and *S. aureus*
   (D) *S. pneumoniae*, nontypable *H. influenzae*, and *Moraxella catarrhalis*
   (E) *S. pneumoniae*, *S. aureus*, and *M. catarrhalis*

113. A newborn has fine facial features, low set ears, prominent occiput, unusual flexion deformity of the fingers, and rocker bottom feet. This newborn most likely has

   (A) cri du chat syndrome
   (B) Turner syndrome
   (C) trisomy 13
   (D) trisomy 18
   (E) trisomy 21

114. Children with chromosomal breakage syndromes are at high risk of which of the following conditions?

   (A) Aniridia
   (B) Malignancy
   (C) Mental retardation
   (D) Microcephaly
   (E) Short stature

115. Each of the following statements about congenital cytomegalovirus infection is correct EXCEPT

   (A) congenital infection can be diagnosed after infancy by culture of the virus from the urine
   (B) intracranial calcifications and chorioamnionitis can result from severe congenital infection
   (C) most congenital infections are asymptomatic
   (D) perinatal infection can also occur through breast milk or blood transfusion
   (E) sensorineural hearing loss is a long-term sequelae of congenital cytomegalovirus infection

**Questions 116–118**

A 6-month-old infant presents with a 2-day history of cough, rhinitis, and fever (temperature to 103°F). On examination, the temperature is 103.6°F, the anterior fontanelle is full, and there is a suggestion of nuchal rigidity.

116. The laboratory studies that should be performed on this child include each of the following EXCEPT

   (A) blood culture
   (B) complete blood count
   (C) examination of the cerebrospinal fluid
   (D) liver function tests
   (E) urine culture

117. If a 6-month-old infant has bacterial meningitis, you would expect to find each of the following on examination of the cerebrospinal fluid (CSF) EXCEPT

   (A) elevated CSF glucose level
   (B) elevated CSF protein level
   (C) Gram stain showing gram-negative, intracellular diplococci
   (D) Gram stain showing gram-positive cocci in pairs
   (E) numerous neutrophils

118. Complications of bacterial meningitis in this infant may include each of the following EXCEPT

   (A) hearing loss
   (B) hydrocephalus
   (C) language delay
   (D) seizures
   (E) subdural hematoma

119. An 18-month-old child presents for a routine health maintenance visit. On examination, the child is found to be pale. On closer questioning of the parent, a history is elicited of anorexia, fatigue, and irritability. A possible diagnosis in this child includes each of the following EXCEPT

   (A) iron deficiency anemia
   (B) lead poisoning
   (C) leukemia
   (D) sickle cell trait
   (E) thalassemia

120. Signs of respiratory distress in a young child include each of the following EXCEPT

   (A) grunting
   (B) intercostal retractions
   (C) nasal flaring
   (D) respiratory rate of 24/min
   (E) supraclavicular retractions

121. Each of the following statements about Graves' disease in children is correct EXCEPT

   (A) antimicrosomal antibodies are usually present
   (B) early symptoms are emotional lability, hyperactivity, and declining school performance
   (C) excessive production of thyroid-stimulating hormone (TSH) results in hyperthyroidism
   (D) Graves' disease is most common in adolescent girls
   (E) lymphocytic infiltration of the retro-orbital tissues results in exophthalmos

## Pediatrics Questions

**122.** Each of the following statements about respiratory distress syndrome (RDS) is correct EXCEPT

(A) corticosteroids administered to the mother prior to delivery can help prevent RDS
(B) continuous positive airway pressure can prevent atelectasis in infants with RDS
(C) RDS is a transient condition with no long-term sequelae
(D) RDS occurs in premature infants
(E) surfactant therapy can be used to prevent and treat RDS

**123.** Each of the following is associated with severe protein-energy malnutrition EXCEPT

(A) electrolyte abnormalities
(B) fractures
(C) hypothermia
(D) severe infection
(E) vitamin A deficiency

**124.** Hypernatremia can occur as a consequence of each of the following EXCEPT

(A) cystic fibrosis
(B) dehydration
(C) diabetes insipidus
(D) improper preparation of infant formulas
(E) salt poisoning

**125.** A 16-month-old infant who presents with a history of having been fed only breast milk and who has had no vitamin D supplementation would be expected to have each of the following clinical manifestations EXCEPT

(A) craniotabes
(B) delayed closure of the fontanelles
(C) edema
(D) fractures
(E) widening of the distal ends of long bones

## PEDIATRICS

**126.** Vesicoureteral reflux can result in each of the following conditions EXCEPT

(A) chronic renal failure
(B) dilatation of the ureters
(C) hypertension
(D) proteinuria
(E) urinary tract infection

**127.** Each of the following statements about neonatal herpes simplex infection is correct EXCEPT

(A) infants suspected of having neonatal herpes simplex infection should be treated with acyclovir
(B) infection is limited to the skin and mucous membranes
(C) measurement of IgG antibodies against herpes simplex virus in the infant does not confirm neonatal infection
(D) the diagnosis is confirmed by the culture of herpes simplex virus
(E) the risk of neonatal infection is higher in women with primary herpes simplex infection

**128.** Each of the following occurs with greater frequency in an infant of a diabetic mother EXCEPT

(A) birth injuries
(B) congenital heart disease
(C) hypoglycemia
(D) respiratory distress syndrome
(E) retinopathy

**129.** Hydrocephalus can be caused by each of the following conditions EXCEPT

(A) aqueductal stenosis
(B) Dandy-Walker cyst
(C) maternal alcohol use
(D) meningitis
(E) subarachnoid hemorrhage

**130.** Each of the following statements about breast milk is true EXCEPT

(A) it is available in an uncontaminated form
(B) it contains factors that promote the growth of nonpathogenic bacteria
(C) it contains more carbohydrates and less protein than cow's milk
(D) it contains secretory IgA
(E) it contains sufficient vitamin D to prevent nutritional rickets

**131.** Each of the following is a characteristic of fetal alcohol syndrome EXCEPT

(A) facial abnormalities
(B) hydrocephalus
(C) intrauterine growth retardation
(D) mental retardation
(E) ventricular septal defect

**132.** Each of the following statements about hemolytic disease of the newborn is correct EXCEPT

(A) antibodies can be directed against ABO or Rh antigens on the fetal red blood cells
(B) anti-Rh immune globulin can prevent Rh incompatibility
(C) congestive heart failure can occur in newborn infants with severe erythroblastosis fetalis
(D) it results from maternal IgM antibodies that cross the placenta
(E) Rh incompatibility occurs when an Rh-negative mother has an Rh-positive fetus

133. In the United States, children less than 2 years of age have a low rate of immunization coverage. Reasons for the lack of coverage include each of the following EXCEPT

(A) lack of public awareness
(B) malpractice litigation
(C) misunderstanding of the contraindications for immunization
(D) poor access to health services
(E) reluctance to give multiple vaccines at the same well-child care visit

134. Each of the following is associated most often with low birth weight EXCEPT

(A) intrauterine growth retardation
(B) maternal hypertension
(C) maternal diabetes mellitus
(D) multiple gestational pregnancies
(E) prematurity

135. Each of the following statements about a newborn's respiratory system is correct EXCEPT

(A) because a newborn is an obligate oral breather, nasal obstruction causes no distress
(B) during inspiration, the thorax moves inward and the abdomen protrudes
(C) short periods of apnea (5 to 10 seconds) are normal
(D) surfactant reduces surface tension and prevents atelectasis
(E) the newborn's respiratory rate is highly variable

136. Causes of short stature include each of the following conditions EXCEPT

(A) chronic renal failure
(B) diabetes mellitus
(C) growth hormone deficiency
(D) inflammatory bowel disease
(E) Turner syndrome

**137.** Characteristics of fetal circulation include each of the following EXCEPT

(A) blood is shunted from the right side of the heart to the left
(B) the ductus arteriosus is patent
(C) the foramen ovale is patent
(D) placental circulation is of low resistance
(E) the pulmonary vascular bed is dilated

**138.** Complications of sickle cell anemia include each of the following EXCEPT

(A) aplastic crisis
(B) dactylitis
(C) gallstones
(D) priapism
(E) thrombocytopenia

**139.** Each of the following statements about congenital adrenal hyperplasia is correct EXCEPT

(A) boys with the simple virilizing form of 21-hydroxylase deficiency can have short stature as adults
(B) children with the salt-losing form of 21-hydroxylase deficiency present as toddlers with subtle signs of hyponatremia
(C) deficiency in cortisol production results in increased secretion of ACTH
(D) girls with the simple virilizing form of 21-hydroxylase deficiency can have ambiguous genitalia
(E) 21-hydroxylase deficiency is the most common enzyme deficiency

**140.** The risk of sudden infant death syndrome (SIDS) is most likely increased in each of the following EXCEPT

(A) boys
(B) families living in poverty
(C) families with a previous child who died of SIDS
(D) supine sleeping position
(E) winter season

# PEDIATRICS

**141.** Each of the following conditions can occur as a result of birth trauma EXCEPT

(A) caput succedaneum
(B) cephalhematoma
(C) clavicular fracture
(D) Erb-Duchenne paralysis
(E) Volkmann contracture

**142.** Each of the following statements about phenylketonuria (PKU) is correct EXCEPT

(A) infants with PKU can have a mousy or misty body odor
(B) infants with PKU develop fair skin, light hair, and dermatitis
(C) PKU can be diagnosed immediately after birth and before milk feedings have begun
(D) the treatment of PKU is dietary reduction of phenylalanine
(E) untreated PKU results in mental retardation

**143.** Each of the following is a correct statement about patent ductus arteriosus (PDA) EXCEPT

(A) a PDA in a full-term infant can usually be closed with indomethacin
(B) infants with a PDA have a wide pulse pressure
(C) pulmonary hypertension is a potential complication of an untreated PDA
(D) the classic murmur of a PDA is a "machinery" murmur
(E) the shunting of blood through a PDA is left to right

**144.** Several laboratory tests are useful in diagnosing HIV infection in children less than 15 months of age. Which test would NOT be helpful in diagnosing HIV in this particular age group?

(A) Anti-HIV IgA antibodies
(B) Anti-HIV IgG antibodies
(C) HIV culture
(D) Polymerase chain reaction
(E) p24 antigen

145. On examination, jaundice is found in a 2-day-old infant. The possible causes of this jaundice include each of the following EXCEPT

   (A) biliary tract obstruction
   (B) hemolysis of red blood cells
   (C) normal immaturity of the conjugation of bilirubin
   (D) sickle cell disease
   (E) sepsis

146. Characteristic features of acute poststreptococcal glomerulonephritis include each of the following EXCEPT

   (A) chronic renal failure
   (B) edema
   (C) gross hematuria
   (D) hypertension
   (E) renal insufficiency

147. Each of the following statements about necrotizing enterocolitis (NEC) is correct EXCEPT

   (A) bloody stools are a sign of NEC
   (B) *Clostridium difficile* is the etiologic agent
   (C) NEC most commonly occurs in the distal ileum and proximal colon
   (D) pneumatosis intestinalis is a pathognomonic radiographic finding
   (E) premature infants are at high risk for NEC

148. Each of the following statements regarding intussusception is correct EXCEPT

   (A) a tender, sausage-shaped mass can be palpated most often in the right upper quadrant
   (B) it can be due to Meckel's diverticulum or Henoch-Schönlein purpura
   (C) usually involves the distal ileum and proximal colon
   (D) signs and symptoms include cramping abdominal pain, vomiting, and blood and mucus in the stool
   (E) upper gastrointestinal barium swallow is both diagnostic and therapeutic

**149.** Each of the following statements regarding Alport syndrome is correct EXCEPT

(A) Alport syndrome can cause chronic renal failure in infants
(B) Alport syndrome is more severe in boys than in girls
(C) children with Alport syndrome can have cataracts
(D) children with Alport syndrome can have sensorineural hearing loss
(E) children with Alport syndrome present with microscopic or gross hematuria

**150.** Failure to pass meconium in the newborn infant can result from each of the following EXCEPT

(A) cystic fibrosis
(B) Hirschsprung's disease
(C) imperforate anus
(D) malrotation
(E) small left colon syndrome

**151.** Each of the following statements regarding spherocytosis is correct EXCEPT

(A) children without a functioning spleen are at risk of pneumococcal sepsis
(B) diagnosis is confirmed by the osmotic fragility test
(C) is due to a defect in the cell wall of red blood cells
(D) splenic infarction and autosplenectomy result in gradual resolution of the anemia
(E) symptoms are anemia, jaundice, and splenomegaly

**152.** Clinical manifestations of diabetic ketoacidosis include each of the following EXCEPT

(A) abdominal pain
(B) dehydration
(C) hyperglycemia
(D) metabolic acidosis with a normal anion gap
(E) respiratory alkalosis

**153.** Signs and symptoms of Kawasaki disease include each of the following EXCEPT

(A) bilateral conjunctival infection without discharge
(B) desquamation of the fingers, toes, and perianal region
(C) glomerulonephritis
(D) lymphadenopathy
(E) prolonged high fever

**154.** Each of the following is used in the management of HIV-infected children EXCEPT

(A) intravenous gamma globulin
(B) live measles vaccine
(C) live polio vaccine
(D) nutritional support
(E) trimethoprim-sulfamethoxazole

**155.** Each of the following statements about hemorrhagic disease of the newborn is correct EXCEPT

(A) intracranial hemorrhage is a rare but serious complication
(B) it should be treated with vitamin K but cannot be prevented
(C) it is due to a transient decrease in vitamin K–dependent factors
(D) it is usually more severe in preterm and breast-fed infants
(E) it usually occurs 2 to 3 days after birth

**156.** A child with beta thalassemia might be expected to have each of the following signs or symptoms EXCEPT

(A) failure to thrive
(B) generalized lymphadenopathy
(C) jaundice
(D) pallor
(E) splenomegaly

**157.** Characteristics of myotonic dystrophy include each of the following EXCEPT

(A) associated with endocrinopathies
(B) associated with immunodeficiencies
(C) autosomal dominant disorder
(D) muscle wasting of the distal muscles of the hands, forearms, and legs
(E) rapid, jerky relaxation of muscle contraction

**158.** Which of the following is NOT a characteristic feature of the nephrotic syndrome?

(A) Edema
(B) Hyperlipidemia
(C) Hypertension
(D) Hypoalbuminemia
(E) Proteinuria greater than 1000 mg/m$^2$/day

**159.** Each of the following is a manifestation of congenital syphilis EXCEPT

(A) anemia and thrombocytopenia
(B) anterior bowing of the shins
(C) chorioretinitis
(D) profuse nasal discharge
(E) saddle nose deformity

**160.** Characteristic signs and symptoms of Henoch-Schönlein purpura include each of the following EXCEPT

(A) arthritis of the knees and ankles
(B) glomerulonephritis
(C) gross or occult gastrointestinal bleeding
(D) purpura over the posterior legs and buttocks
(E) thrombocytopenia

**161.** Each of the following statements regarding severe gastroesophageal reflux in infants is correct EXCEPT

(A) barium swallow examination can demonstrate anatomic abnormalities
(B) chronic esophagitis can cause iron deficiency anemia
(C) common in premature infants
(D) may require pharmacologic therapy or surgery
(E) failure to thrive and recurrent aspiration pneumonia

**162.** Each of the following conditions can occur as a result of congenital rubella infection EXCEPT

(A) cataracts
(B) congenital heart disease
(C) fever
(D) hearing loss
(E) microcephaly

**163.** Clinical manifestations of neurofibromatosis type 1 include each of the following EXCEPT

(A) axillary freckling
(B) café-au-lait spots
(C) Lisch nodules
(D) neuroblastoma
(E) optic gliomas

**164.** Common signs and symptoms of inborn errors of metabolism include each of the following EXCEPT

(A) developmental delay
(B) failure to thrive
(C) persistent vomiting
(D) seizures
(E) sensorineural hearing loss

**165.** Each of the following statements regarding Hodgkin's disease is correct EXCEPT

(A) children treated for Hodgkin's disease are at risk for opportunistic infections
(B) children typically present with an enlarged cervical or supraclavicular node
(C) it has a peak incidence in early childhood
(D) metastatic disease occurs to the lungs, liver, and bone marrow
(E) the Reed-Sternberg cell is the characteristic histologic finding

**166.** Each of the following statements about galactosemia is correct EXCEPT

(A) a tentative diagnosis of galactosemia can be made by documenting the presence of reducing sugars in the urine
(B) infants with galactosemia are at increased risk of gram-negative infection
(C) infants with galactosemia are ill at birth
(D) the disease is due to the toxic accumulation of galactose
(E) vomiting, hypoglycemia, and seizures are symptoms of galactosemia

**167.** Thrombocytopenia is associated with each of the following conditions EXCEPT

(A) disseminated intravascular coagulation (DIC)
(B) hemolytic-uremic syndrome
(C) Henoch-Schönlein purpura
(D) Kasabach-Merritt syndrome
(E) Wiskott-Aldrich syndrome

**168.** Each of the following conditions is highly suggestive of child abuse EXCEPT

(A) "bucket handle" fractures of the long bones
(B) burns to the soles of both feet
(C) fractures in different stages of healing
(D) posterior rib fractures
(E) supracondylar fractures of the elbow

## Pediatrics Questions

**169.** Each of the following is important in the management of the child with insulin-dependent diabetes mellitus (IDDM) EXCEPT

(A) dietary management
(B) exercise
(C) glucose monitoring
(D) health education for the child and family
(E) once-a-day administration of insulin

**170.** A 3-year-old boy presents with a 1-day history of fever, a barking cough, and respiratory distress. On examination, the child appears toxic and is sitting forward and drooling. His temperature is 104.4°F and severe inspiratory stridor and intercostal and subcostal retractions are present. Relative to this patient, each of the following statements is true EXCEPT

(A) immunization against *Haemophilus influenzae* type b might have prevented the patient's condition
(B) examination of the patient's pharynx should not be performed
(C) nasotracheal intubation of the patient may be required
(D) a cold air mist tent is the therapy of choice for this patient
(E) the diagnosis of this patient can be confirmed by lateral radiograph of the neck

**171.** Hemolytic anemia can result from each of the following EXCEPT

(A) hemoglobinopathies
(B) red blood cell enzyme defects
(C) structural abnormalities of the red blood cell
(D) traumatic destruction of red blood cells
(E) vitamin B12 deficiency

172. Hypoglycemia in a child with insulin-dependent diabetes mellitus is caused by each of the following EXCEPT

(A) antibodies to insulin
(B) excessive insulin administration
(C) honeymoon period
(D) Somogyi phenomenon
(E) use of nonhuman insulin preparations

173. A 7-year-old girl presents with a history of fever and sore throat with a duration of 1 day. On examination, the child has a temperature of 102°F and diffusely inflamed tonsils and pharynx. The potential causes of this pharyngitis include each of the following organisms EXCEPT

(A) adenovirus
(B) coxsackievirus
(C) Epstein-Barr virus
(D) herpes simplex virus
(E) group A streptococci

174. Characteristics of Marfan syndrome include each of the following EXCEPT

(A) arachnodactyly
(B) arm span greater than height
(C) dislocation of the lens
(D) frequent fractures of long bones
(E) mitral valve prolapse

175. Adrenocortical insufficiency in children can result from each of the following EXCEPT

(A) Addison's disease
(B) adrenocortical adenomas
(C) congenital adrenal hyperplasia
(D) high-dose corticosteroid therapy
(E) Waterhouse-Friderichsen syndrome

**176.** Each of the following statements regarding simple partial seizures is correct EXCEPT

(A) they are common in children
(B) they are associated with a transient loss of consciousness
(C) they may be confused with tics
(D) they usually consist of clonic or tonic movements of the face, neck, and extremities
(E) they usually last 10 to 20 seconds

**177.** A 1-year-old boy presents with a history of easy bruising of several weeks duration. On examination, multiple ecchymoses are found on the legs, buttocks, and back. Each of the following is a likely diagnosis EXCEPT

(A) child abuse
(B) hemophilia A
(C) Henoch-Schönlein purpura
(D) leukemia
(E) rickets

**178.** Each of the following statements regarding osteomyelitis in children is correct EXCEPT

(A) blood cultures frequently reveal the causative organism
(B) fever invariably is present
(C) most children have a leukocytosis
(D) multifocal osteomyelitis can occur in neonates
(E) radiographs of the bone do not show evidence of infection until 10 to 14 days after the onset

**179.** Which of the following is NOT a cause of pancytopenia?

(A) Androgens
(B) Chloramphenicol
(C) Hepatitis infection
(D) Infiltration of the bone marrow by leukemia
(E) Radiation

180. Risk factors for the development of nonfebrile seizures or idiopathic epilepsy in a child with febrile seizures include each of the following EXCEPT

    (A) children with febrile seizure of greater than 15 minutes
    (B) family history of febrile seizures
    (C) focal seizures
    (D) neurologic abnormalities
    (E) repeated seizures within the same febrile episode

181. Each of the following phrases about sinusitis in children is correct EXCEPT

    (A) associated with severe or prolonged upper respiratory tract infection
    (B) periorbital edema
    (C) orbital cellulitis is a complication
    (D) the diagnosis requires computerized tomography
    (E) *Streptococcus pneumoniae*, nontypable *Haemophilus influenzae*, and *Moraxella catarrhalis* are the most common bacterial pathogens

182. Each of the following disorders is associated with a limp and hip pain in children EXCEPT

    (A) Legg-Calve-Perthes disease
    (B) Osgood-Schlatter disease
    (C) septic arthritis
    (D) slipped capital femoral epiphysis
    (E) toxic synovitis

183. Each of the following statements regarding indirect inguinal hernias is correct EXCEPT

    (A) associated with testicular feminization syndrome
    (B) equally frequent in boys and girls
    (C) incarceration can cause intestinal obstruction
    (D) more common in premature infants
    (E) ovary may be found in the inguinal canal

**184.** Each of the following statements regarding autoimmune thrombocytopenia purpura (ATP) is correct EXCEPT

(A) ATP usually presents several weeks after a minor viral illness
(B) examination of the bone marrow shows a decreased number of megakaryocytes
(C) intracranial hemorrhage is a rare but serious complication
(D) large platelets can be seen on peripheral blood smear
(E) the total platelet count is low and anemia may be present

**185.** A 16-year-old adolescent presents with possible infectious mononucleosis. In this patient, which of the following signs and symptoms would NOT be an indication of this illness?

(A) Atypical lymphocytes
(B) Exudative pharyngitis
(C) Lymphadenopathy
(D) Splenomegaly
(E) Thrombocytopenia

**186.** Classification of acute lymphoblastic leukemia uses each of the following types of analysis EXCEPT

(A) cytologic appearance
(B) DNA fingerprinting
(C) histochemical stains
(D) identification of cell surface antigens
(E) identification of chromosomal translocations

**187.** A 2-month-old infant is diagnosed with DiGeorge anomaly. Which of the following will NOT be found in this patient?

(A) Complement deficiency
(B) Congenital heart disease
(C) Hypocalcemic tetany
(D) Hypoparathyroidism
(E) T-cell dysfunction

188. Each of the following is associated with poor prognosis for children with acute lymphoblastic leukemia (ALL) EXCEPT

   (A) age less than 2 years
   (B) age more than 10 years
   (C) initial white blood cell count greater than 100,000/mm³
   (D) a mediastinal mass
   (E) null cell ALL

189. Which of the following phrases regarding the genetics of cystic fibrosis is NOT correct?

   (A) Gene located on chromosome 9
   (B) Gene codes for a cell membrane protein
   (C) General prevalence of about 1/2500 children of European ancestry
   (D) Inherited as an autosomal recessive trait
   (E) Uncommon in black children

190. Each of the following lesions results in cyanosis EXCEPT

   (A) atrial septal defect
   (B) Eisenmenger syndrome
   (C) tetralogy of Fallot
   (D) transposition of the great vessels
   (E) truncus arteriosus

191. Infectious causes of conjunctivitis in children include each of the following EXCEPT

   (A) adenovirus
   (B) Epstein-Barr virus
   (C) *Haemophilus influenzae*
   (D) measles
   (E) staphylococci

**192.** Common signs and symptoms in children with infratentorial brain tumors include each of the following EXCEPT

(A) ataxia
(B) bilateral ptosis
(C) headache
(D) nystagmus
(E) vomiting

**193.** Each of the following statements regarding varicella-zoster infection is correct EXCEPT

(A) children exposed to varicella in utero are at high risk of herpes zoster
(B) complications of varicella include ataxia
(C) immunocompromised children with varicella can develop disseminated disease
(D) the lesions of varicella are indistinguishable morphologically from those of herpes simplex virus
(E) the lesions of varicella progress through the same stages of development in synchrony

**194.** Each of the following statements regarding Langerhans' cell histiocytoses is correct EXCEPT

(A) cystic bone lesions are common in children with class I histiocytoses
(B) diagnosis is confirmed by biopsy
(C) erythrophagocytic syndromes are part of the histiocytoses
(D) failure to thrive, seborrheic dermatitis, and hepatosplenomegaly are signs and symptoms of type I histiocytoses
(E) they are all highly malignant tumors

**195.** A 6-year-old boy presents with a history of fever, erythema, and swelling of the eye. The diagnosis of orbital or periorbital cellulitis is considered. To distinguish orbital from periorbital cellulitis, each of the following clinical features can be considered EXCEPT

(A) decreased ocular mobility
(B) loss of visual acuity
(C) pain on movement of the eye
(D) periorbital swelling
(E) proptosis

**196.** Each of the following statements regarding neural tube defects is correct EXCEPT

(A) complications of myelomeningoceles include paralysis, hip deformities, and bladder and bowel dysfunction
(B) in myelomeningoceles both the spinal cord and the meninges herniate through the bony defect in the spine
(C) neural tube defects can be detected prenatally through measurement of an elevated alpha-fetoprotein level
(D) neural tube defects can be prevented by folic acid supplementation in the third trimester of pregnancy
(E) the neural tube closes at 3 to 4 weeks of embryonic life

**197.** A 3-year-old girl presents with a history of fever and cough. On examination, she has a temperature of 103°F and inspiratory stridor. This finding is consistent with each of the following conditions EXCEPT

(A) bacterial tracheitis
(B) diphtheria
(C) epiglottitis
(D) esophageal foreign body
(E) laryngotracheobronchitis

198. Clinical manifestations of tuberous sclerosis include each of the following EXCEPT

(A) hypopigmented "ash leaf" lesions
(B) infantile spasms
(C) sclerema
(D) sebaceous adenomas
(E) shagreen patch in the lumbosacral region

199. Each of the following statements regarding complex partial seizures is correct EXCEPT

(A) they are frequently associated with automatisms
(B) they are frequently preceded by an aura
(C) they are manifested by unresponsiveness and staring for 1 to 2 minutes
(D) the characteristic electroencephalogram finding is hypsarrhythmia
(E) they may be followed by generalized seizures

200. Clinical manifestations of measles include each of the following EXCEPT

(A) conjunctivitis
(B) croup
(C) encephalitis
(D) Koplik spots
(E) pharyngeal ulcers

201. Each of the following conditions occurs with increased frequency in children with trisomy 21 EXCEPT

(A) acute lymphocytic leukemia
(B) duodenal atresia
(C) endocardial cushion defects
(D) imperforate anus
(E) pyloric stenosis

202. Each of the following is classified as a movement disorder EXCEPT

(A) ataxia
(B) chorea
(C) dystonia
(D) infantile spasms
(E) tics

**203.** Characteristics of viral meningitis include each of the following EXCEPT

(A) commonly caused by enteroviruses
(B) epidemics occur during summer and fall in the United States
(C) cerebrospinal fluid (CSF) pleocytosis
(D) initial predominance of neutrophils in the CSF
(E) can easily be distinguished from bacterial meningitis

**204.** Each of the following statements regarding febrile infants less than 2 months of age is correct EXCEPT

(A) a complete blood count should be obtained
(B) a delay in the diagnosis of sepsis can be fatal
(C) clinical signs and symptoms can be used to detect serious bacterial infection
(D) cultures of the blood, urine and cerebrospinal fluid should be obtained
(E) parenteral antibiotics should be administered

**205.** Each of the following statements regarding Reye's syndrome is correct EXCEPT

(A) it is associated with aspirin given to children with varicella or influenza
(B) it is caused by mitochondrial dysfunction
(C) it is noted by low serum ammonia levels
(D) it presents with vomiting and mental status changes
(E) it rapidly progresses to seizures and coma

**206.** Severe bilateral intrauterine obstruction of the urinary tract results in each of the following EXCEPT

(A) abnormal facies
(B) azotemia
(C) limb anomalies
(D) oligohydramnios
(E) pulmonary hypoplasia

**Pediatrics Questions**

207. A 4-year-old child presents to the emergency department with a history of a fall from a swing in a playground. The mother reports that the child was unconscious for about 5 minutes. Each of the following statements about this child is correct EXCEPT

    (A) a skull fracture predicts underlying brain injury
    (B) better prognosis for children over 2 years of age than for adults
    (C) headaches and behavioral disturbances may present as late complications
    (D) some degree of retrograde and posttraumatic amnesia may be present
    (E) subdural or epidural hematomas can be early complications

208. Clinical signs and symptoms of coarctation of the aorta include each of the following EXCEPT

    (A) a soft continuous murmur occurring in both systole and diastole
    (B) congestive heart failure
    (C) notching of the inferior border of the ribs visible on chest radiograph
    (D) systolic hypertension in the upper extremities
    (E) weak or absent pulses in the lower extremities

209. Complications of otitis media include each of the following EXCEPT

    (A) cholesteatoma
    (B) conductive hearing loss
    (C) mastoiditis
    (D) persistent effusion
    (E) posterior auricular adenopathy

210. Each of the following statements regarding Duchenne muscular dystrophy is correct EXCEPT

    (A) Gower's sign is usually evident at 3 to 5 years of age
    (B) hypotonia is evident in the first months of life
    (C) it is inherited as an X-linked recessive disorder
    (D) serum creatinine kinase levels are markedly elevated
    (E) the genetic defect involves the gene for dystrophin

211. Streptococcal skin infections include each of the following EXCEPT

    (A) blistering distal dactylitis
    (B) bullous impetigo
    (C) erysipelas
    (D) perianal cellulitis
    (E) periorbital cellulitis

212. Signs and symptoms of group A streptococcal pharyngitis include each of the following EXCEPT

    (A) abdominal pain
    (B) cervical adenopathy
    (C) headache
    (D) vesicles on the tonsillar pillars
    (E) vomiting

213. Each of the following is characteristic of tetralogy of Fallot EXCEPT

    (A) dextroposition of the aorta
    (B) endocardial cushion defect
    (C) pulmonary valve and infundibular stenosis
    (D) right ventricular hypertrophy
    (E) ventricular septal defect

214. A 4-year-old child is diagnosed with group A streptococcal pharyngitis. Early treatment of this condition can prevent each of the following complications EXCEPT

    (A) acute poststreptococcal glomerulonephritis
    (B) cervical adenitis
    (C) peritonsillar abscess
    (D) retropharyngeal abscess
    (E) rheumatic fever

**215.** Each of the following statements regarding atopic dermatitis is correct EXCEPT

(A) it frequently involves the extensor surfaces in infants
(B) it frequently involves the flexural surfaces in older children
(C) it improves with frequent bathing
(D) it may become infected with herpes simplex virus
(E) it results in intense pruritus

**216.** Signs and symptoms of congestive heart failure in infants include each of the following EXCEPT

(A) failure to thrive
(B) heart murmur
(C) poor feeding
(D) tachypnea
(E) sweating during feeding

**217.** Each of the following statements regarding Klinefelter syndrome is correct EXCEPT

(A) behavioral, cognitive, and psychiatric symptoms may occur in early childhood
(B) boys are usually diagnosed when virilization occurs prematurely
(C) it results from nondisjunction during meiosis
(D) mental retardation may be prominent
(E) risk increases with advanced maternal age

**218.** Each of the following statements regarding congenital aganglionic megacolon (Hirschsprung's disease) is correct EXCEPT

(A) barium enema shows a narrow involved segment with an abrupt dilatation where normal colon begins
(B) infants present with difficulty or delay in passing meconium
(C) it is the most common cause of intestinal obstruction in neonates
(D) the presence of diarrhea excludes the diagnosis of this condition
(E) there is absence of ganglion cells within the intestinal wall

219. Each of the following statements regarding the diagnosis of a urinary tract infection is correct EXCEPT

   (A) blood cultures should be obtained in addition to urine cultures in infants with urinary tract infection
   (B) differentiation of cystitis and pyelonephritis can be difficult in infants
   (C) suprapubic puncture may be used to collect a urine specimen from an infant
   (D) the diagnosis requires the careful collection of an uncontaminated urine specimen
   (E) the presence of white blood cells in the urine is diagnostic of a urinary tract infection

220. Enteroviruses can cause each of the following disorders EXCEPT

   (A) conjunctivitis-otitis media syndrome
   (B) hand-foot-mouth syndrome
   (C) herpangina
   (D) myocarditis
   (E) pleurodynia

221. A 5-year-old girl presents with a chief complaint of swelling of the eye. On examination edema and erythema of the conjunctiva and area around the eye are found. The cause of such a red swollen eye includes each of the following EXCEPT

   (A) conjunctivitis
   (B) glaucoma
   (C) orbital cellulitis
   (D) periorbital cellulitis
   (E) sinusitis

222. Each of the following statements regarding the hemolytic-uremic syndrome (HUS) is correct EXCEPT

   (A) children with HUS have a microangiopathic hemolytic anemia
   (B) HUS commonly follows gastroenteritis due to *Escherichia coli* O157:H7
   (C) HUS is the most common cause of chronic renal failure in children
   (D) intravascular coagulation may cause colitis
   (E) thrombocytopenia occurs in children with HUS

**223.** Each of the following statements about vitamin A deficiency is true EXCEPT

(A) corneal clouding and blindness can result from chronic, severe vitamin A deficiency
(B) hyperkeratosis is a sign of vitamin A deficiency
(C) night blindness is a sign of vitamin A deficiency
(D) vitamin A deficiency can occur in children with malabsorption syndromes or liver disease
(E) vitamin A supplementation has no effect on the outcome of measles infection in children

**224.** Each of the following disorders occurs in children with Lyme disease EXCEPT

(A) arthritis
(B) erythema chronicum migrans
(C) facial palsy
(D) myocarditis
(E) purpura

**225.** Risk factors for congenital hip dislocation include each of the following EXCEPT

(A) breech presentation
(B) cerebral palsy
(C) neural tube defects
(D) oligohydramnios
(E) prematurity

**226.** Cataracts in children are associated with each of the following EXCEPT

(A) congenital rubella syndrome
(B) galactosemia
(C) retinopathy of prematurity
(D) trauma
(E) trisomies

**227.** Each of the following statements regarding lead poisoning is correct EXCEPT

(A) a diet low in minerals increases lead absorption
(B) acute lead encephalopathy results in cerebral edema
(C) chronic low levels of lead can cause cognitive and behavioral deficits
(D) lead poisoning should be diagnosed on the basis of clinical signs and symptoms
(E) young children absorb lead more readily than adults

**228.** Each of the following statements regarding fever in children is correct EXCEPT

(A) fever may be an adaptive host response
(B) the height of the fever can be used reliably to distinguish bacterial infection from viral infection
(C) the pattern of fever can be useful in establishing certain diagnoses
(D) the pattern of fever can be useful in monitoring response to therapy
(E) young children appear to tolerate fever better than adults

**229.** Causes of a metabolic acidosis with increased anion gap include each of the following EXCEPT

(A) diabetic ketoacidosis
(B) lactic acidosis
(C) methanol
(D) renal tubular acidosis
(E) starvation ketoacidosis

**230.** Clinical manifestations of mumps include each of the following EXCEPT

(A) erythema of the opening of Stensen's duct
(B) meningoencephalitis
(C) orchitis
(D) parotid swelling
(E) splenomegaly

**231.** Each of the following statements about urea cycle defects is correct EXCEPT

(A) hyperammonemia is the characteristic laboratory finding
(B) ornithine transcarbamylase deficiency is inherited as an autosomal recessive disorder
(C) ornithine transcarbamylase deficiency is the most common urea cycle defect
(D) the urea cycle detoxifies free ammonia
(E) vomiting, lethargy, and seizures are common manifestations of urea cycle defects

**232.** Cocaine use during pregnancy can result in each of the following conditions EXCEPT

(A) cerebral infarction
(B) cocaine withdrawal syndrome in the newborn
(C) intrauterine growth retardation
(D) premature labor
(E) spontaneous abortion

**233.** Autoimmune hemolytic anemia is associated with each of the following EXCEPT

(A) infection with human immunodeficiency virus
(B) lymphoma
(C) rheumatic fever
(D) systemic lupus erythematosus

**234.** Signs of acute otitis media include each of the following EXCEPT

(A) bulging tympanic membrane
(B) failure of the tympanic membrane to move with pneumatic otoscopy
(C) obscured bony landmarks
(D) red auditory canal
(E) red tympanic membrane

235. Each of the following statements about the newborn hematologic system is correct EXCEPT

   (A) hemoglobin F is the predominant hemoglobin
   (B) hemoglobin F binds oxygen at lower pressures than hemoglobin A
   (C) a premature infant has a higher hemoglobin level than a full-term infant
   (D) the hemoglobin level falls to a nadir at 2 to 3 months of age
   (E) the hemoglobin level in a normal full-term infant is 15 to 20 mg/dL

236. Each of the following is a cause of hypopituitarism in children EXCEPT

   (A) bacterial meningitis
   (B) cranial irradiation
   (C) craniopharyngioma
   (D) septo-optic dysplasia
   (E) trauma

237. Neonatal conjunctivitis or keratitis can be caused by each of the following EXCEPT

   (A) cytomegalovirus
   (B) *Chlamydia trachomatis*
   (C) herpes simplex virus
   (D) *Neisseria gonorrhoeae*
   (E) silver nitrate drops

238. Each of the following statements about the syndrome of inappropriate secretion of antidiuretic hormone (SIADH) is correct EXCEPT

   (A) neurologic symptoms can occur with severe hyponatremia
   (B) SIADH is associated with meningitis, trauma, and pneumonia
   (C) therapy is with parenteral fluids high in sodium
   (D) the characteristic laboratory finding is hyponatremia
   (E) the diagnosis is confirmed by demonstrating a less than maximally dilute urine in the face of low serum osmolality

## Pediatrics Questions

**239.** Clinical manifestations of acute lymphoblastic leukemia include each of the following EXCEPT

(A) bone pain
(B) fatigue
(C) fever
(D) jaundice
(E) petechiae

**240.** Each of the following statements regarding chromosomal abnormalities is correct EXCEPT

(A) advanced maternal age is associated with a greater risk of nondisjunction during meiosis
(B) about half of all chromosomal abnormalities in neonates are of the sex chromosomes
(C) monosomies other than Turner syndrome are extremely rare
(D) most trisomies are delivered prematurely but in the third trimester
(E) common chromosomal structural defects are translocations and deletions

**241.** Failure to thrive is a possible manifestation of each of the following conditions EXCEPT

(A) chronic renal failure
(B) congenital heart disease
(C) cystic fibrosis
(D) glucose-6-phosphate dehydrogenase (G6PD) deficiency
(E) neglect

**242.** Each of the following statements regarding von Willebrand disease is correct EXCEPT

(A) bleeding frequently occurs after trauma or surgery
(B) children with it have decreased factor VIII activity
(C) it is classically transmitted as an autosomal dominant disorder
(D) platelet aggregation and adhesiveness are diminished
(E) recurrent hemarthroses and the development of chronic joint disease are common complications

**PEDIATRICS**

243. Each of the following is associated with adverse fetal outcome EXCEPT

    (A) lack of prenatal care
    (B) low maternal socioeconomic and educational status
    (C) maternal colonization with *Escherichia coli*
    (D) oligohydramnios
    (E) polyhydramnios

244. Which of the following is NOT a feature of physiologic hyperbilirubinemia in the newborn?

    (A) It can be more prolonged in breast-fed infants
    (B) It usually peaks on the third day of life
    (C) It is due to an elevated level of conjugated bilirubin that exceeds normal adult levels
    (D) It is due to the normal immaturity of the conjugation of bilirubin
    (E) It typically reaches a maximum of 5 to 6 mg/dL

245. Risk factors for recurrent febrile seizures include each of the following EXCEPT

    (A) age less than 18 months
    (B) family history of febrile seizures
    (C) focal seizures
    (D) shorter duration of fever before the first seizure
    (E) temperature lower than 101°F associated with the first seizure

246. Common laboratory findings in children with inborn errors of metabolism include each of the following EXCEPT

    (A) hyperammonemia
    (B) hypocalcemia
    (C) hypoglycemia
    (D) ketonuria
    (E) metabolic acidosis

**247.** Each of the following is associated with bronchiolitis EXCEPT

(A) wheezing and respiratory distress
(B) winter and early spring
(C) infants and small children
(D) respiratory alkalosis
(E) respiratory syncytial viral infection

**248.** Each of the following is associated with congenital toxoplasmosis EXCEPT

(A) chorioretinitis
(B) intracranial calcifications
(C) mental retardation
(D) most infants are symptomatic at birth
(E) thrombocytopenia

**249.** Life-threatening complications of sickle cell anemia include each of the following EXCEPT

(A) acute chest syndrome
(B) cerebral infarction
(C) painful crises
(D) pneumococcal sepsis
(E) severe hemolytic crisis

**250.** Each of the following is a clinical manifestation of cystic fibrosis EXCEPT

(A) chronic sinusitis
(B) cystic malformations in the lung and liver
(C) malabsorption of fat soluble vitamins
(D) nasal polyps
(E) recurrent pulmonary infections

**251.** Signs of intrapartum asphyxia include each of the following EXCEPT

(A) abnormalities in the fetal heart rate variability
(B) fetal bradycardia
(C) high levels of alpha-fetoprotein in the amniotic fluid
(D) low fetal scalp blood pH
(E) meconium in the amniotic fluid

**252.** Each of the following statements regarding osteogenic sarcoma is correct EXCEPT

(A) children usually present with pain and a mass at the site of the tumor
(B) it is the most common malignant bone tumor in children
(C) it occurs most commonly in adolescents
(D) it usually involves the flat bones such as the pelvis
(E) treatment may require amputation

**253.** Clinical manifestations of Sturge-Weber disease include each of the following EXCEPT

(A) facial nevus
(B) glaucoma
(C) hamartomas of the iris
(D) seizures
(E) unilateral intracranial calcification

**254.** Typical features of supraventricular tachycardia (SVT) in children include each of the following EXCEPT

(A) congestive heart failure can occur
(B) heart rate varies between 200 to 300 beats/min
(C) P waves are usually abnormal
(D) QRS complex is usually narrow
(E) underlying heart disease

**255.** Which of the following reflexes is NOT found in the normal newborn?

(A) Brudzinski
(B) Grasp
(C) Moro
(D) Rooting
(E) Tonic neck

# PEDIATRICS ANSWERS AND DISCUSSION

**1—C (Chapter 16)** An 8-month-old boy with failure to thrive, thrush, lymphadenopathy, and *Pneumocystis carinii* pneumonia most likely has HIV infection.

**2—C (Chapter 9)** Turner syndrome often presents with short stature and primary amenorrhea.

**3—E (Chapter 12)** The patient who presents with fever and malaise, followed by headache, back pain, and asymmetric flaccid paralysis of the lower extremities, most likely has poliomyelitis.

**4—E (Chapter 8)** The most common cause of bacterial pneumonia in children is *Streptococcus pneumoniae*.

**5—B (Chapter 21)** In the United States, the most common cause of death in children is automobile accidents.

**6—D (Chapter 7)** Tuberculosis in children always results from primary infection with *Mycobacterium tuberculosis* rather than a reactivation of latent disease as found in adults. Tuberculosis in a child indicates exposure to an adult with contagious disease and should prompt identification and treatment of the source case. Children with tuberculosis infection, without evidence of the disease, should receive isoniazid prophylaxis for 9 months. Prophylaxis greatly reduces the risk of reactivated tuberculous disease later in life.

**7—E (Chapter 20)** In children, midline cysts of the neck that move with swallowing are most likely thyroglossal duct cysts.

**8—C (Chapter 8)** External otitis media presents with ear pain exacerbated by pressure on the tragus.

**9—D (Chapter 16)** All infants born to HIV-infected women will have antibodies to HIV because of the placental transfer of maternal antibody.

**10—B (Chapter 17)** Slipped capital femoral epiphysis is associated with a fracture through the growth plate. It is most common in obese, adolescent boys and is bilateral in a small proportion of cases. Surgical fixation of the femoral head is urgent.

**11—B (Chapters 6 and 7)** The most serious complication of rubella infection is congenital rubella syndrome.

**12—D (Chapter 10)** Congenital hypothyroidism is most often the result of structural lesions of the thyroid, either thyroid aplasia or ectopic thyroid. Diagnosis is by measurement of low levels of $T_4$ and $T_3$ and elevated levels of thyroid stimulating hormone (TSH). Manifestations of congenital hypothyroidism include coarse facial features, widely open fontanelles, flattened nasal bridge, protruding tongue, hoarse cry, myxedema, constipation, and an umbilical hernia. Treatment is with thyroid hormone (L-thyroxine).

**13—D (Chapter 7)** Fever and petechiae in a child warrant careful evaluation because of the possibility of meningococcemia.

**14—B (Chapter 17)** The metaphyseal ends of long bones are common sites of osteomyelitis, which occurs because blood pools and reduces phagocytic activity in this area.

**15—C (Chapter 2)** Children with cerebral palsy have nonprogressive disorders of motor function as a result of abnormalities of the brain in its early development.

**16—A (Chapter 4)** An infant whose mother is diabetic and who experiences irritability, lethargy, and seizures is suffering from hypocalcemia.

**17—A (Chapter 11)** The most common type of leukemia in children is acute lymphocytic leukemia (ALL), which accounts for approximately 80% of leukemia in children; 15% are acute nonlymphocytic leukemia; and the remainder of cases of leukemia are chronic myelogenous leukemia.

**18—C (Chapter 19)** Orbital cellulitis most commonly results from local extension of infection from the ethmoid sinus because only a thin layer of bone, the lamina papyracea, separates the sinus from the orbit of the eye.

**19—E (Chapter 7)** Cerebral malaria is caused by obstruction of cerebral capillaries by infected erythrocytes. Cerebral malaria can result in the development of seizures, coma, and death.

**20—E (Chapter 15)** Orthostatic proteinuria is a benign syndrome in which protein is found in the urine of children after they have been upright and active for a period of time. However, no proteinuria is found in specimens of the same children after they have been supine (e.g., in bed) for several hours.

**21—C (Chapter 11)** Children with glucose-6-phosphate dehydrogenase (G6PD) deficiency develop a hemolytic anemia after ingestion of a variety of oxidant agents. G6PD is a common, highly variable genetic defect on the X chromosome. Hence, the condition has an X-linked mode of inheritance.

**22—E (Chapter 16)** The basic defect in chronic granulomatous disease (CGD) is caused by impairment of the phagocyte production of superoxide anion, hydrogen peroxide, and hydroxyl radicals so that phagocytes cannot kill such catalase positive organisms as *Staphylococcus aureus*.

**23—D (Chapter 6)** When the mother develops varicella within 5 days before delivery to 2 days after delivery, she has not yet developed protective antibodies to pass on to the infant. Because of this, the newborn is at high risk for developing severe varicella infection and death. To protect the infant from infection, varicella-zoster immunoglobulin (VZIG) should be administered immediately after birth.

# Pediatrics Answers and Discussion

**24—A (Chapter 14)** When nontyphoidal salmonella gastroenteritis occurs in children less than 3 months old, they should be treated with antibiotics.

**25—B (Chapter 20)** An iris or target lesion is characteristic of erythema multiforme. Erythema multiforme is a hypersensitivity reaction to infections or drugs. Herpes simplex is a common precipitating infection.

**26—B (Chapter 11)** The three most common malignancies in children are leukemia, lymphoma, and tumors of the central nervous system. Malignant disease is the principal medical cause of death (following accidental injury and poisoning) in children 1 to 14 years of age.

**27—D (Chapter 16)** Rheumatic fever is a complication of group A streptococcal pharyngitis. It is a systemic disease that represents a nonsuppurative complication of group A beta-hemolytic streptococcal pharyngitis. Rheumatic fever can cause conditions such as arthritis of the ankles and knees, chorea, mitral and aortic insufficiency, and pancarditis. Treatment of children with rheumatic fever includes corticosteroids for those with severe carditis and congestive heart failure; penicillin for the antecedent streptococcal infection and as secondary prophylaxis to prevent subsequent attacks of rheumatic fever; and salicylate therapy for arthritis.

**28—A (Chapter 14)** Meckel's diverticulum can present with acute, painless rectal bleeding caused by erosion of the mucosa of the diverticulum. Rectal bleeding is the most common complication of a Meckel's diverticulum.

**29—C (Chapter 4)** Because of the demands of pregnancy, folic acid supplementation is recommended for most pregnant women during the second and third trimester. Folic acid supplementation reduces the risk of neural tube defects. The Public Health Service has recommended folic acid supplementation for all women likely to become pregnant.

**30—A (Chapter 8)** Airway resistance is inversely proportional to the fourth power of the radius of the airway. In addition, infants have smaller airways.

**31—D (Chapter 13)** A ventricular septal defect may not be apparent until several weeks after birth because the relatively high pulmonary vascular resistance diminishes the left-to-right shunt.

**32—E (Chapter 20)** In children, condylomata acuminata, warts on the genitalia or perianal region, suggest the possibility of sexual abuse.

**33—B (Chapter 4; see also Table 4-2)** A newborn infant evaluated at 1 minute, with a heart rate present but less than 100 beats/min, slow respiratory rate, some flexion of extremities, grimace when suctioned, and blue extremities will have an Apgar score of 5. The

Apgar score is affected by gestational age of the neonate and can be affected by medications taken by the mother. The Apgar score is commonly determined at intervals of 1 and 5 minutes after birth, with normal scores ranging between 8 and 10. Apgar score does not predict cerebral palsy.

**34—B (Chapter 19)** Bullous impetigo is common in the diaper area and should be treated with cleansing, compresses, and topical antibiotics. Acrocyanosis, erythema toxicum, milia, and miliaria are lesions that fade and disappear with time. They do not require therapy.

**35—B (Chapter 5)** IgG antibody crosses the placenta beginning at 20 weeks gestation.

**36—C (Chapter 14)** Children with bacterial gastroenteritis present with blood, mucus, and leukocytes in the stool.

**37—C (Chapter 6)** Suctioning of the airway at birth through an endotracheal tube can prevent meconium aspiration syndrome. Infants who aspirate meconium at delivery can develop such severe respiratory distress and cyanosis as to require mechanical ventilation. The condition also may be complicated by the development of a pneumothorax or pneumomediastinum. Infants with severe meconium aspiration have a high mortality rate.

**38—A (Chapter 11)** An unusual feature of a neuroblastoma is a high rate of spontaneous remission in early infancy. Neuroblastomas are tumors of childhood; 75% of children with these tumors have been identified by the age of 5 years, with a median age at diagnosis of 2 years. The tumor commonly arises in the abdomen. Treatment of neuroblastoma includes surgical resection, chemotherapy, and irradiation.

**39—C (Chapter 3)** The estimated water requirement of a 12-kg child with normal body temperature and normal renal function is 1100 ml. Water requirements vary directly with the body's metabolic rate and estimates of water requirements are based on this relationship. At basal conditions, obligatory water requirements are estimated to be 100 mL/100 calories metabolized. A tripartite, linear relationship is then assumed between metabolic rate and body weight, resulting in the following estimation of water requirements; therefore, 100 mL/kg = first 10 kg of body weight; 50 mL/kg = the next 10 kg of body weight; and 20 mL/kg for additional kg of body weight.

**40—D (Chapter 6)** Retinopathy of prematurity commonly occurs in sick, premature infants. It is a spectrum of vascular abnormalities of the retina, including abnormal vascular proliferation, scarring, and retinal detachment. It occurs in infants in response to several injurious conditions, including hyperoxia.

**41—E (Chapter 15)** Minimal change disease is the most common cause of the nephrotic syndrome in children.

## Pediatrics Answers and Discussion

**42—B (Chapter 11)** The only treatment for thalassemia is frequent blood transfusions, which causes hemosiderosis with the deposit of iron in the heart and liver. Cerebral infarction, pneumococcal sepsis, priapism, and splenic sequestration are all characteristic of sickle cell anemia rather than thalassemia.

**43—B (Chapter 10)** Infants with homocystinuria, an autosomal recessive disorder, develop skeletal abnormalities resembling those associated with Marfan syndrome.

**44—B (Chapter 6)** Premature infants are at risk of intraventricular hemorrhage in the subependymal germinal matrix within the first 3 days of life. The germinal matrix is a highly vascular area of immature neurons and glial cells that is not found in the full-term infant.

**45—D (Chapter 10)** Precocious pseudopuberty is independent of gonadotropin function.

**46—D (Chapter 4)** The syndrome of neonatal systemic lupus erythematosus (SLE) is characterized by heart block and photosensitive skin rash. Infants born to mothers with SLE are at higher risk of developing this disease.

**47—B (Chapter 11)** Anemia in children results from decreased production of red blood cells, increased destruction of red blood cells, or increased loss of red blood cells. Decreased production of red blood cells can result from deficiency of iron, folic acid, and vitamin B12. However, iron deficiency anemia is the most common cause of anemia in children. Characteristics of iron deficiency anemia include decreased serum ferritin, increased red blood cell protoporphyrin level, increased serum iron-binding capacity, and low mean cell volume. An increased red blood cell distribution width in conjunction with a low mean cell volume is strongly indicative of iron deficiency. Factors associated with iron deficiency anemia include early introduction of whole cow's milk, delayed introduction of iron-fortified cereals, prematurity, and low socioeconomic status of the family.

**48—E (Chapter 4)** Pregnant women who have used methadone will most likely deliver an infant who experiences irritability, tremors, high pitched crying, and poor feeding.

**49—C (Chapter 6)** Neonatal bacterial sepsis is most commonly caused by group B beta-hemolytic streptococci. The usual causative agents are those found in the maternal vaginal or gastrointestinal tract. Neonates are especially vulnerable to infections with such gram-negative organisms as *Escherichia coli* and such usually commensal organisms as *Staphylococcus epidermidis*. Neonatal sepsis may be associated with localized infections such as pneumonia or urinary tract infections. Various signs and symptoms may signal the presence of sepsis, including lethargy, poor feeding, jaundice, temperature instability, respiratory distress, or periods of apnea, abdominal distension, hypotonia, and altered cry. Neonatal sepsis is commonly associated with the possibility of several diseases, including meningitis and pneumonia. Because no laboratory or radiographic finding is rapid or reliable enough to substitute for clinical judgment and because of the urgency of the situation, treatment of neonatal sepsis is regularly begun before a causative organism is identified. Broad antibiotic coverage to deal with both gram-negative and gram-positive organisms is commonly used until a definitive bacteriologic diagnosis can be made.

**50—C (Chapter 11)** Red blood cells in children with sickle cell anemia contain 90% hemoglobin S and 2% hemoglobin F. The red blood cells contain no hemoglobin A.

**51—D (Chapter 4; see also Table 4-1)** The use of teratogenic drugs during the period of organogenesis may result in abortion or congenital malformations.

**52—A (Chapter 5)** The normal full-term newborn usually holds the extremities and hips in a flexed posture. The liver and spleen are often palpable at the left and right costal margin. The kidneys are often palpable on deep abdominal palpation. The anterior fontanelle should be patent until it closes between 9 to 18 months of age.

**53—A (Chapter 11)** Infants and young children with sickle cell disease may develop an acute splenic sequestration in which blood pools acutely in the spleen and occasionally in the liver. Children with this condition may rapidly develop vascular shock and require emergency blood transfusions.

**54—D (Chapter 10)** Testicular feminization syndrome may present as an inguinal hernia in a girl; testes are found when the inguinal hernia is diagnosed. This is an X-linked recessive disorder of the androgen receptor in which genetic males have the phenotype of a female with a vaginal pouch and no uterus.

**55—D (Chapter 8)** Retropharyngeal abscesses occur primarily in young children because of the presence of a lymph node chain between the posterior pharyngeal wall and the prevertebral space.

**56—C (Chapter 4)** The ratio of lecithin to sphingomyelin can be used to assess fetal lung maturity. Lung maturity is indicated by a ratio of 2:1 (lecithin:sphingomyelin) and correlates with a greatly diminished probability of respiratory distress syndrome.

**57—E (Chapter 11)** Wilms' tumor is sometimes associated with hemihypertrophy and aniridia. Hypertension can be found in Wilms' tumor, but the hypertension is caused by compression of the renal artery by the tumor. The hypertension found in neuroblastomas is caused by release of catecholamines. Wilms' tumor is a disease of early childhood, with the median age of presentation being 3 years old.

**58—E (Chapter 12)** Craniosynostosis is a condition of premature closure of the cranial sutures. Most affected infants present at birth

## Pediatrics Answers and Discussion

with an abnormal skull, with the shape depending on which specific sutures fused prematurely. The sagittal suture is most commonly involved. Hydrocephalus can result when several sutures close prematurely.

**59—C (Chapter 11)** Children with retinoblastoma usually present with leukokoria, a whitish reflex in the pupil due to growth of the tumor from the retina. Retinoblastoma is the most common malignant tumor of the eye in children.

**60—C (Chapter 12)** Infantile spasms classically present in early infancy as episodes in which the infant's head suddenly drops to the chest, the thighs flex on the abdomen, and the arms adduct and flex on the chest. Extensor, rather than flexor, spasms also occur. Individual episodes may be brief but extremely frequent, following in rapid succession. The EEG shows a characteristically disorganized pattern termed hypsarrhythmia.

**61—E (Chapter 6)** Kernicterus is the deposition of unconjugated bilirubin in the basal ganglia and cerebellum. Clinical manifestations of kernicterus include opisthotonos, seizures, hearing loss, and choreoathetoid cerebral palsy.

**62—C (Chapter 12)** Prolonged use of phenobarbital to prevent the recurrence of a febrile seizure is associated with cognitive and behavioral abnormalities. Hence, its use is not recommended in children with a history of febrile seizures. The use of antipyretics during a febrile illness may prevent a seizure in a child with a history of febrile seizures. Febrile seizures are the most common cause of seizures in children and occur in 3% to 4% of all children. Peak incidence is at 18 months of age, although they occur commonly in infants between the ages of 9 months and 5 years. The episodes are usually of short duration, rarely lasting more than *15 minutes.*

**63—D (Chapter 11)** In full-term infants, iron stores are sufficient for the first 4 months of growth. Premature infants have a higher rate of postnatal growth. Although premature infants have proportionally the same amount of iron per body weight as full-term infants, they have a higher rate of growth and thus a greater propensity to develop iron deficiency anemia.

**64—D (Chapter 12)** *Streptococcus pneumoniae, Haemophilus influenzae* type b, and *Neisseria meningitidis* most often cause bacterial meningitis in children. Risk factors for bacterial meningitis include children of young age (less than 1 year old); defects of the central nervous system (basilar skull fracture); immunodeficiencies (complement deficiencies); and exposure to carriers of pathogenic bacteria in day care centers.

**65—D (Chapter 6)** A maternal marker for the increased risk of transmission of hepatitis B virus to the infant is hepatitis B e antigen. Infants whose mothers are positive for this virus should receive hepatitis B immunoglobulin within 12 hours of birth as well as the initial dose of the hepatitis B vaccine.

**66—E (Chapter 12)** Werdnig-Hoffman disease or spinal muscular atrophy (SMA) type 1, the most severe form of this condition, is found in infancy. Infants with this condition present with generalized hypotonia, weakness, and lack of deep tendon reflexes. Fasciculations, best seen in the tongue, are characteristic. The disease has a poor prognosis, with death usually by 2 years of age.

**67—E (Chapter 12)** There is an urgency in evaluating any child with fever and seizures because of the possibility of meningitis. Many physicians elect to perform a lumbar puncture in young children with a first febrile seizure to exclude the possibility of meningitis.

**68—C (Chapter 8)** The clinical sign that frequently distinguishes upper airway obstruction from lower airway disease is stridor.

**69—D (Chapter 12)** Infantile botulism is the result of ingestion of a preformed *toxin* of *Clostridium botulinum*, not a bacteremia. It is usually found in infants who have been fed contaminated honey, and is characterized by generalized hypotonia, cranial nerve palsies, and respiratory distress.

**70—B (Chapter 12)** The 6-month-old infant who presents with crises consisting of persistent vomiting, irritability, sweating, flushing, and hypertension will be diagnosed with familial dysautonomia (known as Riley-Day syndrome). It is an autosomal recessive trait of individuals of eastern European Jewish descent with onset in infancy. The disease is usually fatal by early childhood.

**71—B (Chapter 11)** Sarcoma botryoides is the result of rhabdomyosarcoma extending into a body cavity such as the vagina or bladder.

**72—C (Chapter 8)** An adolescent who presents with pneumonia, malaise, sore throat, and a positive test for cold hemagglutinins most likely is infected with *Mycoplasma pneumoniae*.

**73—C (Chapter 14)** Acute appendicitis is caused by obstruction of the lumen from a fecalith or calculi or by edema from a bacterial or viral infection. This condition is rare in children under the age of 2. Children with acute appendicitis can have diarrhea or pyuria. The pain of appendicitis is localized to the right lower quadrant.

**74—D (Chapter 8)** Asthma results from increased airway responsiveness and inflammation. Inhaled corticosteroids and alternate-day oral therapy reduce the likelihood of complications from chronic steroid use.

**75—D (Chapter 15)** Poststreptococcal glomerulonephritis must be distinguished from membranoproliferative glomerulonephritis, both of which are associated with low serum complement levels. However, the lower serum complement level found in poststreptococcal glomerulonephritis resolves within about 8 weeks of the onset of the disease. Persistence of hypocomplementemia beyond this period suggests the presence of other forms of glomerulonephritis, particularly membranoproliferative glomerulonephritis.

**76—E (Chapter 13)** The most common congenital heart lesion is a ventricular septal defect. It accounts for approximately one fourth of all cases of congenital heart disease. Ventricular septal defects may be single or multiple and may occur in isolation or with other cardiac lesions, notably tetralogy of Fallot and atrioventricular septal defects. They are characterized by their position and type: membranous or muscular. The severity of symptoms varies with the size of the defect.

**77—E (Chapter 8)** Pertussis, caused by *Bordetella pertussis*, other Bordetella species, and adenovirus, is characterized by repetitive coughs followed by an inspiratory whoop. Marked lymphocytosis is common.

**78—C (Chapter 12)** Chemoprophylaxis with rifampin should be considered for some families of children with meningitis caused by *Haemophilus influenzae* type b.

**79—E (Chapter 13)** Prostaglandin E should be used in infants with congenital heart disease to maintain a patent ductus arteriosus when there is severe restriction to pulmonary blood flow.

**80—B (Chapter 15)** Testicular torsion results from an inadequate fixation of the testicle by the tunica vaginalis, which allows the testicle to rotate and occlude its vascular supply. It is considered a surgical emergency. Defect is often bilateral, hence surgical repair of both testes should be performed. Torsion of the testicular appendix may be confused with testicular torsion.

**81—B (Chapter 13)** Eisenmenger syndrome is best described as a right-to-left shunt through a ventricular septal defect resulting from pulmonary hypertension. A loud single second heart sound is suggestive of pulmonary hypertension.

**82—D (Chapter 12)** Guillain-Barré syndrome is a demyelinating polyneuropathy. It begins with paresthesias of the toes and fingers and progresses to a symmetric, ascending paralysis beginning in the legs and associated with cramping pain and diminished deep tendon reflexes. Examination of the cerebrospinal fluid shows an elevated protein level but few or no cells. Most patients have minor, residual neurologic problems. It is usually less severe in children than in adults.

**83—A (Chapter 8)** A 3-month-old infant with afebrile pneumonitis and eosinophilia is most likely infected with *Chlamydia trachomatis*.

**84—B (Chapter 13)** A widely split second heart sound ($S_2$) that is fixed in both inspiration and expiration is characteristic of an atrial septal defect.

**85—D (Chapter 14)** Pyloric stenosis is due to hypertrophy of the pyloric sphincter and stomach antrum and causes partial obstruction of the stomach. The condition presents in the second or third week of life with projectile, nonbilious vomiting, failure to thrive, and dehydration. After vomiting, the infant appears hungry and anxious to feed again. Because of the protracted vomiting, hypochloremic alkalosis and hypokalemia frequently are present.

**86—C (Chapter 7)** Occult bacteremia is a bacteremia without an obvious focus of infection, and occurs most commonly in children between the ages of 3 months and 2 years of age. It is most commonly caused by *Streptococcus pneumoniae*.

**87—A (Chapter 17)** A positive Ortolani maneuver indicates the presence of dislocation of the hip, in which the femoral head lies out of the acetabulum. A dislocatable hip is one in which the femoral head can be manipulated out of the acetabulum. Legg-Calve-Perthes disease is avascular necrosis of the femoral head and presents with joint stiffness, limp, and pain in the hip, thigh, knee, or groin with a duration of several weeks to months. Slipped capital femoral epiphysis is a condition in which the femoral head is displaced from the femoral neck prior to epiphyseal closure. A fracture through the growth plate allows for the displacement. Subluxation of the hip refers to a condition of malalignment of the femoral head and acetabulum in which the femoral head remains within the joint.

**88—E (Chapter 15)** Undescended testes are especially common in premature infants and are caused by a halt in the normal embryonic migration of the testis into the scrotum, which takes place during the seventh month of gestation. There is a risk of developing testicular malignancy.

**89—A (Chapter 20)** A kerion is a boggy mass associated with tinea capitis. Tinea capitis is a dermatophyte infection of the scalp, characterized by one or multiple pruritic, erythematous, scaly, circular plaques with alopecia. A kerion sometimes accompanies the primary lesion. A keloid is an excessive growth of scar tissue.

**90—C (Chapter 14)** Abdominal pain and bilious vomiting can be caused by intestinal malrotation. Pyloric stenosis causes projectile vomiting; rotavirus gastroenteritis causes vomiting, but not bilious vomiting.

**91—B (Chapter 21)** Protein-polysaccharide conjugate vaccines for *Haemophilus influenzae* allow for the stimulation of humoral immunity in children less than 2 years of age.

**92—E (Chapter 17)** The most common bacterial cause of osteomyelitis in children is *Staphylococcus aureus*.

**93—E (Chapter 9)** Trisomy 21 can occur in younger women because of translocation or paternal nondisjunction. For a small percentage of women whose children have translocation 21, the risk of recurrence in subsequent pregnancies is high.

**94—A (Chapter 15)** Urinary tract obstruction in boys is most commonly caused by posterior urethral valves, which are membranes that obstruct the posterior urethra. Posterior urethral values are associated with vesicoureteral reflex and reflux nephropathy.

**95—B (Chapter 7)** Infants infected with hepatitis B virus are at high risk of developing subsequent cirrhosis or hepatocellular carcinoma. Diagnosis of hepatitis B virus is confirmed serologically.

**96—C (Chapter 14)** Severe diarrhea in infants and young children is most often caused by rotavirus. In the United States, the peak incidence of rotavirus infection is between 3 and 15 months of age and during the winter months. Infants less than 3 months old are most likely protected by passively acquired maternal antibodies.

**97—C (Chapter 17)** Septic arthritis of the hip is particularly dangerous because increased pressure can cause avascular necrosis of the femoral head; *immediate surgical drainage is required.*

**98—B (Chapter 15)** Children less than 8 years of age with the nephrotic syndrome should receive corticosteroid therapy to reduce the proteinuria and reduce infectious complications.

**99—A (Chapter 14)** Lactase deficiency can be confirmed by identifying a reducing sugar in the stool. Most children with gastroenteritis do not require a lactose-free formula. The development of lactase deficiency is common in *adults*, particularly in people of African descent.

**100—D (Chapter 16)** Children with severe combined immunodeficiency (SCID) present early in infancy with failure to thrive, diarrhea, and opportunistic infections such as *Pneumocystis carinii* pneumonia. The most common form of this disorder is X-linked and results from genetic mutations of the interleukin receptors vital to the stimulation and differentiation of both T and B cells.

**101—C (Chapters 11 and 16)** Children treated for leukemia are at increased risk of serious bacterial infection because of neutropenia secondary to chemotherapy for leukemia.

**102—E (Chapter 16; see also Table 16-2)** Systemic symptoms may precede the onset of juvenile rheumatoid arthritis. Treatment is usually with aspirin and nonsteroidal anti-inflammatory drugs (NSAIDs); *corticosteroids are rarely used.*

**103—A (Chapters 9 and 17)** Atlantoaxial instability, which may be congenital or acquired, occurs often in children with trisomy 21.

**104—A (Chapter 19)** Amblyopia is most likely to occur in children with monocular strabismus and those with unilateral cataracts.

**105—D (Chapter 20)** In a young infant, scaling and crusting of the scalp is most likely caused by seborrheic dermatitis, a condition of unknown etiology.

**106—D (Chapter 18)** Sexual abuse of prepubertal girls is suggested by posterior tears and irregularities of the hymen.

**107—A (Chapter 21)** Carbon monoxide poisoning occurs in children exposed to smoke and fire. Carbon monoxide poisoning must be diagnosed by measurement of carboxyhemoglobin. It should be treated with 100% oxygen.

**108—D (Chapter 9)** Fragile X syndrome is a common cause of mental retardation in boys. Heterozygotic females also may be mentally retarded. Males with this syndrome have large testicles.

**109—E (Chapter 7)** A young child with a high fever (40°C) that resolves with the onset of a generalized erythematous rash most likely has roseola. Roseola is caused by infection with human herpesvirus 6 and frequently causes a high fever in children between the ages of 6 months and 2 years. It is transmitted via the respiratory route.

**110—C (Chapter 16)** Boys with X-linked agammaglobulinemia are prone to infection with *Streptococcus pneumoniae* and *Haemophilus influenzae* type b. X-linked agammaglobulinemia (Bruton's disease) is a genetic defect resulting from mutations in a cytoplasmic signal-transducing molecule that results in the lack of B cells and low or absent levels of IgG, IgA, and IgM. Passively acquired maternal IgG protects affected boys during the first year of life. However, subsequently these children present with frequent episodes of otitis media, sinusitis, pneumonia, and skin infections. Treatment consists of regular infusions of intravenous immune globulin.

**111—C (Chapter 7)** The most prevalent nematode infection in the United States is pinworm, caused by infection with the nematode *Enterobius vermicularis*.

**112—D (Chapter 8)** The most common bacterial causes of acute otitis media are *Streptococcus pneumoniae*, nontypable *Haemophilus influenzae*, and *Moraxella catarrhalis*.

**113—D (Chapter 9)** A newborn with fine facial features, low set ears, prominent occiput, unusual flexion deformity of the fingers, and rocker bottom feet most likely has trisomy 18. Most children with trisomy 18 die in early infancy.

**114—B (Chapter 10)** Children with chromosomal breakage syndromes are at high risk of malignancy.

**115—A (Chapter 6)** Most congenital cytomegalovirus (CMV) infections are asymptomatic; diagnosis is made by viral isolation, particularly from the urine or by a positive test for serum IgM anti-CMV antibody. However, after the infant is 3 weeks old, isolation of the virus does not distinguish intrauterine *or congenital* infection from postnatal infection. Perinatal infection can occur through breast milk or by blood transfusion. Long-term sequelae include sensorineural hearing loss and learning disabilities. Severe congenital infection can cause intracranial calcifications and chorioamnionitis.

**116—D (Chapter 12)** The laboratory evaluation of a child with suspected sepsis or meningitis includes cultures of the blood, urine, and spinal fluid. Liver function tests are not indicated in the initial laboratory evaluation of such children.

**117—A (Chapter 12)** Findings in cerebrospinal fluid (CSF) examined from children with bacterial meningitis include elevated CSF protein level and *decreased* CSF glucose level. Gram stain of the CSF may reveal the causative organism.

**118—E (Chapter 12)** Complications of bacterial meningitis include hearing loss, hydrocephalus, language delay, and seizures. *Subdural effusions*, but not subdural hematomas, are complications of bacterial meningitis.

**119—D (Chapter 11)** Pallor is a prominent finding in iron deficiency anemia, leukemia, and thalassemia. Children with lead poisoning commonly also have iron deficiency anemia. Children with *sickle cell trait* are not anemic and therefore do not have pallor.

**120—D (Chapter 1)** Signs of respiratory distress in a young child include grunting, intercostal retractions, nasal flaring, and supraclavicular retractions. In a young child, a respiratory rate of 24 breaths per minute indicates a normal rate.

**121—C (Chapter 10)** Excessive production of *thyroid hormone* (not thyroid-stimulating hormone) results in hyperthyroidism. Graves' disease (diffuse toxic goiter) is most common in girls and presents with symptoms of emotional lability, hyperactivity, and a decline in school performance.

**122—C (Chapter 6)** Respiratory distress syndrome, also known as hyaline membrane disease, is a disease of preterm infants caused by a deficiency of surfactant in the distal airways resulting in severe atelectasis and reduced lung compliance. Found in premature infants, it can be prevented by steroid therapy to the mother prior to delivery as well as the administration of surfactant to the infant at the time of delivery or shortly thereafter.

**123—B (Chapter 2)** Electrolyte abnormalities, hypothermia, severe infection, and vitamin A deficiency are all associated with severe protein-energy malnutrition (PEM).

**124—A (Chapter 3)** Hypernatremia results from excessive oral or parenteral intake or impaired renal excretion. Hypernatremia can occur as a consequence of dehydration, diabetes insipidus, improper preparation of infant formulas, and by salt poisoning. Hypernatremia does not occur as a consequence of cystic fibrosis.

**125—C (Chapter 3)** Infants fed exclusively with breast milk may develop rickets or vitamin D deficiency. Clinical manifestations of rickets, or vitamin D deficiency, include craniotabes (thinning and softening of the skull), delayed closure of the fontanelles, fractures, and widening of the distal ends of long bones. Vitamin D deficiency is characterized by the failure in mineralization of osteoid tissue, typically at the end of long bones. Edema is not associated with rickets.

**126—D (Chapter 15)** Vesicoureteral reflex results from valvular incompetence at the ureterovesicular junction as a result of a shortened segment of ureter within the bladder wall. It is often associated with other genitourinary anomalies. Vesicoureteral reflux can result in chronic renal failure, dilatation of the ureters, hypertension, and urinary tract infections. It does not cause proteinuria.

**127—B (Chapter 6)** The risk of neonatal herpes simplex infection is higher in women with primary herpes simplex infection than in those with recurrent infection. The diagnosis of this disease is confirmed by culture of the virus from the vesicles, nasopharynx, eyes, or body fluids. Culture of the virus is difficult in infants with localized encephalitis. Infants suspected of having this virus should be treated promptly with acyclovir. Infection can result in systemic infection, including the liver and the central nervous system, localized encephalitis, or involvement of the skin and mucous membranes.

**128—E (Chapter 4)** An infant born of a diabetic mother will tend to have more frequent birth injuries, congenital heart disease, hypoglycemia, and respiratory distress syndrome. Retinopathy is associated with low birth weight and oxygen therapy.

**129—C (Chapter 2)** Hydrocephalus, or excess accumulation of cerebrospinal fluid (CSF), is a significant cause of an increased head circumference. It is classified as either obstructive or nonobstructive. Structure abnormalities include stenosis of the aqueduct of Sylvius or compression of the fourth ventricle. Compression of the fourth ventricle occurs in the Chiari malformation and the Dandy-Walker cyst. Nonobstructive, or communicating, hydrocephalus results from failure of absorption of the CSF by the arachnoid villi and can be caused by subarachnoid hemorrhage and by meningitis. Maternal alcohol use is not related to hydrocephalus.

**130—E (Chapter 3)** Breast milk is available in an uncontaminated form (the human body) and contains antibodies against bacterial and viral pathogens. Secretory IgA in human milk is directed against the pathogens in the maternal-infant environment. Breast milk promotes the growth of nonpathogenic flora, all of which protect the infant against infection. Because the breast milk does not contain sufficient vitamin D to prevent nutritional rickets, breast-fed babies should be given 400 IU of vitamin D daily.

**131—B (Chapter 4)** Characteristics of fetal alcohol syndrome include facial abnormalities, intrauterine growth retardation, mental retardation, and ventricular septal defect. Hydrocephalus is not a characteristic of fetal alcohol syndrome.

**132—D (Chapter 6)** Hemolytic disease of the newborn is a common cause of jaundice and a rapidly rising unconjugated bilirubin level. The most common form is isoimmune hemolysis, which is caused by incompatibilities between red blood cell antigens of the mother and the infant. Infants with severe Rh disease or erythroblastosis fetalis

# Pediatrics Answers and Discussion 281

may present with generalized edema and severe congestive heart failure. Maternal IgM antibodies do not cross the placenta.

**133—B (Chapter 21; see also Table 21-3)** In the United States, children less than 2 years of age have a low rate of immunization coverage for several reasons, including lack of public awareness of immunization programs, poor access to health services, misunderstanding of the contraindications for immunization, and reluctance to give multiple vaccines at the same well-child visit.

**134—C (Chapter 4)** Low birth weight, less than 2500 grams, is associated with intrauterine growth retardation, maternal hypertension, multiple gestational pregnancies, and prematurity. Maternal diabetes mellitus is associated with large for gestational age infants.

**135—A (Chapter 5)** Because newborns breathe through their nose, any bilateral nasal obstruction, as in choanal atresia, will cause severe respiratory distress. Newborns breathe almost exclusively through diaphragmatic contraction; therefore, the thorax recedes inward, and the abdomen protrudes during inspiration. The respiratory rate of the newborn is highly variable and may include short periods of apnea. Surfactant is a phospholipid produced after the 20th week of gestation. It lines the alveoli and reduces the surface tension that opposes the expansion of the lung.

**136—B (Chapter 2)** Chronic renal failure, growth hormone deficiency, inflammatory bowel disease, and Turner syndrome are all causes of short stature. Diabetes is not associated with short stature.

**137—E (Chapter 5)** In fetal circulation, right-sided pressure elevation depends on pulmonary vascular resistance caused by pulmonary arteriolar vasoconstriction. In contrast, left-sided pressure remains low because of the low resistance of the placental circulation. The ductus arteriosus and the foramen ovale are patent. At birth, these relationships change and pulmonary vasodilatation increases.

**138—E (Chapter 11)** Complications of sickle cell anemia include aplastic crisis, dactylitis, gallstones, and priapism, which is the result of pooling of blood in the corpora cavernosa. Thrombocytopenia is not a complication of sickle cell anemia.

**139—B (Chapter 10)** Congenital adrenal hyperplasia is most often caused by 21-hydroxylase deficiency. About 75% of cases of 21-hydroxylase deficiency will present with metabolic symptoms of adrenal insufficiency. Infants known as "salt-losers" present within the first few weeks to months of life with failure to thrive, arrhythmias, vomiting, and dehydration, leading to vascular collapse and death. Boys can have short stature as adults; girls can have ambiguous genitalia.

**140—D (Chapter 8)** The risk of sudden infant death syndrome (SIDS) is *not increased* by the infant sleeping in a supine position, although this continues to be a controversial issue. Additional increased risks include families living in poverty, those with a previous child who died of SIDS, the winter season, and prevalence in boys.

**141—E (Chapter 4)** Birth trauma can result in caput succedaneum (edema of the presenting newborn scalp), cephalhematoma (areas of subperiosteal hemorrhage), clavicular fracture, and Erb-Duchenne paralysis. Volkmann contracture is not associated with birth trauma.

**142—C (Chapter 10)** Testing for phenylketonuria should not be performed until the infant *has been fed* several milk feedings containing phenylalanine. Infants with this condition appear normal at birth but gradually develop fair skin, light hair, eczematoid or seborrheic dermatitis, growth retardation, and seizures. A mousy or misty body odor of phenylacetic acid often can be detected. Treatment consists of dietary manipulation in which phenylalanine is reduced and should continue until the child is at least age 6 years or older.

**143—A (Chapter 6)** A patent ductus arteriosus (PDA) in a premature infant is a result of gestational immaturity or hypoxia and is frequently associated with respiratory distress syndrome. This type of PDA often closes spontaneously. However, the prostaglandin inhibitor indomethacin may be used to facilitate closure of a PDA in a *premature infant* but not a full-term infant.

**144—B (Chapter 16)** Anti-HIV IgA antibodies, HIV cultures, polymerase chain reaction (PCR), and P24 antigen have all been used to diagnose HIV infection in children less than 15 months of age. Anti-HIV IgG antibodies are not useful in children less than age 15 months because of the presence of the maternal HIV antibodies in the infant that were transferred via the placenta during the pregnancy.

**145—D (Chapter 6; see also Table 6-1)** Neonatal jaundice can result from biliary tract obstruction, hemolysis of red blood cells, normal immaturity of the conjugation of bilirubin, or sepsis. Neonatal jaundice appears in newborns when the serum bilirubin exceeds 5 mg/dl. Jaundice is not found in newborns with sickle cell anemia; however, children with sickle cell anemia, as with other congenital hemolytic anemias, are often found jaundiced.

**146—A (Chapter 15)** Characteristic features of acute poststreptococcal glomerulonephritis include edema, gross hematuria, hypertension, and renal insufficiency. Chronic renal failure is not a feature of acute poststreptococcal glomerulonephritis.

**147—B (Chapter 6)** Necrotizing enterocolitis (NEC) is a mucosal or transmucosal intestinal necrosis commonly of the distal ileum or proximal colon. Manifestations of NEC include abdominal distension, vomiting, and bloody stools. Abdominal radiographs may demonstrate pneumatosis intestinalis, a pathognomonic finding of intramural gas within the intestinal wall. The etiology of this disease is *unknown*, although it is known that premature infants are at high risk. Other implicating factors include polycythemia, early oral feed-

# Pediatrics Answers and Discussion

ing, and gastrointestinal infection. *Clostridium difficile* is associated with pseudomembranous enterocolitis found in children and is treated with antibiotics.

**148—E (Chapter 14)** Intussusception is a condition in which one portion of the intestine telescopes or invaginates into another, most commonly the distal ileum into the proximal colon. A tender, sausage-shaped mass can be palpated most often in the right upper quadrant. Intussusception can be caused by Meckel's diverticulum, polyp, or Henoch-Schönlein purpura. This condition can be reduced using the hydrostatic pressure of barium introduced into the *rectum* and *colon*, a procedure that is both diagnostic and therapeutic.

**149—A (Chapter 15)** Alport syndrome is the most common form of hereditary nephritis, and it is much more severe in boys than in girls, suggesting an X-linked dominant mode of transmission in some cases. It is not a cause of chronic renal failure in infants. Boys with Alport syndrome may develop chronic renal failure in adolescence or early adulthood.

**150—D (Chapters 5 and 6)** Failure to pass meconium in the newborn infant may occur in several diseases including cystic fibrosis, Hirschsprung's disease, and small left colon syndrome, which occurs in infants of diabetic mothers and infants whose mothers were treated with magnesium sulfate therapy for preeclampsia. Malrotation is not associated with failure to pass meconium.

**151—D (Chapter 11)** Spherocytosis is a hemolytic anemia caused by a defect in the cell wall of red blood cells. Typical symptoms include anemia, jaundice, and splenomegaly. Diagnosis of spherocytosis is confirmed by the osmotic fragility test, which shows normal biconcave red cells swelling when placed in a hypertonic solution. Spherocytes are at maximum volume for their surface area and thus rupture. Treatment of the disease involves splenectomy. However, children who have a splenectomy are at increased risk for serious bacterial sepsis and should receive vaccines that protect against *Haemophilus influenzae* type b and pneumococcus. They also should be placed on prophylactic penicillin.

**152—D (Chapter 10)** Clinical manifestations of diabetic ketoacidosis include abdominal pain, dehydration, hyperglycemia, and a compensatory respiratory alkalosis. Also, metabolic acidosis with an *elevated* anion gap is a clinical manifestation of diabetic ketoacidosis. Complications of diabetic ketoacidosis and its therapy include cerebral edema, hypocalcemia, hypoglycemia, and hypokalemia. Treatment involves fluid and electrolyte replacement, particularly with potassium.

**153—C (Chapter 13)** Kawasaki disease is a generalized vasculitis that occurs in children under the age of 5 years and is of unknown etiology. Signs and symptoms of Kawasaki disease include bilateral conjunctival infection without discharge, desquamation of the fingers, toes, and perianal region, lymphadenopathy, and prolonged high fever. The most serious complication of Kawasaki disease is the development of coronary artery aneurysms. Children with Kawasaki disease are treated with intravenous gamma globulin and salicylates during the acute phase of the disease. Treatment results in the amelioration of symptoms and, if initiated early in the course of disease, in the prevention of coronary artery aneurysms.

**154—C (Chapter 16)** HIV-infected children should *not* be given live polio vaccine but, instead, should be given inactivated polio vaccine (IPV). Live measles vaccine may be given because the risk of the disease, measles, outweighs the risk of live viral vaccines to immunocompromised children. Children infected with HIV can be given intravenous gamma globulin to previous serious bacterial infection, trimethoprim-sulfamethoxazole to prevent *Pneumocystis carinii* pneumonia, and nutritional support.

**155—B (Chapter 6)** Hemorrhagic disease of the newborn *can be prevented* by parenteral administration of 1 mg of vitamin K at birth. Hemorrhagic disease is caused by a transient decrease in vitamin K dependent factors; it is more severe in preterm and breast-fed infants, and usually occurs within 2 to 3 days after birth. Intracranial hemorrhage is a rare but serious complication.

**156—B (Chapter 11)** Children with beta thalassemia present with the typical signs and symptoms of hemolytic anemia, pallor, splenomegaly, jaundice, and failure to thrive. They do not have generalized lymphadenopathy.

**157—E (Chapter 12)** Myotonia is the *slow* relaxation of muscle contraction rather than a rapid relaxation of muscles following contraction.

**158—C (Chapter 15)** Characteristics of the nephrotic syndrome include edema, hyperlipidemia, hypoalbuminemia, and proteinuria of more than 1000 mg/m$^2$/day. Hypertension is not a characteristic feature of the nephrotic syndrome.

**159—C (Chapter 6)** Manifestations of congenital syphilis include anemia and thrombocytopenia, anterior bowing of the shins, profuse nasal discharge, and saddle nose deformity. Chorioretinitis is not associated with congenital syphilis.

**160—E (Chapter 13)** Characteristic signs and symptoms of Henoch-Schönlein purpura include arthritis of the knees and ankles, glomerulonephritis, gross or occult gastrointestinal bleeding, and purpura over the posterior legs and buttocks. Thrombocytopenia is not a sign of Henoch-Schönlein purpura.

**161—C (Chapter 14)** Pharmacologic therapy with metoclopramide and cisapride may be of benefit in moderate to severe cases of gastroesophageal reflux; surgery may be necessary for those cases with recurrent aspiration pneumonia. The disease is associated with Down's syndrome and children with developmental delay. It is not associated with prematurity.

**162—C (Chapter 6)** Congenital rubella infection can cause cataracts, congenital heart disease, hearing loss, and microcephaly. The effect on the fetus depends on the gestational age; thus, congenital heart disease occurs when the gestational age is 9 to 12 weeks; congenital deafness occurs with infection prior to 16 weeks gestation. Fever is not directly associated with congenital rubella infection.

**163—D (Chapter 12)** Clinical manifestations of neurofibromatosis type 1 include axillary freckling café-au-lait spots, Lisch nodules (hamartomas of the iris), optic gliomas, and neurofibromas. Neuroblastoma, a malignant tumor of the sympathetic nervous system, is not associated with neurofibromatosis.

**164—E (Chapter 10)** Common signs and symptoms of inborn errors of metabolism include failure to thrive, developmental delay, lethargy, poor feeding, persistent vomiting, hepatomegaly, and seizures. Sensorineural hearing loss is not associated with inborn errors of metabolism.

**165—C (Chapter 11)** Hodgkin's disease is characterized by the Reed-Sternberg cell. It has a peak incidence in adolescence and *early adulthood* with a second peak after age 50. Children with Hodgkin's disease typically present with an enlarged cervical or supraclavicular node with no evidence of inflammation. Other lymph nodes may be involved. Metastasis occurs to the lungs, liver, and bone marrow. Non-Hodgkin's lymphoma involves the abdomen, bone marrow, lymph nodes of the head and neck, and the meninges. This group of lymphomas occurs more often in young children than does Hodgkin's disease.

**166—C (Chapter 10)** Galactosemia is an autosomal recessive inborn error of carbohydrate metabolism and results from a deficiency of the enzyme galactose-1-phosphate uridyltransferase. The absence of this enzyme causes a gradual and toxic accumulation of galactose in all body tissues. Infants with this condition appear *normal at birth* but develop symptoms when fed milk, which contains galactose. However, they are at increased risk of gram-negative sepsis; they typically present with symptoms such as failure to thrive, vomiting, hypoglycemia, and seizures.

**167—C (Chapter 11)** Disorders associated with thrombocytopenia include disseminated intravascular coagulation, hemolytic-uremic syndrome, Kasabach-Merritt syndrome, and Wiskott-Aldrich syndrome. Henoch-Schönlein purpura is not a disorder associated with thrombocytopenia.

**168—E (Chapter 18)** Conditions that are highly suggestive of child abuse include fractures of the long bones that are characterized by corner fractures and elevation of the periosteum, as well as posterior rib fractures; burns to the soles of both feet, which are unlikely to occur by a child stepping in hot water but which suggest deliberate submersion; and fractures or bruises that are in different stages of healing. Supracondylar fractures of the elbow are not highly suggestive of child abuse.

**169—E (Chapter 10)** Treatment of the child with insulin-dependent diabetes mellitus (IDDM, or type I) includes management of diet, exercise, monitoring glucose, *twice daily* administration of insulin, and social support and health education for the child and parents. IDDM may first manifest with an abrupt onset of diabetic ketoacidosis, triggered by an infection or trauma. Classic symptoms of IDDM include weight loss, polyuria, and polydipsia. It results from an absolute deficiency of endogenous insulin. There is strong evidence that IDDM is the result of autoimmune destruction of pancreatic islet cells, which may be triggered by a viral infection in persons with a genetic predisposition, particularly those with certain HLA types.

**170—D (Chapter 8)** Children with epiglottitis are medical emergencies. The pharynx should not be examined because of the danger of provoking respiratory arrest. A lateral radiograph of the neck will show a swollen epiglottis. The disease is treated with parenteral antibiotic therapy and may require several days of nasotracheal intubation. Cold air mist tents are useful in the treatment of spasmodic croup but not acute epiglottis.

**171—E (Chapter 11)** Hemolytic anemia can result from hemoglobinopathies, red blood cell enzyme defects, structural abnormalities of the red blood cell, and traumatic destruction of red blood cells. Vitamin B12 deficiency causes a megaloblastic anemia rather than a hemolytic anemia.

**172—E (Chapter 10)** Episodes of hypoglycemia may occur in the child with insulin-dependent diabetes mellitus (IDDM). It may be beneficial to change the type of insulin preparation (pork, beef, human).

**173—D (Chapter 8)** Acute pharyngitis in children *can be* caused by adenovirus, coxsackie-virus, Epstein-Barr virus, and group A streptococci. Herpes simplex virus does not cause acute pharyngitis in children.

**174—D (Chapter 17)** Characteristics of Marfan syndrome include arachnodactyly (long, thin fingers); arm span greater than the child's height; ocular abnormalities such as dislocation of the lens, blue sclera, retinal detachment, and severe myopia; and cardiac conditions such as mitral valve prolapse, and aortic root dilatation leading to aortic valve insufficiency. Frequent fractures of long bones is not a characteristic of Marfan syndrome.

**175—B (Chapter 10)** Adrenocortical insufficiency in children can result from Addison's disease, Waterhouse-Friderichsen syndrome, congenital adrenal hyperplasia, or high dose corticosteroid therapy. Adrenocortical insufficiency in children does not result from adrenocortical adenomas.

# Pediatrics Answers and Discussion

**176—B (Chapter 12)** Simple partial seizures are common in children and consist of short episodes (10 to 20 seconds) of clonic or tonic movements of the face, neck, and extremities without impairment of consciousness. They may be confused with tics.

**177—E (Chapter 11)** Hemophilia A is an X-linked disorder of coagulation that may present with easy bruising when the child begins to walk. Leukemia with associated thrombocytopenia may present with bruising. Child abuse is often first suspected with signs of bruising, particularly in such areas as the buttocks and back where trauma is not usual. Henoch-Schönlein purpura typically has a rash that evolves into ecchymotic areas, especially in the extremities and buttocks. Ecchymoses are not typical findings in children with rickets. The characteristic laboratory finding in both hemophilia A and hemophilia B is a prolonged activated partial-thromboplastin time (APTT).

**178—B (Chapter 17)** Fever is usually present in infants with osteomyelitis, but is *not invariably* present in older children with the disease. Most children have a leukocytosis with a left shift and an elevated erythrocyte sedimentation rate. Blood cultures frequently reveal the causative pathogen because the pathogenesis begins with bacteremia. Multifocal osteomyelitis can occur in neonates.

**179—A (Chapter 11)** Pancytopenia is not caused by androgens. However, pancytopenia is caused by chloramphenicol, which induces aplastic pancytopenia in 1 per 24,000 to 60,000 patients; by hepatitis and other viral infections; by infiltration of the bone marrow by leukemia; or by radiation.

**180—B (Chapter 12)** Risk factors for developing nonfebrile seizures or idiopathic epilepsy in a child with febrile seizures include focal seizures, neurologic abnormalities, repeated seizures within the same febrile episode, and those with febrile seizures of prolonged duration (longer than 15 minutes). A family history of febrile seizures is not a risk factor for developing nonfebrile seizures.

**181—D (Chapter 8)** The diagnosis of sinusitis in children seldom requires computerized tomography. Sinusitis presents as a purulent nasal discharge, often in children with a history of a prolonged upper respiratory infection. Orbital cellulitis is a complication of ethmoid sinusitis.

**182—B (Chapter 17)** Legg-Calve-Perthes disease, septic arthritis, slipped capital femoral epiphysis, and toxic synovitis are all associated with a limp and hip pain in children. Osgood-Schlatter disease is associated with pain and swelling at the site of one or both tibial tubercles.

**183—B (Chapter 14)** Indirect inguinal hernias occur in 1% to 3% of children, with 90% occurring in boys. Girls with an inguinal hernia should be suspected of having testicular feminization syndrome, which is found in approximately 1% to 2% of girls with inguinal hernias. In girls, the ovary is likely to herniate into the inguinal canal. Treatment is herniorrhaphy.

**184—B (Chapter 11)** Examination of the bone marrow shows an *increased* number of megakaryocytes in autoimmune thrombocytopenia purpura (ATP). The total platelet count is low and anemia may be present. Large platelets are seen on peripheral blood smear. ATP usually presents several weeks after a minor viral illness.

**185—E (Chapter 7)** Thrombocytopenia is not a sign of infectious mononucleosis in an adolescent. However, signs and symptoms do include exudative pharyngitis, atypical lymphocytes, lymphadenopathy, and splenomegaly. Infectious mononucleosis is caused by a herpesvirus, Epstein-Barr virus, and is transmitted by close personal contact.

**186—B (Chapter 11)** Acute lymphoblastic leukemia is classified with the use of cytologic appearance, histochemical stains, and identification of cell surface antigens and of chromosomal translocations. DNA fingerprinting is not used in this classification.

**187—A (Chapter 16)** Characteristics of DiGeorge anomaly include congenital heart disease, hypocalcemic tetany, hypoparathyroidism, and T-cell dysfunction. Complement deficiency is not associated with DiGeorge anomaly.

**188—E (Chapter 11)** Poor prognosis for children with acute lymphoblastic leukemia is associated with age less than 2 years or greater than 10, initial white blood cell count greater than 100,000/mm$^3$, and the presence of a mediastinal mass. Children with null cell ALL, those without definite markers for either mature T or B cells, have the best prognosis.

**189—A (Chapter 8)** Cystic fibrosis is an inherited multisystem disease, located on the long arm of chromosome 7, and is characterized by chronic lung disease, exocrine gland dysfunction, and malabsorption resulting from an apical membrane ion transport defect.

**190—A (Chapter 13)** An atrial septal defect does not result in cyanosis. Cyanosis, best seen in the nail beds, lips, and mucous membranes, is due to the shunting of deoxygenated blood from the right side of the heart to the systemic circulation. Eisenmenger syndrome causes a right-to-left shunt and thus cyanosis.

**191—B (Chapter 19)** Infectious causes of conjunctivitis in children include adenovirus, *Haemophilus influenzae*, measles, and staphylococci. Epstein-Barr virus does not cause conjunctivitis in children.

**192—B (Chapter 11)** Common signs and symptoms in children with infratentorial brain tumors include ataxia, headache, nystagmus, and vomiting, which indicates increased intracranial pressure resulting from obstructive hydrocephalus. Bilateral ptosis is not associated with this condition. Types of infratentorial brain tumors in children include brain stem gliomas, cerebellar astrocytomas, ependymomas, and medulloblastomas.

# Pediatrics Answers and Discussion

**193—E (Chapter 20)** Varicella, or chickenpox, infection is a common and highly contagious herpesvirus infection. The lesions of varicella characteristically are found in various stages of development, papules, vesicles and crusting lesions, at the same time. Encephalitis and cerebellar ataxia are neurologic complications of varicella.

**194—E (Chapter 11)** Langerhans' cell histiocytoses form a subgroup of histiocytosis syndromes, of which the majority are not malignant. Langerhans' cell histiocytoses are cystic bone lesions common in children with class I histiocytoses. Manifestations of this condition include fever, failure to thrive, pituitary dysfunction, seborrheic dermatitis, and bone marrow suppression resulting in anemia and thrombocytopenia. Diagnosis is confirmed by biopsy.

**195—D (Chapter 19)** Orbital cellulitis can be distinguished from periorbital cellulitis by the following clinical features: decreased ocular mobility, loss of visual acuity, pain on movement of the eye, and proptosis. Periorbital swelling is associated with both periorbital cellulitis and orbital cellulitis.

**196—D (Chapter 12)** Neural tube defects can possibly be prevented by folic acid supplementation begun before conception.

**197—D (Chapter 8)** Upper airway obstruction is common in conditions such as bacterial tracheitis, diphtheria, epiglottitis, and laryngotracheobronchitis. It is not a common condition associated with an esophageal foreign body.

**198—C (Chapter 12)** Clinical manifestations of tuberous sclerosis include hypopigmented "ash leaf" lesions, infantile spasms, sebaceous adenomas appearing around the nose, and a shagreen patch in the lumbosacral region.

**199—D (Chapter 12)** Complex partial seizures are frequently associated with automatisms and are manifest by unresponsiveness and staring for 1 to 2 minutes. The characteristic electroencephalogram (EEG) finding shows temporal lobe sharp waves and focal spikes. The EEG finding of hypsarrhythmia is characteristic of infantile spasms.

**200—E (Chapter 7)** Clinical manifestations of measles include conjunctivitis, croup, encephalitis, and Koplik spots. Pharyngeal ulcers are not associated with measles.

**201—E (Chapter 9)** Pyloric stenosis does not occur with frequency in children with trisomy 21. Conditions that do occur in these children are acute lymphocytic leukemia, duodenal atresia, endocardial cushion defects, and imperforate anus.

**202—D (Chapter 12)** Ataxia, chorea, dystonia, and tics are all classified as movement disorders. Infantile spasms are classified as a seizure disorder.

**203—E (Chapter 12)** Viral meningitis is clinically *difficult* to distinguish from bacterial meningitis. The diagnosis is often one of exclusion based upon the results of culture of the cerebrospinal fluid. Epidemics of aseptic meningitis occur during the summer and fall in the United States.

**204—C (Chapter 7)** The presence of sepsis in a very young infant can be very difficult to diagnose. The clinical signs and symptoms are often so subtle that the clinician cannot rely only on the history and physical examination to detect serious bacterial infection.

**205—C (Chapter 12)** Reye's syndrome is characterized by mitochondrial dysfunction. It begins with vomiting and mental status changes, and can rapidly progress to seizures, coma, and fatty degeneration of the liver. Serum levels of ammonia and liver and muscle enzymes are *elevated.*

**206—B (Chapter 15)** Severe bilateral intrauterine obstruction of the urinary tract results in abnormal facies, limb anomalies, oligohydramnios, and pulmonary hypoplasia. It does not result in azotemia.

**207—A (Chapter 12)** Children over the age of 2 tolerate head injuries better than adults. Children with concussions may have some degree of retrograde or posttraumatic amnesia. Subdural or epidural hematomas are early complications of serious head trauma while headaches and behavioral problems represent late complications. However, the presence of a skull fracture is *not* an excellent predictor of underlying brain injury.

**208—A (Chapter 13)** A soft continuous murmur occurring in both systole and diastole is not a sign or symptom of coarctation of the aorta.

**209—E (Chapter 8)** Complications of otitis media include cholesteatoma, conductive hearing loss, mastoiditis, and persistent effusion. Posterior auricular adenopathy is not a complication of otitis media.

**210—B (Chapter 12)** Hypotonia is *not evident* in the first months of life. Gower's sign is usually evident between the age of 3 and 5 years. The use of the hands upon the legs to reach the upright position is a classic sign of muscular dystrophy.

**211—B (Chapter 20)** Streptococcal skin infections include blistering distal dactylitis, erysipelas, perianal cellulitis, and periorbital cellulitis. Bullous impetigo is caused by staphylococcus rather than streptococcus.

**212—D (Chapter 8)** Signs and symptoms of group A streptococcal pharyngitis include abdominal pain, cervical adenopathy, headache, and vomiting. Vesicles on the tonsillar pillars are not a sign of group A streptococcal pharyngitis.

**213—B (Chapter 13)** Tetralogy of Fallot is characterized by dextroposition of the aorta, pulmonary valve and infundibular stenosis, right

# Pediatrics Answers and Discussion

ventricular hypertrophy, and ventricular septal defect. An endocardial cushion defect is not a characteristic of tetralogy of Fallot. Most children with tetralogy of Fallot present in the first few weeks or months of life with failure to thrive and cyanosis with feeding.

**214—A (Chapter 8)** Early treatment of group A streptococcal pharyngitis can prevent cervical adenitis, peritonsillar abscess, retropharyngeal abscess, and rheumatic fever. Early treatment of group A streptococcal pharyngitis *does not prevent* acute poststreptococcal glomerulonephritis.

**215—C (Chapter 20)** Atopic dermatitis frequently involves the extensor surfaces in infants and the flexural surfaces in older children, causing intense pruritus. It may become infected with herpes simplex virus. Treatment involves avoiding soaps and frequent bathing, both of which dry the skin; use of oils and creams to keep the skin moist after bathing; wet dressing with Burrow solution; and topical corticosteroids.

**216—B (Chapter 13)** Signs and symptoms of congestive heart failure in infants include failure to thrive, poor feeding, tachypnea, and sweating during feeding. Heart murmur is not a sign or symptom of congestive heart failure.

**217—B (Chapter 9)** Klinefelter syndrome usually is diagnosed in boys with *delayed* puberty. Klinefelter syndrome occurs in approximately 1/1000 live male births, resulting from nondisjunction during meiosis. Behavioral, cognitive (mental retardation), and psychiatric symptoms may be prominent in these infants.

**218—D (Chapter 6)** The presence of diarrhea does not exclude the diagnosis of Hirschsprung's disease. Diarrhea may occur and can alternate with periods of constipation.

**219—E (Chapter 15)** The diagnosis of urinary tract infection is confirmed by culture of bacteria from the urine. Suprapubic puncture and catheterization are techniques used to obtain sterile urine specimens in infants and children. Differentiation of cystitis and pyelonephritis can be difficult, particularly in young children. Because pyuria can occur in the absence of urinary tract infection and a urinary tract infection can occur without pyuria, the diagnosis should not be based solely on the presence or absence of leukocytes in the urine.

**220—A (Chapter 7)** Conjunctivitis-otitis media syndrome is not caused by enteroviruses. Several distinct clinical syndromes are caused by enteroviruses, including hand-foot-mouth syndrome, herpangina, myocarditis, and pleurodynia. Enteroviral infections have a seasonal pattern of summer and fall with an incubation period of 3 to 6 days. Children may be infectious for several weeks.

**221—B (Chapter 19)** There are several causes of a red swollen eye in children including conjunctivitis, orbital cellulitis, periorbital cellulitis, and sinusitis. Glaucoma is not associated with a red, swollen eye in children.

**222—C (Chapter 15)** Hemolytic-uremic syndrome (HUS) is the most common cause of *acute* renal failure in children under the age of 4 years. HUS is associated with a preceding upper respiratory infection or bacterial or viral gastroenteritis, especially that resulting from *Escherichia coli* O157:H7.

**223—E (Chapter 3)** Both hyperkeratosis and night blindness are signs of vitamin A deficiency. Chronic vitamin A deficiency can cause corneal clouding and blindness. Malabsorption syndromes or liver disease may be caused by vitamin A deficiency. There is no correlation between vitamin A supplementation and the outcome of measles infection in children.

**224—E (Chapter 7)** Children with Lyme disease may have arthritis, erythema chronicum migrans (annular rash), facial palsy, or myocarditis. Purpura is not associated with Lyme disease.

**225—E (Chapter 17)** Risk factors for congenital hip dislocation include breech presentation, neural tube defects, oligohydramnios, cerebral palsy, and a family history of congenital hip dislocation. Prematurity is not a risk factor for congenital hip dislocation.

**226—C (Chapter 19)** Cataracts in infants and children are associated with congenital infections such as rubella syndrome; metabolic disorders such as galactosemia and mucopolysaccharidoses; and chromosomal abnormalities including trisomy 21, 18, and 13 and Turner syndrome; and trauma. Cataracts are not associated with retinopathy of prematurity.

**227—D (Chapter 21)** Although the symptoms of lead poisoning can be very subtle and early detection is crucial, routine screening using blood lead levels is recommended for all children residing in areas in which they might be exposed to excessive amounts of lead. Typically, children with moderate to severe lead poisoning present with anemia, encephalopathy, and colic. Acute lead encephalopathy can result in cerebral edema. Young children absorb lead more readily than adults.

**228—B (Chapter 7)** Generally, the height of fever does not distinguish bacterial infection from viral infection, although some studies suggest that bacterial infection is more likely with extremes of hyperpyrexia (greater than 41°C). The pattern of fever can be useful in monitoring response to therapy. Fever in children may be an adaptive host response.

**229—D (Chapter 3)** Metabolic acidosis is characterized by a low bicarbonate level and blood pH. The causes of this condition are classified on the basis of changes in the anion gap and include diabetic ketoacidosis, lactic acidosis, toxins such as methanol, and starvation ketoacidosis. Renal tubular acidosis is not a cause of metabolic acidosis with increased anion gap.

**230—E (Chapter 7)** Clinical manifestations of mumps include erythrema of the opening of Stensen's duct, meningoencephalitis, orchitis, and parotid swelling. Splenomegaly is not a clinical manifestation of mumps.

**231—B (Chapter 10)** Ornithine transcarbamylase deficiency is inherited as an X-linked dominant disorder. Manifestations of urea cycle defects in infants include vomiting, lethargy, and seizures.

**232—B (Chapter 4)** Cocaine use during pregnancy can result in cerebral infarction, intrauterine growth retardation, spontaneous abortion, and premature labor. There is no clearly defined withdrawal syndrome found in newborns whose mothers are addicted to cocaine.

**233—C (Chapter 11)** Autoimmune hemolytic anemia is associated with HIV, other viral infections, lymphoma, and systemic lupus erythematosus.

**234—D (Chapter 8)** A red auditory canal is not a sign of acute otitis media but of acute otitis externa. However, bulging tympanic membrane, failure of the tympanic membrane to move with pneumatic otoscopy, obscured bony landmarks, and red tympanic membrane are all signs of acute otitis media.

**235—C (Chapter 5)** The newborn's red blood cells contain hemoglobin F, which binds to oxygen at lower pressures than hemoglobin A (which is found in adult red blood cells). At the age of 2 to 3 months, the hemoglobin level falls to a range of 15 to 20 mg/dL.

**236—A (Chapter 10)** Hypopituitarism in children results from cranial irradiation, craniopharyngioma, trauma, and septo-optic dysplasia. Bacterial meningitis is not associated with hypopituitarism.

**237—A (Chapter 6)** Neonatal conjunctivitis can be caused by inflammation from silver nitrate drops, infection with *Chlamydia trachomatis* or *Neisseria gonorrhoeae*, or herpes simplex virus. Cytomegalovirus is not associated with neonatal conjunctivitis or hepatitis.

**238—C (Chapter 10)** The syndrome of inappropriate secretion of antidiuretic hormone (SIADH) is often asymptomatic. It is characterized by low serum sodium levels. Neurologic symptoms of increasing severity occur with worsening hyponatremia. Therapy involves fluid restriction and treatment of the underlying disorder.

**239—D (Chapter 11)** Clinical manifestations of acute lymphoblastic leukemia include bone pain, fatigue, fever, and petechiae. Jaundice is not associated with acute lymphoblastic leukemia. Without prophylactic treatment, the central nervous system and testes are common sites for relapse of acute lymphoblastic leukemia in children.

**240—D (Chapter 9)** Approximately 50% of all fetuses with trisomy 21 are spontaneously aborted early in pregnancy. Most children with trisomy 18 and trisomy 13 die in early infancy. Advanced maternal age is associated with a greater risk of nondisjunction during meiosis.

**241—D (Chapter 2)** Failure to thrive and growth retardation are among the most common presenting signs of serious disease in children. Failure to thrive is a possible manifestation of chronic renal failure, congenital heart disease, cystic fibrosis, and neglect. G6PD is not associated with failure to thrive.

**242—E (Chapter 11)** Von Willebrand disease is an autosomal dominant disorder caused by a deficiency of functional von Willebrand protein, which transports factor VIII. Children with the disease have decreased factor VIII activity and a prolonged partial thromboplastin time. Platelet aggregation and adhesiveness also are diminished. Recurrent hemarthroses and the development of chronic joint disease are common complications of hemophilia A but are not associated with von Willebrand disease.

**243—C (Chapter 4)** Adverse outcome of pregnancy is associated with lack of prenatal care, low maternal socioeconomic and educational status, oligohydramnios (inadequate amount of amniotic fluid), polyhydramnios (excessive amount of amniotic fluid), extremes of maternal age (older or younger), and diseases such as diabetes mellitus or hypertension. Maternal colonization with *Escherichia coli* is not indicated as a cause of adverse fetal outcome.

**244—C (Chapter 6)** Physiologic hyperbilirubinemia in the newborn is an elevated level of *unconjugated* bilirubin that exceeds normal adult levels. It usually peaks on the third day of life with typical levels reaching a maximum of 5 to 6 mg/dL.

**245—C (Chapter 12)** Risk factors for recurrent febrile seizures include family history of febrile seizures, age less than 18 months, lower temperatures (lower than 101°F), and shorter duration of fever when the first seizure occurred. Focal seizures are not a risk factor for recurrent febrile seizures.

**246—B (Chapter 10)** Hypocalcemia is not a laboratory finding commonly associated with inborn errors of metabolism.

**247—D (Chapter 8)** Bronchiolitis is a winter or early spring viral infection of infants and small children. It is usually caused by respiratory syncytial virus but other viral etiologic agents such as parainfluenza virus and adenovirus can cause this disease. Infants with bronchiolitis can develop *respiratory acidosis*, not respiratory alkalosis.

**248—D (Chapter 6)** Most infants with congenital toxoplasmosis are not symptomatic at birth. However, newborns with severe congenital infection may have hydrocephalus, microcephaly, chorioretinitis, hepatosplenomegaly, and thrombocytopenia.

**249—C (Chapter 11)** Children with sickle cell anemia present with characteristic signs of chronic hemolytic anemia, including reticulocytosis, intermittent indirect hyperbilirubinemia, and moderate-to-severe anemia. Life-threatening complications of sickle cell anemia include acute chest syndrome, which may rapidly progress to respiratory failure. They may suffer an infarction of the brain, resulting in serious brain damage as a result of occlusion of vessels supplying the central nervous system. Children with sickle cell anemia are prone to serious bacterial infections. Although painful crises do occur in children with sickle cell anemia, they are not life-threatening.

**250—B (Chapter 8)** Clinical manifestations of cystic fibrosis include chronic sinusitis, malabsorption of fat soluble vitamins, nasal polyps, and recurrent pulmonary infections. Cystic malformations in the lung and liver are not a manifestation of cystic fibrosis.

**251—C (Chapter 4)** Signs of intrapartum asphyxia include abnormalities in the fetal heart rate variability, fetal bradycardia, low fetal scalp blood pH, and meconium in the amniotic fluid. A high level of alpha-fetoprotein in the amniotic fluid is not a sign of intrapartum asphyxia.

**252—D (Chapter 11)** Osteogenic sarcoma is the most common malignant bone tumor of children. It occurs at the metaphyses of long bones, usually during the adolescent period of accelerated growth. Children usually present with pain and a mass at the site of the tumor. Treatment includes extensive local excision or amputation of the affected limb and intensive chemotherapy with multiple drugs.

**253—C (Chapter 12)** Clinical manifestations of Sturge-Weber disease include facial nevus (port wine stain), glaucoma, seizures, and unilateral intracranial calcification. Children with this condition often have mental retardation as well. Hamartomas of the iris are not a clinical manifestation of Sturge-Weber disease.

**254—E (Chapter 13)** Typical features of supraventricular tachycardia in children include the possibility of congestive heart failure, variable heart rate between 200–300 beats/min, P waves that are usually abnormal, and a QRS complex that is usually narrow. Underlying heart disease is not a typical feature of supraventricular tachycardia.

**255—A (Chapter 5)** Reflexes found in the newborn include the grasp, Moro, rooting, and tonic neck reflexes. The Brudzinski reflex, more commonly known as the Brudzinski sign, involves involuntary flexion of the hips and legs with flexion of the neck, and is found in children with meningitis.

# Pediatrics
## Must-Know Topics

The following are must-know topics discussed in this review. It would be useful for you to formulate outlines of these subjects since knowledge of the related material will be key to your understanding of the subject and material and for passing the examination.

### *History, physical examination, and differential diagnosis*

- Elements of history especially important to children

### *Growth and development*

- Abuse and neglect

- Average size of normal newborn

- Cerebral palsy: definition and types

- Major causes of abnormal growth

    - failure to thrive

    - obesity

    - short stature

    - microcephaly

*(continued)*

- hydrocephaly

- Major theories of psychosocial development

  - Freud

  - Erikson

  - Piaget

- Mental retardation: major categories and causes

- Rate of weight change in normal infant

- Stages of adolescent sexual development

- Use of developmental screening tests

  - Denver Developmental Screening test

  - Draw-a-Man test

- Use and value of growth charts

## Nutrition and metabolism

- Advantages and contraindications of breast-feeding

- Basic water, caloric, and vitamin requirements

- Basic elements and causes of acid-base balance

- Causes of imbalances in sodium, potassium, and glucose levels

- Vitamin and mineral deficiency or excess: causes, signs, and symptoms

## Pregnancy, labor, and delivery

- Apgar score

- Adverse outcomes of pregnancy associated with:
  - maternal age
  - maternal diabetes
  - maternal medication or substance abuse
  - nutrition
  - toxemia

- Causes of intrauterine growth retardation

- Common birth injuries

- Complications of low birth weight and prematurity

- Definitions of gestational age

- Methods and use of fetal assessment

- Risk factors for infant during labor and delivery

- Signs of fetal distress

## Normal newborn

- Common skin lesions in newborns

- Definition and time of disappearance of newborn primitive reflexes

- Physiologic changes in the newborn cardiorespiratory system at birth

*(continued)*

- Status of the newborn renal, hematopoietic, gastrointestinal, and immune systems

- Time of closure of fontanelles

## Diseases of the newborn

- Causes, signs, symptoms, treatment, and complications of:

  - congenital aganglionic megacolon
  - congenital infections
  - hemolytic disease of the newborn
  - HIV infection
  - intraventricular hemorrhage
  - necrotizing enterocolitis
  - neonatal jaundice
  - neonatal sepsis
  - respiratory distress syndrome

## Infectious diseases

- Causes, signs, symptoms, and treatment of:

  - bacteremia and sepsis
  - chickenpox
  - hepatitis
  - hook worm

- infectious mononucleosis
- Lyme disease
- measles
- meningococcemia
- mumps
- pinworms
- Rocky Mountain spotted fever
- roseola
- roundworm
- rubella
- scarlet fever
- tuberculosis

## Diseases of the respiratory system

- Asthma: symptoms, signs, and treatment

- Causes, symptoms, signs, treatment, and complications of:

  - acute otitis media

  - bronchiolitis

  - croup

*(continued)*

- pertussis
- pharyngitis
- pneumonia
- sinusitis

• Cystic fibrosis: epidemiology, genetics, signs and symptoms

## *Genetic disorders*

• Signs and symptoms of:
  - Klinefelter syndrome
  - trisomy 21
  - trisomy 18
  - trisomy 13
  - Turner syndrome

## *Metabolic and endocrine disorders*

• Genetics, symptoms, signs, and complications of metabolic disorders:
  - galactosemia
  - phenylketonuria
  - Tay-Sachs disease
  - urea cycle defects

• Genetics, symptoms, signs, and complications of endocrine disorders:

- adrenal: increased secretion of ACTH

- pancreas: insulin-dependent diabetes; hypoglycemia

- pituitary: diabetes insipidus; hypopituitarism; syndrome of inappropriate antidiuretic hormone secretion (SIADH)

- pubertal disorders

- thyroid: hypothyroidism, hyperthyroidism

## Hematologic and malignant disorders

- Causes, signs, symptoms and treatment of:

  - anemias: iron-deficiency; megaloblastic; hemolytic; thalassemias

  - hemophilias

  - leukemias

  - lymphomas

  - pancytopenia

  - thrombocytopenia

  - tumors of the central nervous system (CNS)

## Disorders of the central nervous system

- Causes, symptoms, signs, laboratory evaluation, and treatment of infections of the CNS: bacterial and viral meningitis

*(continued)*

- Genetics, symptoms, signs of:
  - muscular dystrophy
  - myotonic dystrophy
  - Werdnig-Hoffman syndrome
- Neurocutaneous syndromes: signs and symptoms
- Reye's syndrome: signs and symptoms
- Seizure disorders: typology and definition
- Types of congenital malformations: neural tube defects

## Cardiovascular disorders

- Anatomic description, symptoms, and signs of common congenital cardiac lesions:
  - Tetralogy of Fallot, ventricular septal defect (VSD), atrial septal defect (ASD), coarctation of the aorta, transposition of the great vessels
- Symptoms, signs, and treatment of Kawasaki disease and Henoch-Schönlein purpura

## Gastrointestinal disorders

- Common causes, symptoms and signs of acute gastroenteritis
- Symptoms, signs, and treatment of:
  - appendicitis
  - inguinal hernias

- intussusception
- malrotation and volvulus
- Meckel's diverticulum
- pyloric stenosis
* Symptoms, signs, and treatment of Crohn's disease and ulcerative colitis

## *Genitourinary and renal disorders*

* Causes, symptoms, and signs of:
  - acute poststreptococcal glomerulonephritis
  - hemolytic-uremic syndrome
  - nephrosis
* Predisposing factors and causes of urinary tract infections
* Renal tubular acidosis: types
* Signs and symptoms of common congenital anomalies of the urinary tract

## *Immunologic and rheumatologic disorders*

* Acute rheumatic fever: signs, symptoms, and complications
* HIV infection: symptoms, signs, complications
* Juvenile rheumatoid arthritis: description of types

*(continued)*

- Pathology, symptoms, and signs of:
  - chronic granulomatous disease
  - combined immunodeficiencies: DiGeorge anomaly; Wiskott-Aldrich syndrome; ataxia-telangiectasis

## *Orthopedic disorders*

- Common causes, signs, and symptoms of osteomyelitis and septic arthritis
- Description of common congenital orthopedic anomalies
- Description of common skeletal dysplasias

## *Ophthalmologic disorders*

- Common causes and treatment of conjunctivitis
- Common causes, symptoms, signs, and treatment of periorbital and orbital cellulitis
- Description of common congenital anomalies of the eye: strabismus, glaucoma, dacryostenosis

## *Skin disorders*

- Description of common congenital anomalies of the skin
- Description of symptoms, signs, and treatment of common dermatitis: atopic, seborrheic, erythema multiforme, and acne vulgaris

## Preventive pediatrics

- Immunizations: schedule and contraindications

- Symptoms, signs and treatment of lead poisoning

# Index

Page numbers followed by a *t* refer to tables; those followed by an *f* refer to figures.

Abdomen, examination of, 3
Abdominal pain, with malrotation, 151
ABO incompatibility, 51
Abruptio placentae, 32
Abscess
 brain, with cyanotic congenital heart disease, 141
 peritonsillar, 76
 retropharyngeal, 76
Abuse and neglect, 181–182
 and nonorganic failure to thrive, 9
Achondroplasia, 180
Acid-base disorders, 20–21. *See also* Acidosis; Alkalosis
 metabolic, 20
 mixed, 20
 respiratory, 20
 simple, 20
Acidemia, 20
 and calcium levels, 26
 fetal, 33
Acidosis, 20. *See also* Diabetic ketoacidosis
 lactic, 21
 metabolic, 20–21
  with inborn errors of metabolism, 89
  with increased anion gap, 21
  with normal anion gap, 21
 renal, 165–166
 renal tubular, 21, 165
  proximal, 165–166
 respiratory, 21
Acne vulgaris, 189
Acoustic neuromas, 127
Acquired immunodeficiency syndrome, 170–171. *See also* HIV
Acrocyanosis, 40
Activated partial-thromboplastin time (APTT), prolonged, with hemophilia A and B, 114
Acute cerebellar ataxia, 131
Acute dystonic reactions, 131
Acute hemorrhagic conjunctivitis, 69–70
Acute lymphocytic (lymphoblastic) leukemia (ALL), 115–116
 disseminated molluscum contagiosum with, 191
 null cell, 116
 prognosis, 116
 relapse, 116
 with trisomy 21, 85, 116
Acute nonlymphocytic leukemia (ANLL), 115–117
Addison's disease, 98
Adenosine deaminase deficiency, 168
Adenovirus
 bronchiolitis, 78
 conjunctivitis, 184–185
 epidemic keratoconjunctivitis, 185
 gastroenteritis, 153
 pertussis, 78
 pneumonia, 79
Adolescence, 7–9
Adolescents, interviewing, 1–2
Adrenal crisis, 98

Adrenal disorders, 21, 98–99
Adrenal insufficiency, with myotonic dystrophy, 135
Adrenocortical insufficiency, 98
Adrenocortical tumors, 99
Adrenocorticotropic hormone (ACTH)
 increased secretion of, 98
 for infantile spasms, 129
Agammaglobulinemia, X-linked, 167
Airway resistance, 75
Airway responsiveness, in children, 80
Alcohol, maternal use, effect on fetus and neonate, 30–31
Alkalemia, 20
 and calcium levels, 26
Alkalosis, 20
 metabolic, 21
 respiratory, 21
Alpha-1-antitrypsin deficiency, 82
Alpha-fetoprotein, maternal serum, 31
Alpha-thalassemia, 110
Alport syndrome, 161
Ambiguous genitalia, 99
Amblyopia, 183
Amenorrhea, primary, with Turner syndrome, 86
Amino acid metabolism, disorders of, 90–91
Aminoaciduria, 166
Amniocentesis, 31
Amniotic fluid
 deficiency, 32
 examination, 31
 excessive, 32
 meconium in, 33, 46
Anaerobes, retropharyngeal abscess, 76
Anal dimples, 187
Anal stage, 12
*Ancylostoma duodenale*, 71
Anemia, 105
 Cooley's, 110
 hemolytic. *See* Hemolytic anemia
 iron-deficiency. *See* Iron-deficiency anemia
 megaloblastic, 26, 107
 pernicious, juvenile, 107
 physiologic, 41
Anencephaly, 32, 99–100, 126
Aneurysms, with Kawasaki disease, 146
Angiotensin converting enzyme (ACE) inhibitors, maternal use, effect on fetus and neonate, 30*t*
Anion gap, 20–21
Aniridia, 87
Anisometropia, 183
Anomalous origin of left coronary artery, 144–145
Anthropometric measurements, 3
Antibiotics
 for acute osteomyelitis, 179
 for acute otitis media, 73
 for bacteremia, 62–63
 for bacterial gastroenteritis, 153
 for epiglottitis, 77
 for immunosuppressed patients, 172
 for periorbital cellulitis, 185
 for rheumatic fever, 173
 for sinusitis, 74
 for urinary tract infection, 160

Antidiuretic hormone deficiency, 100
Antineoplastic agents, maternal use, effect on fetus and neonate, 30*t*
Anti-Rh immune globulin (RhoGAM), 51
Anxiety, 21
Aortic stenosis, 144
Apert syndrome, 126
Apgar score, 34, 35*t*
 low, 16, 34
 at 1 minute, 34
 at 5 minutes, 34
Aplastic crises, due to parvovirus B19 infection, 69
Apnea
 neonatal, 46–47, 47*t*
 primary (idiopathic), 47
 secondary, 47
 in young infants, 78
Apparent life-threatening event (ALTE), 83
Appearance, general, of ill child, 3
Appendectomy, 152
Appendicitis, acute, 152
Appropriate-for-gestational age (AGA) infants, 35
APSGN. *See* Glomerulonephritis, acute post-streptococcal
Arachnodactyly, in Marfan's syndrome, 180
Arboviruses, encephalitis, 133
Arrhythmias, 145
 in Marfan's syndrome, 180
Arterial switch (Jatene) procedure, 141
Arthritis, 62
 of Crohn's disease, 154–155
 gonococcal, 179
 with rheumatic fever, 172
 septic, 179
 with ulcerative colitis, 155
*Ascaris lumbricoides*, 70
Ash leaf lesions, 127
Aspergillus infection, in chronic granulomatous disease, 169
Asphyxia, intrapartum, 33
Aspiration pneumonia, with gastroesophageal reflux, 149–150
Aspirin
 contraindications to, 75
 for juvenile rheumatoid arthritis, 174
 and Reye's syndrome, 134
Asthma, 80–81
 diagnosis, 80–81
 treatment, 81
Astrocytomas
 cerebellar, 119
 supratentorial, 119
Astrovirus, gastroenteritis, 153
Asymptomatic bacteriuria, 160
Ataxia, 131
 acute cerebellar, 131
 Friedreich's, 88, 131
Ataxia-telangiectasia, 131, 169
 and non-Hodgkin's lymphoma, 118
Atlantoaxial instability, 175
Atopic dermatitis, 187–188
Atrial septal defect (ASD), 142–143
Atrioventricular septal defects, 142–143
Auditory canal, infection, 74

309

Auscultation, 3
Autoimmune disease, 167–168
    with complement component deficiencies, 169
    endocrine, 102
Autoimmune hemolytic anemias, 111
Autoimmune thrombocytopenic purpura, 113
Automobile accidents, 197
Autonomy versus shame and doubt, 13

Baby bottle caries, 195
Back pain, 178
Bacteremia, 62–63
    acute osteomyelitis and, 178
    arthritis and, 179
    occult, 62t, 62–63
    pneumococcal, 62–63
    transient, 63
Bacteria, nasopharyngeal colonization, 132
Bacterial gastroenteritis, 153
Bacterial infection(s), 61, 62t, 63
    in chronic granulomatous disease, 169
    with complement component deficiencies, 169
    fever in, 61
    in immunosuppressed patients, 172
    with sickle cell anemia, 108
    of skin, 190–191
Bacterial pneumonia, 79
Bacterial tracheitis, 76
Bacterial vaginosis, 59
Balloon atrial septostomy, 141
Barium enema, for intussusception, 151–152
Barr body, 86
Bartter syndrome, 20–21
Basic trust versus mistrust, 13
Becker muscular dystrophy, 135
Beckwith syndrome, 54
Berger disease, 162–163
Beriberi, 25
Beta-agonists, for asthma, 81
Beta-thalassemia, 110
    protective effect against malaria, 71
Bicarbonate, 20–21
Bicycle helmets, 197
Biliary atresia, 25
Bilirubin, elevated levels of, 48
Birth injuries, 33–34
    in infant of diabetic mother, 28
    in large-for-gestational-age infants, 35
Birth length, 6
Birth weight, 42
    average, 5
Blackfan-Diamond syndrome, 105
Blistering distal dactylitis, 190
Blood
    culture, 63
    glucose level, monitoring, 102
    pH, 20
Blood pressure, measurement, 3
Blood transfusions, with thalassemia, 110
Bloom syndrome, 117
Blue dot sign, 158
Blue spells, 140
Body surface area, and metabolic rate, 18
Body water, 17
Bone(s)
    infections, 178–179
    tumors, 122
Bone age, 7
*Bordetella pertussis*, 78
    culture, 78
Bordet-Genou media, 78
Botulism, 137
Brachial plexus palsies, 34
Bradycardia, fetal, 33
Brain
    abscess, with cyanotic congenital heart disease, 141
    inflammation, 133
    injury, with sickle cell anemia, 108

tumors, 115, 118
    infratentorial, 118
    supratentorial, 118
Brain-stem gliomas, 119
Branchial cleft cysts, 187
Breast-feeding, 22, 50, 106
Breast masses, 101
Breech presentation, and congenital dislocation of hip, 176
Bronchiolitis, 78
    and asthma, 80
Bronchopulmonary dysplasia (BOD), 46
Brudzinski sign, 132
Brushfield spots, 85
Bruton's disease, 167
Buccal cellulitis, 190
Bucket handle fracture(s), 181
Bullous impetigo, 190
Buphthalmos, 184
Burkitt lymphoma, 118
Burns, 198

Café-au-lait spots, 127
Caffey disease, 180
Calcium
    imbalances, 26
    requirements, 17t
    serum, 26
    urinary excretion, 161
Calicivirus, gastroenteritis, 153
Caloric requirement, 17t, 21–23
    average daily, 21
*Campylobacter jejuni* gastroenteritis, 153
*Candida* infection, 192–193
    in chronic granulomatous disease, 169
Capillary hemangiomas, 39, 189–190
Caput succedaneum, 33
Carbamazepine, maternal use, effect on fetus and neonate, 30t
Carbohydrate metabolism, disorders, 93
Carbon monoxide poisoning, 197
Carboxyhemoglobin, measurement, 197
Cardiac. *See* Heart
Cardiopulmonary disorders, neonatal, 45–48
Cardiovascular system
    disorders, 139–147
        must-know topics, 304
    neonatal, 41
Carditis, in rheumatic fever, 172–173
Caries, dental, 195
Carpenter syndrome, 126
Catalase, 169
Cataracts, 184
    amblyopia and, 183
    congenital, 184
Catheters, indwelling, and fever, 61
Cat-scratch disease, 66–67
Cavernous hemangiomas, 190
Cavernous sinus thrombosis, 74
Celiac disease, 154
Cellulitis, 62, 190
    buccal, 190
    orbital, 74, 185–186
    perianal streptococcal, 190
    periorbital, 185, 190
Central nervous system
    congenital malformations, 125–126
    depression, 21
    diseases, 54–55
    disorders, 125–137
        must-know topics, 303–304
    infections, 131–134
    myelination, 43
    neonatal, 43
    trauma, 134
    tumors, 118–120
Cephalhematomas, 33
Cerebellar astrocytomas, 119
Cerebral edema, in diabetic ketoacidosis, 103
Cerebral infarction, with intrauterine cocaine exposure, 30

Cerebral palsy, 16
    causes, 16
    classification, 16
    and congenital dislocation of hip, 176
    risk factors for, 16
Cerebrospinal fluid (CSF)
    examination, 132
    excess accumulation of, 10
Cervical adenitis, 75
CGD. *See* Chronic granulomatous disease
Charcot-Marie-Tooth disease, 136–137
Cherry red spot, on macula, 92
Chiari malformation, 10, 126
Chickenpox, 192
Chief complaint, 1
Child abuse and neglect, 181–182
    and nonorganic failure to thrive, 9
*Chlamydia trachomatis*
    conjunctivitis, 56
    infection, ocular involvement, 185
    pneumonia, 80
Choanal atresia, 41
Cholestasis, 49
    neonatal, 82
Cholesteatoma, 73–74
Chordee, 157
Chorea, 131, 173
Chorioamnionitis, 32
Chorionic villus biopsy, 31
Christmas disease, 114–115
Chromosomal abnormalities, 85–88
    and advanced maternal age, 28
    cataracts due to, 184
    and mental retardation, 15t
Chromosome 13
    deletion of long arm of, 87
    retinoblastoma gene, 122–123
Chromosome 5, deletion of short arm of (5p-), 87
Chromosome 11, deletion of short arm of (11p-), 87
Chronic granulomatous disease, 169
Chronic myelogenous leukemia, 115–117
Chronic renal disease, 100
Chronic renal failure, 10, 100
    with reflux nephropathy, 159
Cirrhosis, 90
    childhood, 82
    with chronic hepatitis B virus, 70
Cisapride, for gastroesophageal reflux, 150
Clavicular fracture, during delivery, 34
Cleft lip and palate, 53
Clinical reasoning, 3–4
Clinitest, 93, 154
*Clostridium botulinum*, 137
*Clostridium tetani*, 56
Club feet, 32
Coarctation of the aorta, 144
Cobblestone appearance, in gastrointestinal tract, 155
Cocaine, maternal use, effect on fetus and neonate, 30, 30t
Cognitive function, decreased, in iron-deficient infants, 107
Colostrum, 22
Common ALL antigen (cALLa), 116
Common cold, 75
Common variable immunodeficiency, 168
Complement
    deficiencies, 169
    serum levels, low, 162
Complete congenital heart block, with neonatal lupus erythematosus, 29, 145
Concrete operational stage, 14
Concussions, 134
Condylomata acuminata, 191
Congenital adrenal hyperplasia, 98–99
    salt-losing form, 98
Congenital aganglionic megacolon, 52–53
Congenital anomalies
    genitourinary, 157–159
    in large-for-gestational-age infants, 35

and mental retardation, 15t
ophthalmologic, 183–184
orthopedic, 175–178
respiratory, 74–75
of skin, 187
Congenital aortic stenosis, 144
Congenital dislocation of hip, 176
Congenital heart block, 145
complete, with neonatal lupus erythematosus, 29, 145
Congenital heart disease, 139–145, 140t
acyanotic, 142–145
cyanotic, 139–141
with trisomy 21, 85
with Turner syndrome, 86
Congenital hypothyroidism, 40, 96
newborn screening programs, 96
Congenital lobar emphysema, 75
Congenital pure red cell aplasia, 105
Congenital rubella syndrome, 59, 68, 184
Congenital spherocytosis, 110–111
Congenital varicella syndrome, 58
Congestive heart failure
with coarctation, 144
with iron deficiency, 107
in Marfan's syndrome, 180
in rheumatic fever, 172–173
Conjunctivitis
acute hemorrhagic, 69–70
acute purulent, 184–185
adenoviral, 184–185
*Chlamydia trachomatis*, 56
enteroviral, 184–185
gonococcal, 56
measles and, 184–185
in newborn, 56
Constitutional growth delay, 10
Contact dermatitis, 188
Continuous positive airway pressure (CPAP), 45, 48
Cooley's anemia, 110
Coombs' test, positive direct, for autoimmune hemolytic anemias, 111
Copper, excess accumulation of, 26
Coronavirus, 75
Cor pulmonale, 46
Corticosteroids
and adrenocortical insufficiency, 98
for asthma, 80–81
cataracts caused by, 184
complications with, 81
for Henoch-Schönlein purpura, 147
immunosuppression caused by, 172
for *Pneumocystis carinii* pneumonia, 171
to prevent respiratory distress syndrome, 45
for stimulating red blood cell production, 105
*Corynebacterium diphtheriae*, 77
Coumadin, maternal use, effect on fetus and neonate, 30t
Cow's milk protein allergy, 23, 154
Coxsackievirus A16, 69
Coxsackievirus B1–B5, 69
Cradle cap, 188
Cranial nerve palsies, with diphtheria, 77–78
Cranial sutures, premature closure, 126
Craniopharyngiomas, 99–100, 119–120
Craniosynostosis, 126
Craniotabes, 24–25
Creutzfeldt-Jacob disease, 100
Cri du chat syndrome, 87
Crohn's disease, 154–155
Cromolyn sodium, for asthma, 81
Croup
infectious, 76
spasmodic, 76
Crouzon syndrome, 126
Cryptorchidism, 158
Cryptosporidium gastroenteritis, 153
Currant jelly stools, 151
Cushing syndrome, 21, 99
Cyanotic congenital heart disease, 139–141
Cystic adenomatoid malformation, 75

Cystic fibrosis, 25, 52, 81–82
diagnosis, 82
genetics, 81
signs and symptoms, 81
Cystic fibrosis transmembrane regulator (CFTR), 81
Cystic gliomas, 119
Cystic hygromas, 187
Cystinosis, 166
Cystitis, 160
Cytomegalovirus (CMV) infection
congenital, 58
cataracts due to, 184
in organ transplant recipients, 172
perinatal, 58

Dacryocystitis, 184
Dacryostenosis, 184
Dactylitis, with sickle cell anemia, 108
Dandy-Walker cyst, 10
Dawn phenomena, 103
Deferoxamine, 110
Dehydration, 19
assessment, 19
with gastroenteritis, 152–153
hypernatremic, 19
mild, 19
moderate, 19
severe, 19
signs and symptoms, 19
Delayed puberty, with myotonic dystrophy, 135
Delivery, must-know topics, 301
Demyelinating polyneuropathy, 136
Dennie lines, 188
Dental care, 195
Denver Developmental Screening Test, 14
Dermatitis, 187–189
atopic, 187–188
chronic, 187–188
contact, 188
diaper, 188
candidal, 192–193
seborrheic, 188
Development
abnormal, 14–16
must-know topics, 297–299
normal, 10
Developmental disability, 14–16
Developmental history, 2
Developmental milestones, 11, 11t–13t
Developmental screening tests, 14
Dextrose, in parenteral solutions, 18
Diabetes insipidus, 19, 100, 119
nephrogenic, 100
Diabetes mellitus
complications, long-term, 103
honeymoon period, 102–103
insulin-dependent (IDDM), 19
maternal, 28
with myotonic dystrophy, 135
Diabetic ketoacidosis (DKA), 102–103
treatment, 103
Diaper dermatitis, 188
candidal, 192–193
Diarrhea, 21
with appendicitis, 152
in disaccharidase deficiency, 154
with neuroblastoma, 120
in viral gastroenteritis, 153
Diencephalic syndrome, 120
Dietary history, 2
Diethylstilbestrol, maternal use, effect on fetus and neonate, 30t
Differential diagnosis, generating, 3–4
DiGeorge anomaly, 97, 168
Diphtheria, 76–78
immunization, 198, 199t–200t
Diphtheria toxoid vaccine, 78
Disaccharidase deficiency, 154
Disseminated intravascular coagulation (DIC), 113
Down syndrome. See Trisomy 21

Draw-a-man test, 14
Drowning, 198
Drugs, in breast milk, 22
DTaP vaccine
characteristics, 200t
recommended schedule for, 199t
DTP vaccine
characteristics, 200t
recommended schedule for, 199t
Duchenne muscular dystrophy, 134–135
Ductus arteriosus, 41
closure, failure of, 48
Dumbbell tumors, 120
Duodenal atresia, 32
with trisomy 21, 85
Dystonia musculorum deformans, 131
Dystonias, 131
Dystrophin, 134–135

Eagle-Barrett syndrome, 159
Ear(s)
disorders, 73–74
pain, exacerbated by pressure on tragus, 74
Early antigen, 69
Ebstein anomaly, 141
EBV nuclear antigens (EBNA), 69
Eclampsia, 29
Ectopic testes, 158
Eczema herpeticum, 187
Eisenmenger syndrome, 141–142
Electroencephalogram (EEG), 128
Electrolytes, 18–19
Electronic fetal monitoring, 33
Emesis, for poisoning, 196
Emphysema
congenital lobar, 75
early onset, 82
Empyema, with staphylococcal pneumonia, 79
Encephalitis, 133
Encephalocele, 126
Endocardial cushion defects, 143
with trisomy 21, 85
Endocarditis
bacterial
in Marfan's syndrome, 180
prophylaxis, 143
with ventricular septal defect, 142
Endocrine diseases (endocrinopathies), 135
and mental retardation, 15t
must-know topics, 302–303
Endotracheal tube, surfactant administration via, 45–46
Energy deficiency, 9
*Enterobius vermicularis*, 70
Enterocolitis, 52–53
Enterovirus 70, 69
Enteroviruses
conjunctivitis, 184–185
encephalitis, 133
nonpolio, 69
syndromes caused by, 69
Enzyme deficiencies, 154
Eosinophilic granuloma, 123
Epidemic keratoconjunctivitis, 185
Epiglottitis, 76–77
Epilepsy, 128
benign partial, with centrotemporal spikes, 129
idiopathic, 130
myoclonic
of childhood, 130
juvenile, 130
Epstein-Barr virus (EBV), 69
Epstein pearls, 40
Erb-Duchenne paralysis, 34
Erikson, Erik, stages of psychosocial development, 13
Erysipelas, 190
Erythema chronicum migrans, 66
Erythema infectiosum, 68–69
Erythema multiforme, 188–189
Erythema toxicum, 39

# INDEX

*Erythroblastosis fetalis*, 50
Erythrocyte sedimentation rate, elevated, with Kawasaki disease, 146
Erythromycin, for pertussis, 78
*Escherichia coli*
    gastroenteritis, 153
    meningitis, 132
    neonatal sepsis, 55–56
    osteomyelitis, 178
    urinary tract infection, 160
Esophageal atresia, 53
Esophageal foreign bodies, 149
Esophageal pH, monitoring, with gastroesophageal reflux, 150
Esophagitis, chronic, 150
Ethanol, maternal use, effect on fetus and neonate, 30*t*
Evans syndrome, 111
Ewing's sarcoma, 122
Exchange transfusion, 51
Exercise, and asthma, 80
Exercise-induced proteinuria, 161
Extensor spasms, 129
External auditory canal, neonatal, 40
Extracellular fluid, in newborn, 42
Extracellular water, 17
Extracorporeal membrane oxygenation (ECMO), 48
Eye(s), infections, 184–186

Fabry disease, 92–93
Factor VIII
    antibodies to, 114
    concentrates, 114
    deficiency, 113–114
    replacement, 114
Factor II, decreased, 25
Factor VII, decreased, 25
Factor IX deficiency, 114–115
Failure to thrive, 9
    with inborn errors of metabolism, 89
    nonorganic, 9
Familial dysautonomia, 137
Family history, 2
Fanconi pancytopenia, 112, 117
Fanconi syndrome, 90, 166
Fasciculation, in tongue, 135
Febrile seizures, 130
Femoral head
    avascular necrosis, 176–177
    fracture through growth plate, 176–177
Fetal alcohol syndrome, 30–31
Fetal assessment, 31–32
Fetal circulation, 41
Fetal distress, 33
Fetal-fetal transfusion, 29
Fetal heart rate, 33
Fetal hemoglobin, hereditary persistence of, 109
Fetal lung fluid, delayed resorption of, 46
Fetal lung maturity, assessment, 31–32
Fetoscopy, 31
Fetus
    head circumference, intrauterine growth curves for, 37
    intrauterine cocaine exposure, 30
    length, intrauterine growth curves for, 37
    weight, intrauterine growth curves for, 37
Fever, 21, 61, 130
    in acute osteomyelitis, 178
    in bacterial infection, 61
    in immunosuppressed patients, 172
    with periorbital cellulitis, 185
    and petechiae, 63
    proteinuria with, 161
    in septic arthritis, 179
    with urinary tract infection, 160
    and viral infections, 61
Fever syndromes, in children, 62*t*
Fifth disease, 68–69
Fine motor development, 11, 12*t*
Fluid and electrolyte replacement, in diabetic ketoacidosis, 103
Fluoride, supplementation, 22

Folic acid
    deficiency, 26, 107
    supplementation, in pregnancy, 31, 125
Fontanelle(s), 40
    anterior, 40
    bulging, 24, 40
    closure, 40
        delayed, 24–25
    posterior, 40
Foramen ovale, 41
Formal operational stage, 14
Fracture(s), 179
    bucket handle, 181
    clavicular, during delivery, 34
    femoral, through growth plate, 176–177
    greenstick, 179
    healing, 34
Fragile X syndrome, 87–88
Free T3, elevation, with hyperthyroidism, 97
Free T4, elevation, with hyperthyroidism, 97
Freud, Sigmund, theory of psychosocial development, 11–12
Friedreich's ataxia, 88, 131
Fructose intolerance, hereditary, 93, 166
Full-term infant, 35
Fungal infection(s)
    in immunosuppressed patients, 172
    of skin, 192–193

Galactose, removal from diet, 93
Galactosemia, 23, 166
    cataracts due to, 184
    classic, 93
Galactose-1-phosphate uridyltransferase deficiency, 93
Gamma globulin, with Kawasaki disease, 146
*Gardnerella vaginalis* vaginosis, 59
Gastroenteritis
    acute, 152–153
    bacterial, 153
    dehydration secondary to, therapy for, 19
    viral, 153
Gastroesophageal reflux, 149–150
    and asthma, 80
Gastrointestinal disorders, 149–156
    must-know topics, 304–305
    neonatal, 52–54
Gastrointestinal tract
    cobblestone appearance, 155
    neonatal, 42
Gaucher disease, 92
Genetic anticipation, 88
Genetic disorders, 85–88
    multifactorial, 88
    must-know topics, 303
Genital stage, 12
Genitourinary disorders, 157–160
    congenital anomalies, 157–159
    must-know topics, 305
Germinal matrix, 54
Gestational age, 34–36
    assessment, 34–35, 36f
GFR. *See* Glomerular filtration rate
*Giardia lamblia* gastroenteritis, 153
Gilles de la Tourette syndrome, 131
Gingivostomatitis, acute herpetic, 191
Glaucoma, 184
Gliadin intolerance, 154
Gliomas
    brain-stem, 119
    supratentorial, 119
Globin chain synthesis, genetic defects of, 109
Glomerular filtration rate
    neonatal, 42
    in renal failure, 165
Glomerulonephritis
    membranoproliferative, 162, 164
    poststreptococcal, 76, 162
Glucose, disorders, 20
Glucose-6-phosphatase (G6P) deficiency, 94
Glucose-6-phosphate dehydrogenase (G6PD) deficiency, 108–109, 111–112
    protective effect against malaria, 71

Glucosuria, 102, 166
Gluten-sensitive enteropathy, 154
Glycogen storage disease, 20, 94
    type Ia, 94
    type II, 94
    type V, 94
    type VI, 94
Glycosylated hemoglobin, 102
Goiter, 97
Gonadoblastomas, 87
Gonococcal arthritis, 179
Goodenough draw-a-man test, 14
Gower's sign, 135
Granuloma, umbilical, 54
Grasp reflex, 43
Graves' disease, 97
Greenstick fracture, 179
Gross motor development, 11, 11*t*
Growth
    abnormal patterns, 9–10
    definition, 5
    in embryonic and fetal period, 5
    must-know topics, 297–299
    normal, 5–9
    patterns, 6–7
    in puberty, 5, 7
    rate, 5
    standards, 6
Growth charts, 6–7
Growth hormone
    deficiency, 10, 99–100
    recombinant, therapy with, 99–100
Growth retardation, 9
    with hypopituitarism, 99–100
Guillain-Barré syndrome, 136

*Haemophilus influenzae*
    acute purulent conjunctivitis, 184–185
    infection, in X-linked agammaglobulinemia, 167
    meningitis, 132
    and orbital cellulitis, 186
    otitis media, 73
    sinusitis, 74
    type b
        acute osteomyelitis, 178
        bacteremia, 62
        cellulitis, 190
        conjugate vaccine, 199*t*, 200*t*, 201
        epiglottitis, 77
        infection, in IgG subclass deficiencies, 168
        meningitis, 132
        periorbital cellulitis, 185
        pneumonia, 79
        septic arthritis, 179
        vaccine, 132
Hand and foot syndrome, with sickle cell anemia, 108
Hand-foot-mouth syndrome, 69
Hand-Schüller-Christian disease, 123
Hashimoto thyroiditis, 97
Head
    circumference, 6
        intrauterine growth curves for, 37
        measurement, 3
        normal, 6
    examination of, 3
    injuries, 134
        complications, 134
        and mental retardation, 15*t*
    neonatal, 40
Hearing loss
    conductive, 73
    sensorineural, 133
    with Turner syndrome, 86
Heart
    disease, congenital. *See* Congenital heart disease
    failure. *See also* Congestive heart failure
        signs and symptoms, 142
    malformations, in infant of diabetic mother, 28

# INDEX

Heart block
  congenital, 145
    complete, with neonatal lupus erythematosus, 29, 145
    with diphtheria, 77–78
Heart murmur(s)
  with coarctation, 144
  functional, 3
  innocent, 3
  transient neonatal, 41
  with ventricular septal defect, 142
Heart rate, in children, age-specific, 4t
Height, 6
  estimation, 6
  measurement, 3
Hemangiomas, 189–190
  capillary, 39, 189–190
  cavernous, 190
Hemarthroses, with hemophilia, 114
Hematocrit, normal values in children, 106t
Hematologic disorders, 105–123
  must-know topics, 303
  neonatal, 48
Hematologic values, normal, 106t
Hematopoietic system, neonatal, 41
Hematuria, 161
  glomerular and nonglomerular, differentiation, 161t
Hemoglobin (Hg), normal values in children, 106t
Hemoglobin Bart's, 110
Hemoglobin F, 41
Hemoglobin H disease, 110
Hemoglobin S, 108–109
  with beta and alpha thalassemia, 109
  in combination with other hemoglobinopathies, 109
  and hemoglobin C, 109
Hemolytic anemia, 50, 107–112
  autoimmune, 111
  chronic, 108–109
  in erythroblastosis fetalis, 50
Hemolytic disease of the newborn, 50–51
Hemolytic-uremic syndrome, 163
Hemophilia, 113–115
  A, 113–114
  B, 114–115
Hemorrhagic disease of the newborn, 51
Henoch-Schönlein purpura, 146–147, 151, 163
Hepatic disorders, neonatal, 48
Hepatitis, 70
Hepatitis A virus, 70
Hepatitis B immune globulin, 59
Hepatitis B virus, 70
  e antigen, 58–59
  maternal screening during pregnancy for, 57
  perinatal transmission, 58–59
  vaccine, 59, 201
    characteristics, 200t
    recommended schedule for, 199t
Hepatitis E virus, 70
Hepatobiliary disease, neonatal, 48–49
Hepatocellular carcinoma, with chronic hepatitis B virus, 70
Hepatolenticular degeneration, 26
Hereditary fructose intolerance, 93, 166
Hereditary nephritis, 161
Hernia(s)
  hiatal, 150
  incarcerated, 156, 158
  inguinal
    in girls, 155
    hydrocele with, 157
    incarceration, undescended testes and, 158
    indirect, 155–158
  umbilical, 54
Herniorrhaphy, 156
Heroin, maternal use, effect on fetus and neonate, 29–30, 30t
Herpangina, 69
Herpes encephalitis, 133
Herpes simplex virus
  erythema multiforme and, 188–189
  infection, 191
  keratoconjunctivitis, 185
  perinatal infection, 57
Herpes zoster, 192
Herpetic gingivostomatitis, acute, 191
β-Hexosaminidase A deficiency, 92
Hiatal hernia, 150
Hip
  congenital dislocation of, 176
  dislocatable, 176
  dislocated, 176
  subluxation, 176
Hirschsprung's disease, 52–53
Histiocytosis
  class I, 123
  class II, 123
  class III, 123
Histiocytosis syndromes, 123
Histiocytosis X, 123
History
  developmental, 2
  dietary, 2
  past medical, 2
  of pediatrics, 1–2
  of present illness, 1–2
HIV
  antibody, placental transfer, 170
  infection, 111, 113, 170–171
    disseminated molluscum contagiosum with, 191
    gastroenteritis in, 153
    in hemophiliacs, 114–115
    and immunization, 171
    maternal, perinatal outcome, 58
    and non-Hodgkin's lymphoma, 117
    organ involvement, 170
    perinatally acquired, 170
    *Pneumocystis carinii* pneumonia in, 170–171
    risk factors for, 170
    seborrhea with, 188
  maternal screening during pregnancy for, 57
  transmission, 170
    in breast-feeding, 22
    maternal-infant, prevention, 171
    perinatal, 58
  type 1, 170–171
HIV encephalopathy, 171
Hodgkin's disease, 117
  histologic subtypes, 117
  prognosis, 117
  treatment, 117
Homocystinuria, 90–91
Homovanillic acid (HVA), urinary, 120–121
Homozygous beta⁺-thalassemia, 110
Homozygous beta⁰-thalassemia, 110
Honey, contaminated, and botulism, 137
Hookworm infection, 70
Hormone deficiencies, 20
Human immunodeficiency virus. *See* HIV
Human papillomavirus. *See* Papillomavirus
Humoral immune deficiencies, 167
Hunter syndrome (MPS II), 95
Huntington's disease, 88
Hurler syndrome (MPS IH), 95
HUS. *See* Hemolytic-uremic syndrome
Hutchinson teeth, 57
Hyaline membrane disease, 45
Hydrocarbon pneumonia, 80
Hydroceles, 157
Hydrocephalus, 10, 126
  nonobstructive or communicating, 10
  obstructive, 10
Hydronephrosis, 159–160
Hydrops fetalis, 50, 110
11β-Hydroxylase deficiency, 98
21-Hydroxylase deficiency, 98
  simple virilizing form, 99
Hyperaldosteronism, 21
Hyperammonemia, with inborn errors of metabolism, 89
Hyperbilirubinemia, 29
  conjugated, 49
  in infant of diabetic mother, 28
  neonatal, treatment, 51
  physiologic, 49–50
  unconjugated, 49t
Hypercalcemia, 26, 100
Hypercalciuria, idiopathic, 161
Hyperglycemia, 20, 102
Hyperinsulinism, 20
Hyperkalemia, 19–20
Hypermagnesemia, 26
Hypernatremia, 19
Hypersplenism, with thalassemia, 110
Hypervitaminosis A, 24
Hypervitaminosis D, 25
Hypoalbuminemia
  in nephrotic syndrome, 163
Hypocalcemia, 26
  with hypoparathyroidism, 98
  in infant of diabetic mother, 28
  signs and symptoms, 98
Hypogammaglobulinemia, with myotonic dystrophy, 135
Hypoglycemia, 20
  causes, 20
  in diabetes, 102
  with inborn errors of metabolism, 89
  neonatal, 28
  risk factors for, 20
  sequelae, 20
Hypokalemia, 20
Hypomagnesemia, 26
Hyponatremia, 19
Hypoparathyroidism, 97–98
Hypopituitarism, 99–100
Hypoplastic left heart syndrome, 141
Hypospadias, 157
Hypothyroidism
  congenital, 40, 96
  with myotonic dystrophy, 135
  neonatal screening for, 89
Hypoventilation, with metabolic alkalosis, 21
Hypoxemia, 21
  fetal, 33
Hypoxia
  fetal, 33
  and mental retardation, 15t
Hypsarrhythmia, 129

Identity versus role confusion, 13
Idiopathic scoliosis, 177–178
Idiopathic thrombocytopenic purpura (ITP), 113
IgA deficiency, 167–168
IgA nephropathy, 162–163
IgG antibodies, maternal, 42, 50
IgG subclass deficiencies, 167–168
Immunization(s), 198–201
  contraindications to, 200–201, 201t
  HIV-infected (AIDS) patients and, 171
  recommended schedule for, 199t
  varicella, 192
Immunization history, 2
Immunodeficiencies
  acquired, 170–172
  with myotonic dystrophy, 135
  primary, 167–169
  white blood cell, 169
Immunoglobulin. *See also* IgA; IgG
  for immunocompromised children exposed to measles, 67
Immunologic disorders, 167–174
  must-know topics, 307–308
Immunologic system, neonatal, 42
Immunosuppression, acquired, 171–172
Imperforate anus, 42
  with trisomy 21, 85
Impetigo, 190
Inborn errors of metabolism, 10, 89
  and mental retardation, 15t
Indirect inguinal hernia, 155–158
Indomethacin, for patent ductus arteriosus (PDA), 48
Industry versus inferiority, 13

# INDEX

Infant(s)
  of diabetic mothers, 28, 35
  urinary tract infection in, 160
Infant feeding, 22–23
Infant formulas
  commercially prepared, 22–23
  milk-based, 23
  protein hydrolysate, 23
  soy, 23
  soy-based, 23
Infantile spasms, 129
  cryptogenic, 129
Infant mortality rate, 27
Infection(s)
  of auditory canal, 74
  bacterial, 61, 62t, 63
    in chronic granulomatous disease, 169
    with complement component deficiencies, 169
    fever in, 61
    in immunosuppressed patients, 172
    with sickle cell anemia, 108
    of skin, 190–191
  of bones, 178–179
  central nervous system, 131–134
    and mental retardation, 15t
  congenital, 56–60
  of eye, 184–186
  fungal
    in immunosuppressed patients, 172
    of skin, 192–193
  of joints, 178–179
  in neonate, 42
  opportunistic, 167
  pyogenic, 167
  sexually transmitted, 181–182
  umbilical, 53–54
  urinary tract, 55, 159–160
  viral, of skin, 191–192
Infectious croup, 76
Infectious diseases, 61–71
  must-know topics, 300–301
  pediatric, general principles of, 61
Infectious mononucleosis, 69
Infertility, undescended testes and, 158
Inflammatory bowel disease, 10
Influenza vaccine, 201
  characteristics, 200t
Inguinal hernia
  in girls, 155
  hydrocele with, 157
  incarceration, undescended testes and, 158
  indirect, 155–158
  testes found in girl with, 101
Initiative versus guilt, 13
Insulin
  antibodies to, 103
  in treatment of diabetes mellitus, 102–103
Insulin-dependent diabetes mellitus (IDDM) (type I diabetes), 102
Intestinal malrotation, 151
Intestinal obstruction
  due to meconium plug, 52, 81
  in neonates, 52–53
Intestinal volvulus, 151
Intracellular fluid, 17
Intracranial hemorrhage, with intrauterine cocaine exposure, 30
Intracranial pressure, increased, with ependymomas, 119
Intraocular pressure, elevation, 184
Intrauterine growth retardation, 36
  causes, 35
  with intrauterine cocaine exposure, 30
Intraventricular hemorrhage, 54
Intrinsic factor, absence of, 107
Intussusception, 151–152
  with Meckel's diverticulum, 151
Ipecac, 196
Iron
  absorption, 106
  in breast milk, 106
  in cow's milk, 106
  requirements, 17t
    during adolescence, 106
    supplementation, 22, 106
    in pregnancy, 31
Iron deficiency anemia, 105–107
  with hookworm infection, 71
  laboratory findings in, 107
  in premature infants, 106
  treatment, 107
Isoimmune hemolysis, 50–51
Isoniazid
  hepatitis due to, 65
  prophylaxis, 64
  for pulmonary tuberculosis, 65
Isotretinoin, maternal use, effect on fetus and neonate, 30t

Jaundice
  breast-milk, 50
  in hemolytic disease of the newborn, 50
  neonatal, 43, 48–49
    causes of, 49t
    with congenital hypothyroidism, 96
  physiologic, 49–50
  with urinary tract infection, 160
Joint infections, 178–179
JRA. See Juvenile rheumatoid arthritis
Juvenile rheumatoid arthritis, 173–174
  pauciarticular type I, 173–174, 174t
  polyarticular, 174, 174t
  rheumatoid factor-negative, 174
  rheumatoid factor-positive, 174
  systemic onset, 174, 174t

Kartagener syndrome, 82
Kasabach-Merritt syndrome, 113, 190
Kawasaki disease, 145–146
Keratoconjunctivitis, epidemic, 185
Kerion, 193
Kernicterus, 29, 51
Kernig signs, 132
Ketoacidosis, 21. See also Diabetic ketoacidosis
Ketonuria, with inborn errors of metabolism, 89
Kidney(s)
  disease, 160–166
    chronic, 100
    must-know topics, 305
    polycystic, 161–162
    failure. See Renal failure
    in Henoch-Schönlein purpura, 146–147
    hereditary cystic disease, 161–162
Klinefelter syndrome, 87
Klippel-Feil syndrome, 175
Klippel-Trenaunay-Weber syndrome, 190
Klumpke paralysis, 34
Koplik spots, 67
Korotkoff sound, 3
Krabbe disease, 93
Kugelberg-Welander disease, 136
Kussmaul respirations, 103
Kwashiorkor, 9

Labor
  must-know topics, 299
  precipitous, 32
  premature, 32–33
  risk factors during, 32
Lactase deficiency, 23, 154
Lactic acidosis, 21
Langerhans' cell histiocytosis, 99–100, 123
  seborrhea with, 188
Language development, 11, 12t
Large-for-gestational age (SGA) infants, 35
Laryngomalacia, 74
Laryngotracheobronchitis, 76–77
Latency stage, 12
Laurence-Moon-Biedl syndrome, 9
Lead poisoning, 196–197
Left coronary artery, anomalous origin, 144–145
Legg-Calve-Perthes disease, 177
Leiner disease, 188
Length
  birth (neonatal), 6
  fetal, intrauterine growth curves for, 37
Lennox-Gastaut syndrome, 130
Lesch-Nyhan syndrome, 96, 164
Leterrer-Siwe disease, 123
Leukemia(s), 113, 115–117
  immunodeficiency in, 172
Leukocytosis
  in acute osteomyelitis, 178
  with appendicitis, 152
  with periorbital cellulitis, 185
Leukokoria, with retinoblastoma, 123
Lice, 193
LIP. See Lymphoid interstitial pneumonitis
Lisch nodules, 127
Listeria monocytogenes, neonatal sepsis, 55
Littre hernia, 151
Liver
  disease, 20
  hereditary cystic disease, 161–162
  neonatal, 43
Low-birth-weight infants, 35
  clinical management of, 27
  survival of, 27
Lowe syndrome, 166
Lumbosacral agenesis, in infant of diabetic mother, 28
Lung, obstructive disease of, 21
Lyme disease, 65–66
  meningitis, 133
Lymphocytic thyroiditis, 97
Lymphoid interstitial pneumonitis, in HIV-infected (AIDS) patients, 171
Lymphoma(s), 111, 113, 115, 117–118

Macrocephaly, in absence of hydrocephalus, 10
Magnesium, imbalances, 26
Magnesium sulfate
  maternal use, effect on fetus and neonate, 30t
  therapy, for preeclampsia, 52
Maintenance hydration, 19
Malaria, 71
  cerebral, 71
  congenital, 71
Malassezia furfur, 193
Malignancy, 105–123
  must-know topics, 303
Malrotation, 151
Mantoux skin test, positive, 64, 65t
Maple syrup urine disease (MSUD), 91
Marasmic kwashiorkor, 9
Marasmus, 9
Marfan's syndrome, 180
Maroteaux-Lamy syndrome (MPS VI), 95
Mastoiditis, 73–74
Maternal age, extremes of, 28
McArdle syndrome, 94
McCune-Albright syndrome, 101
Mean corpuscular hemoglobin concentration (MCHC), normal values, 106t
Mean corpuscular volume (MCV), normal values, 106t
Measles, 67
  conjunctivitis, 184–185
  encephalitis, 133
  immunization, 67, 198
  recommended schedule for, 199t
Mechanical ventilation, 45–46
Meckel's diverticulum, 150–151
Meconium, 42
Meconium aspiration syndrome, 46–47
Meconium ileus, 52, 81
Meconium peritonitis, 52
Meconium staining, of amniotic fluid, 33, 46
Medulloblastomas, 118
Megaloblastic anemias, 26, 107
Meiosis, nondisjunction during, 85, 87
Membranoproliferative glomerulonephritis, 162, 164
Menarche, age at, 8
Meningitis, 55, 62, 131–133
  aseptic, 133
  bacterial, 131–132
    chemoprophylaxis, 133

# INDEX

diagnosis, 132
  short-term complications, 132–133
  clinical presentation, 132
  long-term sequelae, 133
  tuberculous, 64
  viral, 133
Meningocele, 126
Meningococcal bacteremia, 62
Meningococcal infections, 132
Meningococcemia, 63
Meningococci and W-135 vaccine, characteristics, 200t
Meningoencephalitis, mumps, 68
Mental retardation, 14–16
  in boys, 87
  causes, 15t, 16
  educable, 16
  severely retarded, 16
  trainable, 16
Metabolic acidosis, 20–21
  with inborn errors of metabolism, 89
  with increased anion gap, 21
  with normal anion gap, 21
Metabolic alkalosis, 21
Metabolic disorders, must-know topics, 302–303
Metabolic rate
  and body weight, 18
  and water requirements, 18
Metabolism, 17–26
  must-know topics, 298
Metatarsus adductus, 175
Methadone, maternal use, effect on fetus and neonate, 29–30, 30t
Methimazole, for hyperthyroidism, 97
Methionine, dietary restriction of, 91
Metoclopramide, for gastroesophageal reflux, 150
Microcephaly, 10
  acquired, 10
  with chromosomal abnormalities, 10
  genetic, 10
Middle ear, examination of, 3
Milia, 39
Miliaria, 39
Milk
  human, advantages of, 22
  intolerance, 23, 154
  IgE mediated, 23
Mineral imbalances, 26
Mineral requirements, 17t
Minimal change disease, 163–164
Mitochondrial encephalomyelopathies, 88
Mitral insufficiency, 143
Mixed gonadal dysgenesis, 87
MMR vaccine
  characteristics, 200t
  recommended schedule for, 199t
Molars, permanent, eruption, 7
Molluscum contagiosum, 191
Mongolian spots, 39
*Moraxella catarrhalis*
  otitis media, 73
  sinusitis, 74
Morgan folds, 188
Moro reflex, 43
Morquio syndrome (MPS IV), 95
Movement disorders, 131
MPGN. *See* Membranoproliferative glomerulonephritis
Mucocutaneous lymph node syndrome, 145–146
Mucopolysaccharidoses, 94–96
  cataracts due to, 184
Multifactorial genetic defects, 88
Multiple pregnancies, 29
Mumps, 67–68
  asymptomatic, 68
  encephalitis, 133
  immunization, 198
  recommended schedule for, 199t
Muscular dystrophies, 134–135
Myasthenia gravis, 137
*Mycobacterium avium* complex infection, in HIV-infected (AIDS) patients, 171

*Mycoplasma hominis* vaginosis, 59
*Mycoplasma pneumoniae*, 79
Myelination, 43
Myelomeningoceles, 125–126
Myocarditis, 69
  with diphtheria, 77–78
Myopathies, genetic progressive, 134
Myotonic dystrophy, 88, 135

Nasal flaring, 3
Nasopharyngeal colonization, 132
Nasopharyngitis, acute, 75
*Necator americanus*, 71
Neck, examination of, 3
Necrotizing enterocolitis (NEC), 52, 55
Neglect, 181–182
*Neisseria gonorrhoeae*, conjunctivitis, 56
*Neisseria meningitidis*
  bacteremia, 62
  meningitis, 132
Nematode infection, 70–71
Neonatal lupus erythematosus, 28–29, 145
Neonatal mortality, rate, 27
  and birth rate, 35
Neonatal ocular prophylaxis, 56
Neonatal sepsis, 32
  group B streptococcus, 31
  signs and symptoms, 55
  treatment of, 55–56
Nephritis, hereditary, 161
Nephroblastoma, 121
Nephrosis, 163–164
Nephrotic syndrome, 163
Neural tube defects, 125
  and congenital dislocation of hip, 176
  prevention, 31
Neuroblastoma, 115, 120–121
  diagnosis, 120
  presenting symptoms, 120
  spontaneous regression in early infancy, 120
  treatment, 120
Neurocutaneous syndromes, 126–127
Neurofibromas, 127
Neurofibromatosis, 126–127
  type 1, 126–127
  type 2, 127
Neurogenic bladder, 160
Neuroimaging, 128
Neurological diseases, and mental retardation, 15t
Neuromuscular disorders, 21, 134–137
Neutropenia, 172
Newborn
  anatomy and physiology, 39–43
  classification, 34–37
  diseases of, 45–60
    must-know topics, 300
  head circumference, 6
  infection in
    acquired, 55
    congenital, 56–60
  length, 6
  normal, 39–43
    must-know topics, 299–300
  transient hyperammonemia of, 91
  transient myasthenia gravis, 137
  transient tachypnea of, 46
  weight, 5
Niacin deficiency, 25
Niemann-Pick disease, 92
Night blindness, 24
Nikolsky sign, 191
Nipples, supernumerary, 187
Nitroblue tetrazolium test, 169
Non-Hodgkin's lymphoma (NHL), 117–118
Nonsteroidal anti-inflammatory drugs, for juvenile rheumatoid arthritis, 174
Noonan syndrome, 86–87
Normal saline, 18
Norwalk virus, gastroenteritis, 153
Nuchal rigidity, 132
Nutrition, 17–26
  must-know topics, 298
  requirements, for infants and children, 17t

Obesity, 9
Object concept, 14
Obstructive hydrocephalus
  with cerebellar astrocytomas, 119
  with ependymomas, 119
Obstructive uropathy, 159
Occult bacteremia, 62t, 62–63
Oculocerebral syndrome, 166
Oligohydramnios, 32, 160–161
  and congenital dislocation of hip, 176
  with urinary tract obstruction, 159
Omphalocele, 54
Omphalomesenteric duct, 151
Ophthalmologic disorders, 183–186
  congenital anomalies, 183–184
  must-know topics, 306
Opportunistic infections, 167
Opsoclonus-myoclonus, with neuroblastoma, 120
Oral fluid therapy, for dehydration, 19
Oral stage, 11–12
Orbital cellulitis, 74, 185–186
Orchitis, mumps, 68
Organic acidemias, 91
Organ transplant recipients, immunosuppression in, 172
Ornithine transcarbamylase (OTC) deficiency, 91
Orotic aciduria, 96
Orthopedic disorders, 175–180
  congenital anomalies, 175–178
  must-know topics, 306
Orthopedic trauma, 179–180
Orthostatic proteinuria, 161
Ortolani maneuver, 176
Osgood-Schlatter disease, 177
Osler-Weber-Rendu disease, 190
Osmolality, 17
Osmotic fragility test, 111
Ossification centers, 7
Osteogenesis imperfecta, 180
Osteogenic sarcoma, 122–123
Osteomyelitis, 55, 62
  acute, 178–179
  with sickle cell anemia, 108
Ostium primum defects, 142–143
Ostium secundum defects, 142
Otitis-conjunctivitis syndrome, 184
Otitis media, 75
  acute, 73–74
    complications, 73
  bacterial, 73–74
  external, 74
  with residual or persistent effusion, 73
  with Turner syndrome, 86
  in X-linked agammaglobulinemia, 167

Palmar crease, 85
Pancarditis, with rheumatic fever, 172
Pancreas, disorders of, 102–103
Pancreatic enzymes, oral, in management of cystic fibrosis, 82
Pancreatic islet cells, autoimmune destruction of, 102
Pancytopenia, 112
Papilledema, 118
Papillomavirus, 191
  transmission to newborns, 59
Parainfluenza virus, 77
  bronchiolitis, 78
  pneumonia, 79
Paralytic poliomyelitis, 136
Paraphimosis, 157
Parasitic infestations, 70–71
  of skin, 193
Parathyroid glands, aplasia or hypoplasia, 97
Parenteral solutions, 18
Parinaud syndrome, 120
Parotid gland swelling, 67–68
Paroxysmal atrial tachycardia (PAT), 145
Paroxysmal hypercyanotic attacks, 140
Parvovirus B19 infection, 68–69
  maternal, fetal effects, 59
  with sickle cell anemia, 109
  with spherocytosis, 111

Pastia lines, 64
Past medical history, 2
Patent ductus arteriosus (PDA), 48
　in premature infant, 48
　in term infant, 48
Pediatrics, historical perspective on, 1–2
Pediculosis capitis, 193
Pediculosis pubis, 193
Pellagra, 25
Penicillin
　prophylactic, 111
　for rheumatic fever, 173
　for streptococcal pharyngitis, 76
Pentamidine, for *Pneumocystis carinii* pneumonia, 171
Perianal streptococcal cellulitis, 190
Periodontal disease, 195
Periorbital cellulitis, 185, 190
Peritonsillar abscess, 76
Periumbilical pain, with appendicitis, 152
Periventricular leukomalacia, 54
Pernicious anemia, juvenile, 107
Peroneal muscular atrophy, 136–137
Peroxisomal disorder, 91–92
Persistent fetal circulation (PFC), 48
Pertussis, 78
　catarrhal stage, 78
　convalescent stage, 78
　immunization, 198, 199t–200t
　paroxysmal stage, 78
Petechiae, with fever, 61, 62t
pH, fetal, 33
Phallic stage, 12
Pharyngitis, 75–76
　streptococcal, 75–76
　　epidemiology, 172
　　and rheumatic fever, 172
Phenylalanine hydroxylase deficiency, 90
Phenylketonuria (PKU)
　dietary manipulation in, 90
　genetics, 90
　neonatal screening for, 89
　pregnant women with, 90
　signs and symptoms, 90
　treatment, 90
Phenytoin, maternal use, effect on fetus and neonate, 30t
Phimosis, 157
Phosphaturia, 166
Photosensitive skin rash, with neonatal lupus erythematosus, 29
Phototherapy, 51
Physical abuse, 181
Physical examination, pediatric, 2–4
Piaget, Jean, theory of development, 13–14
Pica, 196
Pinworm, 70
Pituitary disorders, 99–100
Pityriasis alba, 189
Pityriasis rosea, 189
Placenta previa, 32
Plasma osmolality, in acute renal failure, 165t
*Plasmodium falciparum*, 71
Platelet count, normal values in children, 106t
Pleurodynia, 69
Pneumatoceles, with staphylococcal pneumonia, 79
Pneumatosis intestinalis, 52
Pneumococcal pneumonia, 79
Pneumococcal vaccine, 201
　characteristics, 200t
Pneumococci, 63
　acute purulent conjunctivitis, 184–185
　bacteremia, 62
　infections, prevention, with sickle cell anemia, 109
　periorbital cellulitis, 185
*Pneumocystis carinii* pneumonia
　in HIV-infected (AIDS) patients, 170–171
　in severe combined immunodeficiency, 168
Pneumomediastinum, 46

Pneumonia, 55, 62, 79–80
　aspiration, with gastroesophageal reflux, 149–150
　bacterial, 79
　*Chlamydia trachomatis*, 80
　*Haemophilus influenzae* type b, 79
　hydrocarbon, 80
　mycoplasmal, 79
　pneumococcal, 79
　staphylococcal, 79
　viral, 79
　in X-linked agammaglobulinemia, 167
Pneumonitis
　chlamydia, 56
　lymphoid interstitial, in HIV-infected (AIDS) patients, 171
Pneumothorax, 46
Poisoning, 196–197
　carbon monoxide, 197
　lead, 196–97
　prevention, 197
Poliomyelitis, 136, 198
Polio vaccine
　inactivated, characteristics, 200t
　oral, characteristics, 200t
　recommended schedule for, 199t
Polycystic kidney disease, 161–162
Polycythemia
　with cyanotic congenital heart disease, 141
　in infant of diabetic mother, 28
Polyhydramnios, 32
Polyneuropathy, 136
Pompe disease, 94
Posterior urethral valves, 159
Postinflammatory pigmentary changes, 188
Postterm infant, 35
Posture, of normal full-term infant, 39
Potassium
　deficiency, 100
　disorders, 19–20
　requirements, 18
Potter syndrome, 160–161
　with urinary tract obstruction, 159
Prader-Willi syndrome, 9
Preauricular sinuses and pits, 187
Precocious pseudopuberty, 100–101
Precocious puberty, 100–101
　true, 100–101
Preeclampsia, 29
Pregnancy, 28–32
　adverse outcomes, risk factors for, 28
　maternal nutrition in, 31
　maternal use of medication in, 29
　must-know topics, 299
Premature infants, 32–33
　clinical management of, 27
　retinopathy of prematurity (ROP) in, 54
Preoperational period, 14
Presacral dimples, 187
Preterm infant
　definition of, 35
　intraventricular hemorrhage, 54
Preventive pediatrics, 195–201
　must-know topics, 309
Priapism, with sickle cell anemia, 108
Primary ciliary dyskinesis, 82
Primary sexual characteristics, development, 7–8
Prolonged rupture of the membranes (PROM), 32–34
*Propionibacterium acnes*, 189
Proptosis, unilateral, with neuroblastoma, 120
Propylthiouracil
　for hyperthyroidism, 97
　maternal use, effect on fetus and neonate, 30t
Prostaglandin E, to keep ductus arteriosus open, 140–141
Protein
　deficiency, 9
　requirements, 17t
Protein-energy malnutrition (PEM), 9
Protein hydrolysate formulas, 23
Protein-polysaccharide conjugate vaccines, 201

Proteinuria
　exercise-induced, 161
　in nephrotic syndrome, 163
　orthostatic, 161
Prothrombin, decreased, 25
Prune-belly syndrome, 159
Pseudohermaphroditism, 99
*Pseudomonas*, infection, in chronic granulomatous disease, 169
*Pseudomonas aeruginosa*
　external otitis, 74
　pulmonary colonization with, 82
*Pseudomonas cepacia*, pulmonary colonization with, 82
Pseudoparalysis
　in acute osteomyelitis, 178
　in septic arthritis, 179
Pseudotumor cerebri, 24
Psychosocial assessment, 195
Psychosocial development, 11–14
Puberty, 7
　delayed, with myotonic dystrophy, 135
　disorders of, 100
　growth during, 5, 7
　onset
　　in boys, 8
　　in girls, 8
　precocious, 100–101
　true, 100–101
Pulmonary hypertension, 142–144
Pulmonary hypoplasia, 32
　with urinary tract obstruction, 159
Pulmonary sequestration, 75
Pulmonary valve stenosis, 144
Pulmonary vascular obstructive disease, with trisomy 21, 85
Pulmonic stenosis, 3
Pure red cell aplasia, congenital, 105
Pyelonephritis, 160
Pyloric stenosis, 20–21, 150
Pyloromyotomy, 150
Pyrazinamide, for pulmonary tuberculosis, 65
Pyridoxine deficiency, 26
Pyruvate kinase deficiency, 112
Pyuria, 160
　with appendicitis, 152

Radial head subluxation, 179–180
Rapid plasma reagin (RPR), 57
Rashkind procedure, 141
Rectal bleeding, with Meckel's diverticulum, 150
Red blood cell macrocytosis, with Fanconi syndrome, 112
Red blood cells, cell wall defect, 110–111
Red strawberry tongue, 64
Reed-Sternberg cell, 117
Reflexes, primitive, 43
Reflux nephropathy, 158–159
Regional enteritis, 154–155
Rehydration, 19
Renal acidosis, 165–166
Renal calculi, 164
Renal disease, 160–166
　chronic, 100
　must-know topics, 305
Renal failure
　acute, 164–165
　　in intrinsic renal disease, 164, 165t
　　prerenal causes, 164, 165t
　chronic, 10, 100
　　with reflux nephropathy, 159
　　with chronic urinary tract obstruction, 159
　glomerular filtration rate in, 165
Renal system, neonatal, 42
Renal tubular acidosis, 21, 165
　proximal, 165–166
Renal tubular dysfunction, 90
Respiratory acidosis, 21
Respiratory alkalosis, 21
Respiratory disease, 73–83
　must-know topics, 303–304
　signs of, 3

# INDEX

Respiratory distress syndrome (RDS), 41, 45–46
  clinical features, 45
  complications, 46
  incidence, 45
  in infant of diabetic mother, 28
  mortality rate, 45
  surfactant therapy, 46
  therapy for, 45
Respiratory papillomatosis, 59
Respiratory rates, in children, age-specific, 4*t*
Respiratory syncytial virus (RSV)
  bronchiolitis, 78
  pneumonia, 79
Respiratory tract
  congenital anomalies, 74–75
  infections, 75
    neonatal, 40–41
  obstruction, with diphtheria, 77–78
Reticulocyte count, normal values in children, 106*t*
Retina, vascular abnormalities of, 54
Retinoblastoma, 87, 115, 122–123
Retinopathy, in hemoglobin SC disease, 109
Retinopathy of prematurity (ROP), 54–55
Retractions, 3
Retropharyngeal abscess, 76
Review of systems, 2
Reye's syndrome, 75, 133–134
Rhabdomyosarcoma(s), 115, 121–122
Rhagades, 57
Rheumatic fever, 76, 172–173
  diagnosis, Duckett Jones criteria for, 172, 173*t*
Rheumatoid arthritis, juvenile, 173–174
Rheumatologic disorders, 172–174
  must-know topics, 305–306
Rh factor, 50
Rh incompatibility, 50
Rhinoviruses, 75
Ribavirin, for bronchiolitis, 78
Rickets, 24–25
  clinical manifestations, 24–25
  vitamin D-resistant, 90
Rickettsial infections, 66–67
*Rickettsia rickettsii*, 66
Rifampin
  prophylaxis, with *Haemophilus influenzae* type b meningitis, 132
  for pulmonary tuberculosis, 65
Riley-Day syndrome, 137
*Rochalimaea henselae*, 66
Rocky Mountain spotted fever (RMSF), 66
Rooting reflex, 43
Roseola, 68
Rotavirus gastroenteritis, 153
Round worm infection, 70–71
RTA. See Renal tubular acidosis
Rubella, 68
  congenital, 59, 68
    cataracts due to, 184
  immunization, 198, 199*t*–200*t*
  maternal screening during pregnancy for, 57
Rule of fours, 183

Saber shins, 57
Saddle nose deformity, 57
Salicylates
  for Kawasaki disease, 146
  for rheumatic fever, 173
  toxicity, 21
*Salmonella*
  acute osteomyelitis caused by, 178
  bacteremia, 62
  infection, in chronic granulomatous disease, 169
*Salmonella enteritidis*, gastroenteritis, 153
Sandhoff disease, 92
Sanfilippo syndrome (MPS III), 95
Sarcoma botryoides, 121–122
*Sarcoptes scabiei*, 193
Scabies, 193
Scarlet fever, 63–64
SCFE. *See* Slipped capital femoral epiphysis
Scheie syndrome (MPS IS), 95

School performance, 2
SCID. See Severe combined immunodeficiency
Scoliosis, 177
  idiopathic, 177–178
  in Marfan's syndrome, 180
Scurvy, 25
Seborrheic dermatitis, 188
Secondary sex characteristics, development, 7
Secretory IgA, in human milk, 22
Seizure(s)
  absence, 129
  atonic, 129
  classification of, 128*t*
  febrile, 130
  with fever, 62*t*
  generalized, 127, 129
  generalized-onset, 128*t*
  with inborn errors of metabolism, 89
  myoclonic, 129–130
  nonfebrile, 130
  partial, 127, 128*t*, 128–129
    complex, 128
    simple, 128
  recurrent, 127–128
  tonic-clonic, 129
Seizure disorders, 127–130
Selenium deficiency, 26
Seminoma, undescended testes and, 158
Sensorimotor period, 13–14
Sepsis. *See also* Infection(s)
  with burns, 198
  group B streptococcal, 55
  neonatal, 55
  in young infants, 61
Septic arthritis, 179
Septic shock, 63
Septo-optic dysplasia, 99–100
*Serratia marcescens* infection, in chronic granulomatous disease, 169
Severe combined immunodeficiency (SCID), 168
  and non-Hodgkin's lymphoma, 117
Sex chromosome abnormalities, 86–87
Sexual abuse, 181–182, 191
Sexual characteristics
  primary, development, 7–8
  secondary, development, 7
Sexually transmitted infections, 181–182
Sexual maturity ratings, 7, 8*t*
*Shigella* gastroenteritis, 153
Short bowel syndrome, 52
Short stature, 10, 119
  causes of, 10
  genetic or familial, 10
  growth hormone therapy, 100
  with mixed gonadal dysgenesis, 87
  with Turner syndrome, 86
Sickle cell anemia, 108–109
  acute chest syndrome, 108
  acute osteomyelitis with, 178
  acute splenic sequestration with, 108
  cerebral infarcts with, 108
  complications, 108–109
  genetics, 108
  painful crises, 108
  splenic infarcts with, 108
Sickle cell trait, 109
  protective effect against malaria, 71
Silver nitrate, inflammation from, 56
Single gene defects, 88–89
Sinuses
  development, 7
  disorders, 73–74
  preauricular, 187
Sinusitis, 74–75
  and asthma, 80
  and orbital cellulitis, 185–186
  in X-linked agammaglobulinemia, 167
Skeletal dysplasias, 180
Skeletal muscle, soft tissue sarcoma, 121–122
Skin
  congenital anomalies, 187
  disorders, 187–193
    must-know topics, 306

  infections
    bacterial, 190–191
    fungal, 192–193
    viral, 191–192
    in X-linked agammaglobulinemia, 167
    neonatal, 39–40
  parasitic infestations, 193
  postinflammatory pigmentary changes, 188
  vascular lesions, 189–190
Slapped-cheek appearance, 69
Slipped capital femoral epiphysis, 176–177
Small-for-gestational age (SGA) infants, 35
Small left colon syndrome, 52
  in infant of diabetic mother, 28
Social development, 11, 13*t*
Social history, 2
Sodium
  disorders, 19–20
  excessive losses of, 19
  fractional excretion, 164, 165*t*
  in parenteral solutions, 18
  requirements, 18
  urinary excretion, in acute renal failure, 165*t*
Soft tissue tumors, 115
Solid food, introduction of, 23
Somogyi phenomenon, 103
Sotos' syndrome, 10
Soy-based formulas, 23
Spasmodic croup, 76
Spherocytosis, 110–111
  congenital, 110–111
Sphingolipidoses, 92–93
Spina bifida occulta, 125
Spinal muscular atrophy (SMA), 88, 135–136
Spirochetal infection, 65–66
Splenectomy, in spherocytosis, 111
Splenomegaly, in hemoglobin sc disease, 109
Sprengel deformity, 175
Staphylococcal pneumonia, 79
Staphylococcal scalded skin syndrome, 190–191
Staphylococci, acute purulent conjunctivitis, 184–185
*Staphylococcus aureus*
  impetigo, 190
  infection, in chronic granulomatous disease, 169
  orbital cellulitis, 186
  osteomyelitis, 178–179
  periorbital cellulitis, 185
  pulmonary colonization with, 82
  retropharyngeal abscess, 76
  septic arthritis, 179
Startle reflex, 43
Status asthmaticus, 80–81
Steeple sign, 77
Stevens-Johnson syndrome, 188–189
Still's murmur, 3
Stomach, partial obstruction, 150
Strabismus, 183
Strawberry nevi, 189–190
Strawberry tongue
  with Kawasaki disease, 146
  of scarlet fever, 64
Streak gonads, 86
Streptococci
  acute purulent conjunctivitis, 184–185
  group A, 63
    nasopharyngitis, 75
    periorbital cellulitis, 185
  group A beta-hemolytic
    impetigo, 190
    nephritogenic, 162
    pharyngitis, 75–76, 172
    retropharyngeal abscess, 76
    and rheumatic fever, 172
  group B, maternal colonization with, 31
  group B beta-hemolytic
    meningitis, 132
    neonatal sepsis, 55–56
  and orbital cellulitis, 186
  skin infections, 190

*Streptococcus pneumoniae*
  bacteremia, 62
  infection
    in IgG subclass deficiencies, 167–168
    in X-linked agammaglobulinemia, 167
  meningitis, 132
  orbital cellulitis, 186
  otitis media, 73
  pneumonia, 62
  sinusitis, 74
Sturge-Weber disease, 127
Substance abuse, maternal, effect on fetus and neonate, 29–30, 30t
Sudden infant death syndrome (SIDS), 83
Sulfonamides, maternal use, effect on fetus and neonate, 30t
Supraventricular tachycardia (SVT), 145
Surfactant
  administration, 45
  deficiency, 41
  pulmonary, 40–41
Sweat chloride levels, 82
Sweating, with neuroblastoma, 120
Swimmer's ear, 74
Sydenham chorea, 131, 173
Syndactyly, 126
Syndrome of inappropriate antidiuretic hormone (SIADH), 100, 132–133
Synovitis, toxic, 177
Syphilis, 57
  congenital, 57
    cataracts due to, 184
  maternal screening during pregnancy for, 57
Systemic lupus erythematosus (SLE), 111, 113
  with complement component deficiencies, 169
  maternal, 28–29
    and congenital heart block, 29, 145

Tachycardia, fetal, 33
Tachypnea, 3
Talipes equinovarus, 176
Tanner stages, 7, 8t
Tay-Sachs disease, 92
Technetium-99m scan, with Meckel's diverticulum, 150
Teeth, 7
  deciduous, eruption, 7
Teratogenic drugs, 29
Testes
  ectopic, 158
  undescended, 158
Testicular appendix, torsion, 158
Testicular feminization syndrome, 101, 155
Testicular malignancy, undescended testes and, 158
Testicular torsion, 158
Tetanospasmin, 56
Tetanus
  immunization, 198, 199t–200t
  neonatal, 56
Tetanus immune globulin, 56
Tetanus toxoid, recommended schedule for, 199t
Tetany, of hypocalcemia, 26
Tetracycline, maternal use, effect on fetus and neonate, 30t
Tetralogy of Fallot, 139–140
  pink, 139
Thalassemia intermedia, 110
Thalassemia major, 110
Thalassemias, 109–110
Thalassemia trait, 110
Thalidomide, maternal use, effect on fetus and neonate, 30t
Theophylline
  for asthma, 81
  for premature infants with idiopathic apnea, 48
  toxicity, 81
Thiamin deficiency, 25
Throat, examination of, 3
Thrombocytopenia, 113
  autoimmune, 113
  disorders associated with, 113

Thrombocytopenia absent radius (TAR) syndrome, 113
Thrombocytosis, with Kawasaki disease, 146
Thrush, 192–193
Thymus, aplasia or hypoplasia, 97
Thyroglossal duct cysts, 187
Thyroid
  aplasia, 96
  congenital structural lesions, 96
  disorders, 96–98
  ectopic (lingual), 96
Thyroid hormone, replacement therapy, 96–97
Thyroiditis, lymphocytic, 97
Thyroid-stimulating hormone (TSH), decreased, with hyperthyroidism, 97
Thyroxine (T4), elevation, with hyperthyroidism, 97
Tics, 131
Tinea capitis, 193
Tinea corporis, 193
Tinea cruris, 193
Tinea pedis, 193
Tinea versicolor, 193
Tonic neck reflex, 43
Tonsillitis, 75
TORCH infections, 57
Total parenteral nutrition, 45
Toxemia of pregnancy, 29
Toxic epidermal necrolysis, 191
Toxic goiter, 97
Toxic megacolon, 155
Toxic synovitis, 177
Toxins, 20–21
  and mental retardation, 15t
Toxoplasmosis
  congenital, 60
    cataracts due to, 184
  serologic diagnosis, 60
Tracheoesophageal atresia, 32, 53
Tracheoesophageal fistula, 53
Tracheomalacia, 74
Trachoma, 185
Transient hyperammonemia of the newborn, 91
Transient neonatal myasthenia gravis, 137
Transient tachypnea of newborn, 46
Transient tic disorder, 131
Transposition of the great vessels, 141
Trauma
  cataracts caused by, 184
  central nervous system, 134
  orthopedic, 179–180
Triiodothyronine (T3), elevation, with hyperthyroidism, 97
Trimethoprim-sulfamethoxazole, for *Pneumocystis carinii* pneumonia, 170–171
Trinucleotide repeats, 88, 135
Trisomies, and advanced maternal age, 28
Trisomy 13, 86
  cataracts in, 184
Trisomy 18, 86
  cataracts in, 184
Trisomy 21 (Down syndrome), 32, 85, 116, 143–144
  and acute lymphoblastic leukemia, 85, 116
  cataracts in, 184
Truncus arteriosus, 141
Tuberculin skin reaction, 64
Tuberculosis
  in children, 64–65
  congenital, 64
  extrapulmonary, 64
  meningitis, 133
  miliary, 64
Tuberculous infection, children with, 64
Tuberous sclerosis, 127
Turner syndrome, 10, 86, 100
  cataracts in, 184
Turner syndrome phenotype, 86
Twin pregnancies, 29
Tympanic membrane, 40
  examination of, 3
  red, bulging, 73
Tympanostomy tubes, 73

Tyrosinemia, 166
Tyrosinemia type I, 90

Ulcerative colitis, 155
Ultrasound
  to confirm expected date of delivery, 34
  of fetus, 31–32
Umbilical artery, single, 40
Umbilical cord
  neonatal, routine care of, 40
  normal, 40
Umbilical hernias, 54
Umbilicus, 53–54
  infection, 53–54
Undescended testes, 158
Urea cycle defects, 91
Urethral obstruction, chronic, 159
Urinary tract
  anomalies, with Turner syndrome, 86
  infection, 55, 160
    with obstruction, 159–160
  obstruction, 159–160
    chronic, 159
    prenatal, 159
Urine
  culture, 160
  osmolality, in acute renal failure, 165t
  specimen collection, 160
Urolithiasis, 164
Uteroplacental insufficiency, 33

Vaccine(s)
  childhood, characteristics, 200t
  contraindications to, 200–201, 201t
    in HIV-infected (AIDS) patients, 171
  indicated, in HIV-infected (AIDS) patients, 171
Vaccine-preventable diseases, 198–201
Valproic acid, maternal use, effect on fetus and neonate, 30t
Vanillylmandelic acid (VMA), urinary, 120–121
Varicella, 192
  congenital, 58
  infection, in immunosuppressed patients, 172
  vaccine, 192, 201
    characteristics, 200t
Varicella-zoster immunoglobulin (VZIG), 58, 192
Varicella-zoster infection
  maternal, 58
  neonatal, 58
Vasculitis, 145–147
Venereal Disease Research Laboratory (VDRL), 57
Venous hums, 3
Ventricular septal defect (VSD), 139, 142
  with trisomy 21, 85
Very-low-birth weight infants, 35–36
Vesicoureteral reflux, 158–160
  primary, 158
  secondary, 158
Viral capsid antigen (VCA), antibodies against, 69
Viral gastroenteritis, 153
Viral hepatitis, 70
Viral infections, 67–70
  of skin, 191–192
Viral meningitis, 133
Viral pneumonia, 79
Virilization, 99
Visual acuity, 183
  of newborn, 40
Visual disturbances, 119–120
Vital signs
  measurement, 3
  normal, 4t
Vitamin A
  deficiency, 24
  excessive intake, during pregnancy, 31
  requirements, 17t
  treatment, for measles, 67
Vitamin B6 deficiency, 26
Vitamin B12 deficiency, 26, 107

Vitamin C
  deficiency, 25
  requirements, 17t
Vitamin D
  deficiency, 24–25
  requirements, 17t
  supplementation, 22, 24
  toxic syndrome, 25
Vitamin E
  deficiency, 25
  supplementation, 25
Vitamin K
  administration, at birth, 25, 51
  deficiency, 25, 51
Vitamin K-dependent factors, decrease in, 51
Vitamins, 23–26
  imbalances, 24–26
  water-soluble, deficiency, 25–26
Volkmann contracture, 179
Volvulus, intestinal, 151
Vomiting
  with malrotation, 151
  projectile, 150
  protracted, 21
Von Gierke disease, 94

Von-Hippel-Lindau disease, 127
Von Recklinghausen disease, 126–127
Von Willebrand disease, 115
VZIG. *See* Varicella-zoster immunoglobulin

Warts, 191
Water
  metabolism, 17–18
  requirements, 17–18
Waterhouse-Friderichsen syndrome, 98
Weight, 5–6
  estimation, 6
  fetal, intrauterine growth curves for, 37
  gain, normal, 5–6
  measurement, 3
Well-child visits, 195
Werdnig-Hoffmann disease, 135
Wharton jelly, 40
White blood cells (WBC)
  count, elevated, with ALL, 116
  immune deficiencies, 169
  normal values in children, 106t
White strawberry tongue, of scarlet fever, 64
Whooping cough, 78
Williams syndrome, 144

Wilms' tumor, 87, 115, 121
Wilson disease, 26, 131, 166
Wiskott-Aldrich syndrome, 113, 168–169
  and non-Hodgkin's lymphoma, 118
Wolfe-Parkinson-White syndrome, 145
Women, Infants, and Children (WIC) program, 105

X chromosome, single, 86
X-linked adrenoleukodystrophy (ALD), 91–92
  childhood cerebral form, 92
X-linked agammaglobulinemia, 167
  and non-Hodgkin's lymphoma, 117–118
45,X karyotype, 86
45,X/46,XX karyotype, 86
47,XXX karyotype, 87
45,X/46,XY karyotype, 86
47,XXY karyotype, 87
48,XXY karyotype, 87
47,XYY karyotype, 87

*Yersinia enterocolitica* gastroenteritis, 153

Zinc deficiency, 26

# Rypins' Intensive Reviews

*Series Editor: Edward D. Frohlich, MD*

Behavioral Science
Internal Medicine
Surgery
Psychiatry and Behavioral Medicine
Pharmacology
Pediatrics

**FUTURE VOLUMES**

Physiology
Anatomy
Biochemistry
Microbiology
Pathology
Obstetrics and Gynecology
Community Health